Women with
Physical Disabilities

This book is printed on recycled paper.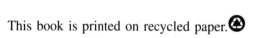

Women with Physical Disabilities

Achieving and Maintaining Health and Well-Being

edited by

Danuta M. Krotoski, Ph.D.
National Institute of Child Health and Human Development
National Institutes of Health

Margaret A. Nosek, Ph.D.
Baylor College of Medicine

and

Margaret A. Turk, M.D.
State University of New York at Syracuse

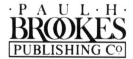

·P·A·U·L·H·
BROOKES
PUBLISHING Co

Baltimore • London • Toronto • Sydney

Paul H. Brookes Publishing Co.
Post Office Box 10624
Baltimore, Maryland 21285-0624

Typeset by PRO-IMAGE Corporation, York, Pennsylvania.
Manufactured in the United States of America by
BookCrafters, Chelsea, Michigan.

Library of Congress Cataloging-in-Publication Data

Women with physical disabilities : achieving and maintaining health
  and well-being / edited by Danuta M. Krotoski, Margaret A. Nosek,
  and Margaret A. Turk.
       p. cm.
  Includes bibliographical references and index.
  ISBN 1-55766-234-7
  1. Physically handicapped women—Health and hygiene.
2. Physically handicapped women—Medical care. I. Krotoski, Danuta
M. II. Nosek, Margaret Ann.   III. Turk, Margaret A.
  RA564.88.W65   1996
  613'.04244'087—dc20   95-50962
                                                                  CIP

British Library Cataloguing-in-Publication data are available from the British
Library.

Contents

Contributors

Barbara M. Altman, Ph.D.
Service Fellow
Agency for Health Care Policy and
  Research
2101 East Jefferson, Suite 500
Rockville, Maryland 20852

Carolyn M. Baum, Ph.D., O.T.R.
Elias Michael Director and Assistant
  Professor of Occupational Therapy
  and Neurology
Washington University School of
  Medicine
Program in Occupational Therapy
Box 8066, 660 South Euclid
St. Louis, Missouri 63110

Carol J. Bennett, M.D.
Associate Professor of Urology
University of Southern California
Chief of Urology
Rancho Los Amigos Medical Center
7601 East Imperial Highway
JPI Building
Neurotrauma Suite, 3rd Floor
Downey, California 90242

Deborah L. Bernal, M.D.
Liaison Councilor to the National
  Medical Association
American Academy of Physical
  Medicine and Rehabilitation
P.O. Box 31296
Washington, DC 20030

Jan M.H. Brewer, R.N., Ph.D.
Director of Nursing
Research and Quality/Risk
  Management
Administrator, Quality Resources
Department of Nursing
Hospital Administration
Rancho Los Amigos Medical Center
7601 East Imperial Highway
Downey, California 90242

Michael B. Chancellor, M.D.
Associate Professor of Urology
Director of Neuro-Urology and Female
  Urology
Thomas Jefferson University
Department of Urology
Thomas Jefferson University Hospital
1025 Walnut Street
Philadelphia, Pennsylvania 19107-5083

George P. Chrousos, M.D.
Chief, Pediatric Endocrinology Section
Developmental Endocrinology Branch
Director
Pediatric Endocrinology Training
  Program
NICHD
National Institutes of Health
Building 10, Room 10N262
9000 Rockville Pike
Bethesda, Maryland 20892

Nancy Clarke, M.Ed., C.R.C.
Doctoral Student
Department of Counseling, Educational
Psychology, and Special Education
Michigan State University
332 Erickson Hall
East Lansing, Michigan 48824-1034

**Graham H. Creasey, M.D.,
F.R.C.S.Ed.**
Physician
Spinal Cord Injury Unit
MetroHealth Center for Rehabilitation
2500 MetroHealth Drive, Room S1159
Cleveland, Ohio 44109

Nancy M. Crewe, Ph.D.
Professor
Department of Counseling, Educational
Psychology, and Special Education
Michigan State University
332 Erickson Hall
East Lansing, Michigan 48824-1034

Karen P. DePauw, Ph.D.
Associate Dean, Graduate School
Washington State University–Pullman
French Administration Room 324
Pullman, Washington 99164-1030

Marcus J. Fuhrer, Ph.D.
Director, NCMRR
National Institutes of Health
Building 61E, Room 2A03
6100 Executive Boulevard, MSC-7510
9000 Rockville Pike
Bethesda, Maryland 20892-7510

Lynn H. Gerber, M.D.
Chief, Department of Rehabilitation
Medicine
Warren Grant Magnuson Clinical
Center
National Institutes of Health
Building 10, Room 6S235
9000 Rockville Pike
Bethesda, Maryland 20892

Carol J. Gill, Ph.D.
President
Chicago Institute of Disability
Research
455 South Frontage Road, Suite 116
Burr Ridge, Illinois 60521

Karen A. Hart, Ph.D.
Assistant Professor of Physical
Medicine and Rehabilitation
Vice-President for Education
Baylor College of Medicine
The Institute for Rehabilitation and
Research
1333 Moursund Avenue
Houston, Texas 77030

Jeanne E. Hicks, M.D.
Deputy Chief
Department of Rehabilitation Medicine
National Institutes of Health
Building 10, Room 6S235
9000 Rockville Pike
Bethesda, Maryland 20892

Amie B. Jackson, M.D.
Chair of Department of Physical
Medicine and Rehabilitation
University of Alabama at Birmingham
Spain Rehabilitation Center
Department of Rehabilitation Medicine,
Room 190
1717 Sixth Avenue South
Birmingham, Alabama 35294

Megan Kirshbaum, Ph.D.
Director
Research and Training Center on
Families of Adults with Disabilities
Through the Looking Glass
2198 Sixth Street, Suite 100
Berkeley, California 94710-2204

Barry R. Komisaruk, Ph.D.
Professor II
Department of Psychobiology
Rutgers–The State University of New
Jersey
101 Warren Street
Newark, New Jersey 07102

Danuta M. Krotoski, Ph.D.
Chief, Basic Rehabilitation Medicine
  Research Group
National Center for Medical
  Rehabilitation Research, NICHD
National Institutes of Health
Building 61E, Room 2A03
9000 Rockville Pike
Bethesda, Maryland 20892

L. Keith Lloyd, M.D.
Professor of Urology
University of Alabama at Birmingham
Division of Urology
Medical Education Building, Suite 606
1813 Sixth Avenue South
Birmingham, Alabama 35294-3296

Margaret A. Nosek, Ph.D.
Associate Professor of Physical
  Medicine and Rehabilitation
Baylor College of Medicine
Center for Research on Women with
  Disabilities
1333 Moursund Avenue
Houston, Texas 77030

Corbett Joan O'Toole
Director
Disabled Women's Alliance
555 Pierce Street #936-E
Albany, California 94706

George D. Patrick, Ph.D.
Chief, Recreation Therapy Section
Department of Rehabilitation Medicine
National Institutes of Health
Clinical Center
Building 10, Room 14SD214
9000 Rockville Pike
Bethesda, Maryland 20892

**P. Sonya Perduta-Fulginiti, R.N.,
  M.S., C.R.R.N.**
Health Sciences Coordinator
New England Regional Spinal Cord
  Injury Center
Boston University Medical Center
  Hospital
88 East Newton Street
Boston, Massachusetts 02118

Marilyn Pires, R.N., M.S., C.R.R.N.
Clinical Nurse Specialist–Spinal Cord
  Injury
Department of Nursing
Rancho Los Amigos Medical Center
7601 East Imperial Highway
Downey, California 90242

Salman S. Razi, M.D.
Research Fellow
Department of Urology
University of Southern California
Rancho Los Amigos Medical Center
7601 East Imperial Highway
Downey, California 90242

Eleanor Richards, Ph.D., R.N., C.S.
Assistant Professor of Nursing
Henry P. Becton School of Nursing
Fairleigh Dickinson University
1000 River Road
Teaneck, New Jersey 07666

Diana H. Rintala, Ph.D.
Assistant Professor of Psychology
Department of Physical Medicine and
  Rehabilitation
Baylor College of Medicine
The Institute for Rehabilitation and
  Research
3555 Timmons, Suite 820
Houston, Texas 77027

Judith G. Rogers, O.T.R.
Through the Looking Glass
2198 Sixth Street, Suite 100
Berkeley, California 94710-2204

Sunny Roller, M.A.
Diversity Coordinator
University of Michigan Medical Center
Medical Campus Department of
  Human Resources
NIE02
300 North Ingalls Building
Ann Arbor, Michigan 48109-0420

Harilyn Rousso, M.S.W., B.C.D.
Executive Director
Disabilities Unlimited Consulting
  Services
3 East 10th Street, Suite 4B
New York, New York 10003

Marsha Saxton, Ph.D.
Founder/Director
The Project on Women and Disability
c/o Massachusetts Office on Disability
1 Ashburton Place #1305
Boston, Massachusetts 02108

Mitchell Tepper, M.P.H.
Doctoral Student in Human Sexuality
  Education
Graduate School of Education
University of Pennsylvania
3700 Walnut Street
Philadelphia, Pennsylvania 19104

Roberta B. Trieschmann, Ph.D.
Consulting Psychologist
President, RBT Associates, Inc.
P.O. Box 5566
Scottsdale, Arizona 85261

Constantine Tsigos, M.D., Ph.D.
Research Associate
Laboratory of Experimental Physiology
Athens Medical School
75 Mikias Asias Street
Goudi 15-27 Athens
GREECE

Margaret A. Turk, M.D.
Associate Professor
Department of Physical Medicine and
  Rehabilitation and Pediatrics
Health Sciences Center
State University of New York at
  Syracuse
750 East Adams Street, Room 7405
Syracuse, New York 13210

Barbara Faye Waxman
Director
National Disability and Reproductive
  Health Access Project
Los Angeles Family Planning Council
19907 Beekman Place
Cupertino, California 95014

Sandra Welner, M.D.
Primary Care Gynecologist
  Specializing in Gynecologic Care of
  Women with Disabilities
8484 Sixteenth Street
Suite 707
Silver Spring, Maryland 20910

**Beverly Whipple, Ph.D., R.N.,
  F.A.A.N.**
Associate Professor
College of Nursing
Rutgers–The State University of New
  Jersey
180 University Avenue
Newark, New Jersey 07102

Mary N. Young, R.N., M.S.
Urological Nursing Coordinator
Department of Nursing
Rancho Los Amigos Medical Center
7601 East Imperial Highway, 132HB
Downey, California 90242

Foreword

The focus in the 1990s on women's health has emphasized the fact that the natural history of disease and effectiveness of current interventions differ in women and men. Until the 1990s, the medical treatment of women was extrapolated from research done primarily on male subjects. Although a host of new studies address this critical gap in knowledge, little research focuses on the unique health needs of women with disabilities. This volume, based on the conference, "The Health of Women with Physical Disabilities: Setting a Research Agenda for the '90's," held in May 1994, responds to this gap in our knowledge. It was sponsored by the National Center for Medical Rehabilitation Research, among others. By highlighting four specific health care issues that are of particular concern to women with disabilities, the editors and contributors hope that these topics will receive their due research attention and will lead to increased research on the health of women with disabilities.

The National Center for Medical Rehabilitation Research (NCMRR) was established in 1990 within the National Institute of Child Health and Human Development (NICHD), at the National Institutes of Health (NIH) for the conduct and support of research that will lead to improved functioning in activities of daily living and enhanced quality of life of persons with disabilities. The National Advisory Board on Medical Rehabilitation Research (NABMRR), in its *Research Plan for the National Center for Medical Rehabilitation Research,* placed research on the health of women with disabilities and other underserved populations as a high priority. At the same time, the NIH established the Office for Research on Women's Health, whose mission is to support and extend research in women's health and stimulate more women researchers to ask questions related to this field. The conference responded to the high priority placed on improving women's health through the conduct and support of research and the dissemination of health information.

A major concern of women in regard to their health is the quality of their lives. In terms of becoming sick, convalescing, coping with disease or disability, what they are concerned with is maintaining health so that they can carry on with their lives. Medical rehabilitation research has as its primary focus the improvement of function in persons with disabilities, and it provides a relevant scientific framework in which to conduct research on the complex nature of women's health concerns and to gain knowledge that will assist them in carrying on with their lives.

The *Research Plan for the National Center for Medical Rehabilitation Research* describes one conceptual model that has proved highly useful in the conduct of inquiry into disability and the rehabilitation process. This model is presented in Chapter 19. The unique feature of the model is that it focuses research questions on the whole person, in this case the woman with a disability, over her life span, and it evaluates the impact of both personal background factors and quality-of-life issues as the rehabilitation process proceeds. This model contrasts, for instance, with models whose focus is a cell, a disease, or an assistive device. It identifies five domains of science relevant to rehabilitation research, ranging from pathophysiology to society. The model thus provides a framework by which to measure functional improvement within the domains in relation to the woman with a disability.

Examining research needs from this holistic perspective calls upon collaboration among researchers from various disciplines (e.g., health care providers, bioengineers, social scientists, economists), so that the cumulative knowledge gained reflects the full scope of the unique concerns of women with disabilities. Five domains for the study of disabilities—pathophysiology, impairment, functional limitation, disability, and societal limitation—guide the conduct of research, regardless of whether the research is based on the cellular, organic, personal, or societal point of view. In structuring this conference, the organizers were guided by this model, and each session explored opportunities for research in all domains.

The recommendations for a research agenda for women with disabilities in this book address fitness and well-being, stress, sexuality, and bowel and bladder management. It is hoped that this volume will stimulate further interest in investigating the issues central to the health of women with disabilities and that a rising level of interest will lead to initiatives to support research into selected problems.

The *Research Plan for the National Center for Medical Rehabilitation Research* stresses the "urgent and immediate need for development of an appropriate model of rehabilitation that addresses a woman's unique role physically, and also addresses her needs within the structure of her own environment" (p. 57). The present volume reflects the commitment of the NABMRR and the cosponsoring organizations to respond to that need.

Dorothy L. Gordon, D.N.Sc., R.N., F.A.A.N.
Chair, National Advisory Board on Medical Rehabilitation Research, 1994–1995
The Johns Hopkins University School of Nursing
Baltimore, Maryland

REFERENCE

National Institutes of Health. (1993). *Research plan for the National Center for Medical Rehabilitation Research.* NIH Publication No. 93-3509. Bethesda, MD: Author.

Preface

The proportion of women with physical disabilities in the population of the United States is substantial and growing. According to the 1992 census, 26,020,000 women have been reported to have disability-related work limitations. This represents 20% of all women, an extraordinary number. Although women with disabilities make up a large proportion of our population, information is sparse about their characteristics, the barriers they face in their daily lives, their special health problems and health care needs, and their quality of life. In some locations, they have organized to advocate for changes in health care delivery, but the impact on a national level has not been reflective of their numbers. Such invisibility has led to a lack of awareness of, or attention to, their physical, psychological, social, and economic needs. This book presents the result of a conference entitled The Health of Women with Physical Disabilities: Setting a Research Agenda for the '90's that was held in May 1994 in Bethesda, Maryland. It has been written to highlight the unique experiences and health needs of women with disabilities. With the establishment, within the National Institute of Child Health and Human Development, at the National Institutes of Health, of the National Center for Medical Rehabilitation Research (NCMRR), together with the Office of Research on Women's Health, there is a new focus on research that will lead to improved health and quality of life for women with disabilities.

In organizing the conference, members of the Advisory Board of the NCMRR and researchers and clinicians with and without disabilities identified topics of interest that would have the greatest potential impact on improving and enhancing the quality of life of women with physical disabilities. Four areas were identified for discussion: sexuality, bowel and bladder management, stress, and physical fitness. No previous conference had addressed these specific needs or brought together federal and private agencies and foundations to develop a research agenda in these areas for the coming decade.

Within each topic area, panels were designed to represent many points of view. First and foremost was the point of view of women with physical disabilities. Their presentations supplied grounding in the reality of everyday problems and provided the context within which all the information and recommendations had to be integrated. Second were clinicians who brought to the forum the essential issues of treatment options available and yet to be developed. Their input provided the medical context and the reality of the systems, both political and bureaucratic, that delimit health care. Third were researchers, many of whom were women with disabilities, who identified the various psychological, behavioral, social, physiological, and environmental factors at play within each of these areas. Other researchers provided overviews of basic and clinical science. Each panel concluded their discussion by formulating recommendations for research and practice. This book represents the content and tone of these presentations, with the addition of substantial supporting documentation.

The material contained in this book is designed to meet the needs of four potential audiences. The first audience is women with disabilities, who will recognize many of the experiences presented and thereby validate their own experiences. They may find new information and perspectives that can be used to make changes in their own lives and fuel advocacy for change in their communities. The second group, health care providers, will be able to expand their clinical knowledge base and their awareness of the practical, quality-of-life needs that are unique to women with disabilities. By gaining a broader understanding of the issues in this volume, they will also be empowered to initiate change from within health care systems. Third, researchers will expand their perspective of how their specialty fits within the context of the lives of women with disabilities. They will gain insights into new methodologies and paradigms for analysis that can be used to enlarge the scope of their investigations and ensure that their findings will have practical application. The recommendations for further research contained within each section and chapter provide guidelines for investigators and those who establish priorities for research funding. Finally, we hope to reach other members of the community, such as families and friends of women with disabilities, who may find this a compendium of useful information to solve problems in their own lives and spheres of influence, to enable them to be more effective consumers of health care, and to help them play a role in increasing access and changing health care policy to be more inclusive and responsive to the needs of all women.

This book is divided into five sections. The first provides the foundation for the four topics of special interest. This section presents the life experiences of a woman with a physical disability, an explanation of wellness within the context of disability, an overview of the characteristics of the population of women with disabilities, and a special look at the effect of combining disability status with cultural minority status. The remaining four sections reflect the broad range of discussions around each of the topics of special interest. Each of these sections differs in the degree to which it addresses clinical and psychosocial issues, depending in many ways on the development of that field. The section on sexuality and reproduction is rich with personal experiences, but demonstrates the critical need for more research into medical issues of contraception, obstetrics, and parenting, as well as the interpersonal issues of relationships and self-development. The interrelationship of stress and its impact on physiology has been identified in clinical settings only in the mid-1990s and may explain the increased level of depression and stress-related disorders seen in women with disabilities. The section not only provides information on practical approaches to stress management but also serves as a model for reducing the negative effects of stressful interactions. The section on bowel and bladder management analyzes a field that has grown primarily in response to the needs of men. It explores the appropriateness of using traditional techniques in treating the problems of women and provides information in considerable detail on new gender-specific methods of bowel and bladder management. Finally, the need for research on exercise and nutrition programs that will enhance wellness and fitness is described from both the physiological and psychosocial perspectives in the section on fitness.

It is our hope, as well as that of the NCMRR and all of the participants, that, with the publication of this book, we have provided a foundation for a better understanding of the health needs of women with physical disabilities and created momentum for the vigorous pursuit of answers to the many questions that have been raised and of changes in health care systems toward more universal access.

Acknowledgments

This volume would not have been possible without the enthusiastic input of many individuals. The willingness of the authors and other participants in the conference to share their knowledge and experience contributed to the outstanding dialogue reflected in this volume.

The editors would like to thank Dr. David B. Gray, whose tireless efforts toward establishing the National Center for Medical Rehabilitation Research and concern for the sexuality and quality of life of both women and men with disabilities stimulated the idea for the conference on which this volume is based. We would also like to thank the members of the National Advisory Board for Medical Rehabilitation Research, especially Drs. Dorothy Gordon (Johns Hopkins University), Theodore Cole (University of Michigan), and Sylvia Walker (Howard University), and Ms. Rebecca Ogle, who enthusiastically helped plan and design the framework for this volume. We are also indebted to Dr. Virginia Cain, then of the Office of Research on Women's Health, Dr. Laura James of the National Institute for Nursing Research, Dr. Barbara Altman of the Agency for Health Care Policy Research, and Dr. Lawrence Johnston of the Paralyzed Veterans of America for their support, both programmatic and financial. We would also like to acknowledge Dr. Duane Alexander, Director of the National Institute of Child Health and Human Development, whose enthusiastic support for research that targets the special health needs of all women allowed us to develop a program that addresses the specific needs of women with disabilities as identified by the women themselves.

Finally, this volume would not have become a reality without the guidance and support provided by the professionals at Paul H. Brookes Publishing Co. We are indebted to Theresa Donnelly and Paul Klemt for their long-standing support, guidance, and patience through the editing process.

Women with
Physical Disabilities

WOMEN WITH PHYSICAL DISABILITIES

Overriding Issues

Danuta M. Krotoski,
Margaret A. Nosek, and Margaret A. Turk

In discussing the health of women with disabilities, it is first important to recognize the scope of experiences they have as women, as women with disabilities, and as consumers of health care. It is also important to have demographic data letting us know who and where these women are, how they are able to gain access to health care, and how that affects their well-being and daily functioning. Finally, it is important to know how their socioeconomic status and ethnicity affect their experiences.

Women with disabilities have become more vocal in taking charge of their lives and their bodies. They are becoming not only more active partners with health care providers but also active members of the research and health care community, identifying their needs, and developing more appropriate approaches to interventions. The goal of this section is to set the stage for the reader, to place the topics addressed in the other sections in the context of personal experience and an understanding of the population of women with disabilities as a whole.

The most poignant means of transmitting information is the use of personal examples, such as those Carol Gill shares in Chapter 1. She very eloquently communicates to the reader the change in society's perception of women with disabilities as they take back responsibility for their own bodies and their own lives. In doing so, they are making important changes in society. Gill very correctly notes that the level of disability experienced by each woman is determined not only by her physical condition but also by her environment, both architectural and attitudinal. She clearly notes that health care providers must look at women with disabilities as women

1

rather than as medical problems. Women should not be defined by their primary disabling condition, but should be seen as women who have health concerns like those of other women. She affirms the fact that women with disabilities are now taking control of their own health care and are now moving to direct and participate in research that will address their own health needs. As she states in the chapter, "We are women. We are disabled. We are proud. And we are here."

Margaret Nosek (Chapter 2) provides insights into the development of holistic wellness models that take into account the needs of the entire individual. She provides a model in which individuals are viewed as being along a continuum of wellness that has many dimensions, including having a sense of control over their fate. Where individuals lie along the continuum toward wellness is determined by their feelings of competence and resilience, their interaction with wellness-enhancing social systems, and empowering policies and environmental conditions. The model that she has used includes wellness lifestyle program components, such as self-awareness, health awareness, wellness skills, and wellness resources, as well as behavioral outcomes. She describes the wellness qualities of women with physical disabilities that she had identified in her own research.

How are women with disabilities faring, and how are they obtaining health care? Barbara Altman (Chapter 3) and Deborah Bernal (Chapter 4) provide demographic information regarding the impact of disability among women and the effects that race and ethnicity bring to bear on this population. Available statistical information regarding the risks, causes, and consequences at the national level is very limited. Altman presents new information about women with disabilities by consolidating analyses of a number of national primary databases. Her chapter provides information on the sociodemographic distribution of women with disabilities, focusing on age, income, work outcomes, and use of services of health care providers. She also provides data identifying the major causes of disability among women of all ages. Using this information, she develops a model for estimating the causes and consequences of disability and determining the risk that an underlying impairment will lead to activity limitations. The data she has collected point to the need for further carefully designed studies that will permit the examination of conditions that have low prevalence in the general population, thus providing researchers and policy makers with a better measure of the impact of disability on health status, employment, and quality of life. Such studies would greatly benefit from the inclusion of women with disabilities in the development of the measurement instruments to ensure that relevant data are collected.

Bernal emphasizes the fact that women from ethnic minorities are more likely to have a disability than their majority counterparts, particularly if they are African American or Hispanic. She proposes that first there should be greater focus on research that examines the causes and prevention of disability in minority populations. It is essential that this research be culturally sensitive and include factors related to quality of life. Second, she recommends that there be efforts to increase the number and integration of minority female health professionals and researchers in order to address these issues.

chapter 1

Becoming Visible
Personal Health
Experiences of Women with Disabilities

Carol J. Gill

Whenever we find a forum, women with disabilities increasingly describe our experiences forthrightly. A true story illustrates how vivid and poignant that expression can be. At a seminar that recently took place at a health center for women with disabilities, a panel addressed the subject of the day: "Images—how to define and project the image that's right for you."

A psychologist on the panel began to speak about self-esteem and how women can feel good about themselves. Her discussion was a bit on the academic side, and after a while, the women with disabilities in the audience grew restless. Finally a few asked the psychologist what she knew specifically about how they, as women with disabilities, could have self-esteem and positive relationships when they experience so much social rejection. The psychologist responded by stressing that "different" does not mean "inferior." To illustrate her point, she used an analogy that can be described as "the metaphor of the pies." She explained that if several different people go to a restaurant and choose dessert, some will prefer the lemon meringue pie and some the banana cream pie and so on. Because one pie is selected and the other is not, that does not mean one is inferior to the other. Pies are different; women are different. A hand shot up in the back of the room. A middle-age African American woman with a visible physical disability quickly brought the discussion back to basics. She asked, "But what if you are considered a smashed pie?"

That wonderfully gutsy question cuts right to the heart of the experience of women with disabilities. Indeed, it is one thing to be put on display and told if you are good, you might get chosen as the tastier, prettier dish. Women have been placed in that demeaning position for centuries. It is quite another thing, however, never even to make it to the display case, to be overlooked as defective, to be dismissed, thrown away from the start. That is the dominant social experience that women with disabilities are expressing as we get together and exchange notes. That is the experience we are working to change for ourselves and for our daughters—our daughters, that is, via culture: the next generation of women with disabilities.

Living in a society that devalues you is very hard. The personal stories of countless women with disabilities underscore how stressful it is to be socially devalued. What makes a devalued status even more stressful is to feel invisible. When you are repeatedly overlooked or dismissed, it adds another layer to your oppression. The message is that not only are you inferior, but it does not matter, because *you* are not important enough to matter.

Since the mid-1970s, women from diverse cultural backgrounds have written and spoken extensively about their devaluation in a male-oriented society. They have rejected the narrow roles and opportunities imposed on them. Lately they have protested their invisibility in the health service system, both in treatment options and in the research that guides those treatments. They have been very effective. The huge National Institutes of Health (NIH) research project on women's health is evidence that women are being heard and seen in the medical system as never before.

It is only since 1993, though, that women with disabilities have begun to gain visibility in asserting our rights, especially in the area of health services. Why has it taken so long for us to be recognized?

We live in a society that, in many ways, has little faith in us. We are invalidated two ways: As people with disabilities, we are often stereotyped as dependent and nonproductive; as women, we are judged incompetent to perform women's work. The verdict is double incompetence. A television series many years ago opened each week with a court-martial scene. After the main character was stripped of his military identity—from his stripes and epaulets down to his buttons—he was banished to oblivion as a nonperson. Similarly, women with disabilities are stripped of our roles. We are not expected to be workers, romantic partners, caregivers, or mothers. Socially, we are in limbo—not quite children, but not adults; not men, but not real women either. It is difficult to get your bearings and struggle out from under that kind of unremitting yet subtle oppression, because it steals from you the very sense of self you need in order to fight.

CHANGING PERCEPTIONS

As women with disabilities began to talk and write about this situation in the late 1970s and early 1980s, and as we began to gain insight into our social invalidation, we were eager to share it with our sisters without disabilities in the women's movement. However, many of us hit a wall there. We attended National Organization for Women (NOW) conferences; we marched in pro-choice parades. But when we tried to talk about our issues, all too often we met with a stunning absence of connection. Sometimes we were surprised and overwhelmed by the extent of our invisibility to other women.

In 1992, for example, some colleagues and I tried to participate in a conference on women's health policy. We looked at the conference brochure and felt encouraged by the organizers' expressed commitment to diversity and innovation. Before long, however, we sensed that we were perhaps a little more diverse and innovative than they anticipated. In a 3-day conference with concurrent presentations, less than 1 hour was devoted to women with disabilities, and that was our presentation! Although our talk emphasized policy and social issues affecting women with disabilities, we were grouped with presenters doing research on specific illnesses, as though disability were primarily a medical treatment problem not at all defined by social and cultural forces.

There were numerous access problems, including economic access, encountered at the conference. It was frustrating and hurtful to realize we were not expected to be at this meeting that proposed to address the health concerns of all women. I remember laughing defensively with my co-presenters over lunch about how invisible we felt. I thought of the words of Bonnie Klein (1992), who wrote an article in *Ms.* magazine about feeling excluded by the women's movement after becoming disabled. I wanted to tell everyone at the conference what Klein told her friends in the movement about her membership in the community of women with disabilities. "We are who you are," she said. I wanted the conference women to know I was who they were—I was a woman, and my issues were legitimate women's issues.

Klein's brave article in *Ms.* is just one example of the way we have been asserting our visibility to other women. We have begun to challenge the disability phobia we find in the women's movement. We realize we have been unwelcome partly because disability is associated with stereotypes of weakness and dependence. These are the very images and unfair stereotypes that feminist women have been trying to live down, so there may be some fear of "devaluation by association" with us. Also, many women have worked hard to liberate themselves from the socially imposed role of caregiver to children and to aging or ill family members. I believe we who have disabilities may threaten women who fear losing ground, women who fear being forced back into these roles and who then see us as part of their oppression.

In truth, women with disabilities are as concerned as anyone else about the oppression of women in helping roles. That is why we are fighting for personal assistance funding to be part of the national health plan. Also, the sheer tensile strength of women with disabilities should refute any notions that we are weak, but it takes time to counter bad press. We have been working hard and collectively to introduce our real selves to the women's community, and it is paying off. Two years after that conference on women's health where I felt so marginalized, the same organizers did a follow-up conference. They took our input to heart and incorporated disability in a substantial way, inviting us to speak for ourselves about our issues. Also, since 1993, many of my women friends with disabilities and I have been increasingly invited to contribute to women's anthologies, conferences, and women's studies programs.

THE MEDICAL COMMUNITY'S RESPONSE

The women's community has certainly not been the only place or the primary place where our womanness has been overlooked. The medical service system is a place where we have frequently felt invisible as women. In the 1990s, the medical field has made efforts to give physicians more training on cultural issues in treatment. The concern is that doctors cannot give people the best treatment if they fail to understand their patients' lives, values, and view of the world. Women have been debating whether there should be a new women's specialty within medicine to treat women in a context of better knowledge of their social and cultural reality. Some women say yes, that would be wonderful, and others say no, because that is letting medicine off the hook—all clinicians should learn about women's issues.

There is an analogous debate in the community of women with disabilities. Some of us want to consult only doctors who specialize in disability, while some of us want all physicians to learn about our issues and make their health services accessible and welcoming to us. Many of us are disturbed by how little doctors and other health professionals actually learn about our lives during their training. The result is that we often get passed from one professional to another. When we approach physicians in our community for prenatal exams and other services, we are often told to go to rehabilitation medicine where the doctors are "used to" people like us.

Consequently, we are often banished from our neighborhood health centers and sent to rehabilitation doctors even when our health needs have little to do with our disabilities. Besides being inconvenient, this practice is unfairly segregating. It keeps us separated from our sisters without disabilities in the community. Furthermore, in truth, rehabilitation doctors do not always know what to do with us either. Perhaps this is because until recently, rehabilitation medicine focused primarily on the needs of men with disabilities—traditionally seen as the workers and soldiers and athletes who need to be fixed—while the needs of women with disabilities have been less visible. As a result, rehabilitation specialists have often been forced to prescribe treatments for us (including contraception or treatment for osteoporosis) by extrapolating from research done on women without disabilities or men with disabilities. Clearly, this is not an ideal approach.

Many women with disabilities tell me they have felt invisible in medical settings in another way. One of the complaints I hear most often is, "They treat me like a medical condition instead of like a woman." Usually that complaint is followed by a disturbing story. Sometimes the stories are about violated privacy, such as medical exams performed with curtains carelessly left open and doors ajar or women's bodies placed on clinical display for medical educational purposes. The latter is an experience so traumatic and haunting to many women with disabilities that they have written about it extensively and named it. They call it "public stripping" (Blumberg, 1990). Sometimes the stories are about being treated as genderless, having questions about sexuality brushed off, or receiving X rays without lead shields because no one thinks about protecting our reproductive potential.

The women who share these stories are absolutely correct in drawing their conclusions. We have been viewed too much in terms of our diagnoses and too little in terms of our personhood. Part of the problem is that medicine has not yet accepted that we have redefined disability in a way that reflects our reality. Increasingly, scholars and activists with disabilities are rejecting the traditional view of disability that says we are physically defective and need fixing or care (Hahn, 1982). Instead, we are asserting that we are a legitimate cultural minority. We are pointing out the fact that most of our problems are caused not by our bodies but by a society that refuses to accommodate our differences. We are trying to tell the health service system that, for most of us, our medical needs are only a small part of our disability experience. The larger, more pressing problems we have are social and political.

We want our health service providers and researchers to know this fact about our lives so it informs their judgments and decisions about us. Only by knowing more about our actual experience can they view our physical problems in proper perspective.

We want them to know, for example, that we may need a lot of information about sexuality and reproductive health options because society limits our knowledge and choices in these areas. We want them to be alert to signs of assault in women and girls with disabilities because our social devaluation places us at high risk for abuse, even from those we rely on for assistance in daily activities. We want our health professionals to know that women with disabilities, particularly women of color with disabilities, are among the most impoverished and socially isolated of all minority groups and that this adds to the enormous stress level in our lives. We want them to know that if we fall in love, the stress may escalate because those of us who rely on government-funded health coverage for our wheelchairs and ventilators may have it ripped away from us as soon as we marry. Many of us spend each day worrying about paying bills, finding the equipment and assistance we need, finding accessible housing, finding transportation, and finding love. Moreover, when we "burn out" from our stress and devaluation, it is important for our health professionals to know why we might be depressed so that we can receive appropriate psychological support and suicide intervention.

There are countless real-life examples that can illustrate the health needs of women with disabilities. For instance, a woman named Lois has good reason to feel passionate about accessible quality health services for all women. During a routine physical, her doctor suggested it was time for her to get a baseline mammogram. When she called her hospital to arrange it and mentioned that she was a paraplegic, they asked her if she could stand. Lois said no, she used a wheelchair. "Then we can't do it," they said. When Lois called her doctor's office to ask for guidance, she discovered her doctor had just been taken in to have heart surgery. Because her breast exam in the doctor's office had revealed no problem, Lois decided to wait.

A while later, she had to be hospitalized for treatment of a decubitus ulcer. During the presurgical exam, a lump was discovered in her breast. Under doctor's orders, a mammogram was performed in the same hospital that had refused to serve her before. Sadly, the lump, already palpable in size, was malignant, and she had a mastectomy. Had her cancer been diagnosed earlier, her treatment options may have been different. Lois wanted her real first name used in this account. She shares her story whenever she feels it might convince others of the need for accessible services, hopeful that other women with disabilities can be spared her outcome.

We must learn more about the access problems encountered by women with disabilities. We must continue to support research that asks the right questions to document the health experiences of women with disabilities as well as programs that are teaching them how to act on their rights to health service access.

SEXUALITY AND REPRODUCTIVE HEALTH

Sexuality and reproductive health constitute another area full of compelling stories. Since 1993, far too many stories have surfaced about women with disabilities having their babies taken from them in custody battles when others impugn their fitness as mothers. One woman told of how her mother and doctor worked together to sedate her and subject her to an abortion without her knowledge. Later, when she brought her first baby to term, her mother went to court to ask that her daughter be denied custody on the basis of disability. After a long, exhausting struggle, the young woman won her child back and has successfully raised three additional children. In fact, she has managed to produce something quite remarkable for a parent: polite and happy teenagers!

There are positive stories, too, concerning reproductive rights. A young woman with very extensive physical disabilities who had a tracheostomy and used a ventilator talked at a sexuality and disability conference about her personal exploration of sexuality. She was getting support and guidance in her quest from a very respectful psychotherapist who honored and affirmed her right to be sexual. At one point in her story, she mentioned that although she realized her life span would be shortened by her condition, she felt at peace because she had finally been able to get to know her total self, including her sensual self.

I recently heard the same theme of gender validation and respect for our bodies from a friend who uses a wheelchair. She phoned to say what a great afternoon she had experienced the day before. When I asked her to elaborate, she told me she had gone to a gynecologist for a pelvic exam—hardly most women's idea of fun! What she found so exciting, though, was the fact that after 20 years of such exams, she had found a gynecological clinic specializing in access for women with disabilities and had felt acknowledged as a woman for the first time. She was effusive about the accessible examining chair, the discreet and respectful assistance she received, and the doctor who allowed her to remain in control and who encouraged her to watch the exam in a mirror. She said the most exciting part was being treated like she was not strange, or defective, or a problem. She had never experienced this attitude of acceptance in a gynecological clinic before. She said it would almost be worth getting a yeast infection so she could go back!

What a contrast to my last gynecological exam at a university hospital's women's clinic. After fighting over the phone just to get in the door at all due to access problems, the doctor remarked to me repeatedly that I must be extraordinary to be so happy, given the severity of my condition. I told her it was anything but extraordinary. I told her that happiness had more to do with relationships and other sources of fulfillment than it does with the extent of one's disability. She said she disagreed with me. Later, I discovered she was the medical director of genetic services at the clinic. One of her jobs was to counsel parents about the possibility of having a child with a disability. I remembered that current research shows that physicians overestimate the negative impact of disability on family life. I shudder to think about what this OB/GYN is telling her patients about bringing people like me into their lives.

Physicians and other health professionals must receive more information about our value and full lives as women with disabilities so we may all leave clinics feeling like *women* rather than medical *problems*. Gynecologists and obstetricians, in particular, must be trained to affirm our gender and sexuality by offering us more complete information and a full array of reproductive health options.

FIGHTING HOPELESSNESS

There are, of course, women with disabilities who are anything but happy, and I am extremely concerned about them. I am very troubled, for instance, that, until he was publicly criticized for his gender preferences, Jack Kevorkian's clients were all middle-age or older women with disabilities and chronic illnesses. We know that depression affects women more than men, and some researchers feel the social pressures on women to be perfect, along with their lack of options, diminished power, and experiences of abuse, account for much of their despair. Osgood and Eisenhandler (1994) wrote about the phenomenon of "acquiescent suicide" as a problem in women who come to believe they should die because they are socially useless and powerless. Considering that many women with disabilities are denied a meaningful role in life, are left without economic power or social supports, and are bombarded with messages that they fall short of society's standards for womanhood, they may very well be at high risk for depression and suicide. Yet informal accounts suggest that women with disabilities who despair are often denied access to adequate suicide intervention sensitive to their cultural issues.

In this regard, the words of Sherry Miller—the woman with multiple sclerosis who became Kevorkian's third public "patient"—are chilling. She said she wanted to die because she felt useless, having to be helped with daily activities (Hirsley & Thomas, 1991). In blaming herself for her problems, Miller's words contrast sharply with the tragic last words of Lynn Thompson, a quadriplegic woman who killed herself after someone turned her in to Social Security for hiding a couple hundred dollars she had earned by working at home. Social Security officials told her that, because she had worked, she would lose the funding she needed to live in her home, thereby consigning her to a nursing home. She left a tape recording to explain her suicide. Referring to the Social Security Administration's ruling, she said, "That was the straw that broke the camel's back" (Hewitt, 1977).

How many women with disabilities are being similarly broken by their social circumstances and their loss of roles? How many will die through assisted suicide before we have any adequate research addressing the despair of women with disabilities?

THE REALITY OF ABUSE

The abuse of women with disabilities is a subject unto itself. It is hard to pick one story here; sadly, there are so many. One of my friends in high school walked with crutches because of polio and won awards for singing opera. After graduation, I attended her wedding, where she sang a love song to her handsome athletic groom. Shortly after the birth of their second child, I received the shocking news that my friend had killed herself after a long series of brutal beatings by her husband. The psychiatrist who had been treating her for postpartum depression had never thought about the possibility of domestic violence and had completely missed the true source of her despair. I also know a woman with cerebral palsy who was sexually assaulted by strangers twice in one week—first, by the driver of the bus she rode to her sheltered workshop, and second, by the plumber who came to fix a drain in her apartment.

For too long, health and social service systems have relied on haphazard anecdotal evidence to understand abuse of women with disabilities. We must have better research on incidence, contributing factors, prevention, and treatment if women with disabilities and their health service providers are to receive the information and services required to heal from violence and to avoid further harm.

A concern expressed more and more by women with disabilities is our desire to care for our bodies through health maintenance and fitness efforts. Apparently, a lot of us like our bodies and want to be around for a long time. This calls for more research focused on physical health maintenance. However, mental health maintenance must not take a back seat. We need more information regarding how we can feel good about ourselves and maintain positive body image and self-esteem when the world tells us to hate our disabled parts—when, in effect, we are treated like smashed pies. Some women with physical disabilities so minor they could be overlooked by an untrained observer are emotionally devastated by negative body image. Conversely, there are others who resist devaluation, such as the vibrant woman I met at a disability rights meeting who was born without legs or arms but who clearly loves her body. She, in fact, celebrates her body by wearing bracelets on her stumps and making fashion statements in pretty clothes and big hats. We must study the factors underlying such contrasting reactions because self-esteem is so critical in mediating women's power to resist stress and oppression in their lives.

GROWING OPTIMISM

This is a miraculous time for women with disabilities, given our history. We are finding ourselves and each other as never before. We are joining forces across the country and across generations to take our rightful place in society, including the health services system and health research. In the last 2–3 years, we have been designing programs and forming new organizations as well as honoring pioneering programs that were initiated by the women with disabilities activists who led the way. We know our greatest power to get what we need is not by doing it alone but through cooperation and collaboration—skills that are hallmarks of the culture of both women and people with disabilities.

Much of what we are seeking is inclusion in good research. We want more information about our physiology and the effects of different treatments and preventive approaches. We want contraception research and pregnancy information, and we want to know how to care for ourselves as we age. We want new options developed that are healthier for us and amenable to our control. We also want to learn about the effects of stress in our lives and how to remain emotionally healthy. Furthermore, we need substantial research on health policy to document how such policies affect women with disabilities and to recommend needed changes.

What we do not need, however, is medical, mental health, or policy research framed in a manner that views the disability experience primarily and simply as a medical defect in the individual that needs to be cured or normalized. The traditional medical model is narrow, biased, and just plain wrong. It ignores the sociocultural reality and complexity of our problems. It asks the wrong questions and yields answers that have not been helpful to most of us in our lives.

As women with disabilities think about our inclusion in research, we are thinking big. We are referring to inclusion on all levels. Our goal is to have a major role in framing the questions, setting the funding priorities, participating as subjects, and disseminating the results. Already we have become more active in conducting and interpreting research ourselves. I am pleased to be one of many women researchers with disabilities across the continent studying disability health issues.

One note of caution: It is important when doing research on the health of women with disabilities to expend the effort necessary to find us. We are a larger community than many think. A lot of research has relied on samples of those of us who are most visible: white heterosexual women with physical disabilities who are functioning in the world and who can speak or write without difficulty. Less represented are women with multiple disabilities, blind women, and women with hearing or cognitive disabilities or communication differences. Many of us remain hidden—some in institutions, some isolated at home or in economically oppressed inner cities or rural areas, some who may be professionals and who may not be thought of as "consumers" or proper subjects of this kind of research, and some with disabilities that are hidden. However, if researchers fail to make the extra effort to find us, their results will not represent our community.

CONCLUSIONS

Who are we and where are we? These are key questions, and the answers are complex. We are mothers and daughters, teachers, and students. Regardless of what society may think, we are also caregivers and, too often, nursing home inmates. We are doctors and sometimes we are patients; we are employed as cooks and CEOs, but too many of us are unemployed. We are from all racial, ethnic, and cultural backgrounds, lesbian and heterosexual. We are rich but more often poor. We are happy and loved but often isolated and sometimes, tragically, suicidal. The critical point is that we are complex individuals. Increasingly, we are a diverse community, but a real community, emerging from our imposed invisibility. What we are saying is this: We are women. We are disabled. We are proud. And we are here.

REFERENCES

Blumberg, L. (1990). Public stripping. *Disability Rag, 11,* 18–20.

Hahn, H. (1982). Disability and rehabilitation policy: Is paternalistic neglect really benign? *Public Administration Review, 43,* 385–389.

Hewitt, D. (Producer). (1977, October 1). *60 Minutes.* New York: CBS.

Hirsley, M., & Thomas, K. (1991, October 25). "Doctor Death" puts new focus on right-to-die debate. *Chicago Tribune,* Sec. 1, pp. 1, 23.

Klein, B.S. (1992, November/December). We are who you are: Feminism and disability. *Ms., 3,* 70–74.

Osgood, N.J., & Eisenhandler, S.A. (1994). Gender and assisted and acquiescent suicide: A suicidologist's perspective. *Issues in Law and Medicine, 9,* 361–374.

chapter 2

Wellness Among Women with Physical Disabilities

Margaret A. Nosek

Wellness and disability, used in the same sentence, could seriously disrupt the status quo in health care. Traditionally, disability has been equated with illness. Indeed, many children and adults with disabilities were relegated to hospital wards for the long term when I was growing up in the 1950s because society was simply not equipped to deal with disability as a normal part of life. This had very little to do with disease states; it had to do with attitudes and physical barriers. With Congressional passage of such liberating laws as the Architectural Barriers Act of 1968 (PL 90-480), the Education for All Handicapped Children Act of 1975 (PL 94-142) (now known as the Individuals with Disabilities Education Act, PL 101-476), Section 504 of the Rehabilitation Act (PL 93-112), which was finally implemented in 1977, and our crowning glory, the Americans with Disabilities Act of 1990 (PL 101-336), we have begun tearing down these physical barriers. Barriers of attitude, however, need much more than a jackhammer and cement to bring them down. Although we are experiencing some progress in removing discrimination on the basis of disability in education, employment, and public services, the mind-set of medical professionals is more deeply rooted in tradition and has been slower to respond. There is a new wave of change in medical practice, however, that focuses on wellness and the whole person. This chapter presents the notion of wellness in disability as an operating principle and reviews the findings of our study of the population most damaged by traditional medical stereotypes, namely, women.

This work is supported by The National Institutes of Health, Public Health Service, National Institute of Child Health and Human Development, Grant HD30166-01. A full report of this study was published by Nosek, M.A., Howland, C.A., Young, M.E., Georgiou, D., Rintala, D.H., Foley, C.C., Bennett, J.L., & Smith, Q. (1994). Wellness models and sexuality among women with physical disabilities. *Journal of Applied Rehabilitation Counseling, 25*(1), 50–58.

When disability is equated with illness, all of the associations made with illness are called into play. Persons who are ill, for example, are exempt from normal responsibilities, are not expected to be productive, are perceived as victims of a horrible disease process, and are expected to comply with the orders of persons who are experts in that disease process (DeJong, 1979). For women, this has the effect of neutralizing their femininity, creating the perception they are gender-free (Adcock & Newbigging, 1990; Danek, 1992; Lesh & Marshall, 1984), have no need for intimacy and sexual expression and are incapable of being a sexual partner (Hanna & Rogovsky, 1991, 1992), and have no need for reproductive health care services. One woman with a severe physical disability who was interviewed for our study commented, "I always felt like a neutral sex. It's like I'm not a woman, not a man, I don't know what I am because I was never approached like a woman." The current grassroots emergence of publications targeting women with disabilities (e.g., *ABLED, It's OK!*) and the growing national network of advocacy organizations of women with disabilities (e.g., WISE in Baltimore, Maryland; the New Jersey Coalition of Women with Disabilities; the Networking Project for Disabled Women and Girls in New York) signals a rising rebellion against the asexual, medical stereotype. This chapter describes a study of women with disabilities and analyzes the data from a wellness perspective.

WELLNESS MODELS

A brief look at the literature on wellness models will help set the stage for our discussion of wellness among women with physical disabilities. A good starting point is perhaps the most well-known definition of health that was stated in the preamble of the World Health Organization (WHO) charter: "Health is a state of complete physical, mental, and social well-being and not merely the absence of disease or infirmity" (quoted in Antonovsky, 1979, p. 52). In our work, we adopted a wellness orientation to sexuality for women with physical disabilities by focusing on achieving optimal sexual functioning rather than on identifying sexual dysfunction. Wellness models have evolved as positive, health-oriented alternatives to the disease orientation of the biomedical model. Most models have in common an integration of some combination of psychological (including emotional and intellectual), social, career, environmental, spiritual, and physical areas of well-being. They speak about harmony, coherence, purpose, feelings of belonging, control, competence, and resilience. Details on some of the models that we found helpful in our study of women with physical disabilities follow.

Most wellness models tend to emphasize the role of harmony (Neuman, 1982) or sense of coherence (Antonovsky, 1979, 1987) in maintaining wellness. Individuals cannot be labeled "ill" or "well," but instead exist somewhere along a continuum between these two poles at any given time. In the Neuman system model (1982), disharmony among an individual's biological, psychological, sociocultural, spiritual, and developmental components reduces wellness. This model is applicable to older adults or to those with physical disabilities because the presence of chronic conditions does not disqualify individuals from wellness as long as they are able to maintain harmony. The Neuman model depicts the individual as having a basic survival core surrounded by three levels of defense against environmental stressors:

1. Lines of resistance—homeostatic mechanisms that attempt to stabilize and maintain the individual's normal line of defense
2. Normal lines of defense—stability factors developed over time, including intelligence, coping abilities, outlook on life, and problem-solving abilities
3. Flexible lines of defense—protective buffers for preventing stressors from breaking through the line of defense

The sense of coherence integral to Antonovsky's Salutogenic Model (1979, 1987) is somewhat comparable to Neuman's concept of harmony. Sense of coherence is defined as

> a global orientation that expresses the extent to which one has a pervasive, enduring though dynamic feeling of confidence that one's internal and external environments are predictable and that there is a high probability that things will work out as well as can reasonably be expected. (Antonovsky, 1979, p. 184)

Antonovsky developed and defined this concept by analyzing in-depth qualitative interviews of 51 persons who were functioning well after having survived severe trauma such as severe disability or the Holocaust. The common characteristics of those functioning well were that they perceived their life activities as meaningful and considered their life events comprehensible and manageable, characteristics that Antonovsky defined as a sense of coherence. In contrast to perceived control or locus of control, events are not necessarily perceived as being under one's own control, but under some kind of control that is comprehensible rather than bewildering. Antonovsky's Salutogenic model also includes psychosocial and physical/biochemical stressors that are countered by generalized resistance resources—that is, sets of meaningful, coherent life experiences to determine where one is on the ease/dis-ease continuum. In this model, people who have a strong sense of coherence manage tension effectively and resist health breakdown.

Cowen's (1991) notion of wellness blends ingredients of both Antonovsky's and Neuman's models of wellness. Just as sense of coherence is integral to Antonovsky's model of wellness, Cowen (1991) includes "having a sense of control over one's fate, a feeling of purpose and belongingness, and a basic satisfaction with oneself and one's existence" (p. 404) as essential indicators of wellness. Where individuals lie along the continuum toward wellness is determined by the extent to which they possess competence and resilience while encountering wellness-enhancing social systems and empowering policies and conditions. These concepts are reminiscent of the defenses against stressors in Neuman's model of wellness. Included in Cowen's concept of competence are life competencies such as interpersonal communication, problem solving, assertiveness, and anger-control skills as well as competence at school or on the job. Resilience refers to the ability to cope with stressful life events and circumstances. Although resilience has been studied in reference to survivors of war and children who survive family violence, it is seldom applied to women with disabilities. Social institutions such as schools and worksites that pose unintended barriers to wellness should be changed, as should social systems that disempower groups such as ethnic minorities and people with disabilities by depriving them of power, justice, and opportunity. Conversely, individuals are empowered by promoting policies and conditions that enable people to gain control over their lives. The simultaneous presence of competence and empowerment increase individuals' perceived control over their own destinies (Cowen, 1991). Perceived control is a vital component of independence for people with disabilities (Nosek & Fuhrer, 1992).

The wellness model developed by Abood and Mundy (1986) has been applied to people with disabilities (Abood & Burkhead, 1988), supporting the belief that a separate wellness model should not be created for people with disabilities; instead, general wellness models and corresponding programs should include them as well. This model consists of wellness lifestyle program components such as self-awareness, health awareness, wellness skills, and wellness resources, as well as behavioral outcomes for each component. Individuals are expected to move toward an integrated lifestyle that is personally appropriate, which includes self-definition of goals.

Witmer and Sweeney (1992) view wellness as being expressed through five life tasks:

1. Spirituality, which consists of oneness, purpose, optimism, and values
2. Self-regulation, which comprises sense of worth, sense of control, realistic beliefs, spontaneous and emotional responsiveness, intellectual stimulation, problem solving, creativity, sense of humor, physical fitness, and nutrition
3. Work, which provides economic sustenance as well as serving psychological and social functions
4. Friendship, which enables connection with the human community

5. Love, by which health is nurtured in marriage or intimate relationships through trust, caring, and companionship

Our study of sexuality in women with physical disabilities deals primarily with the life tasks of self-regulation, friendship, and love.

DESCRIPTION OF THE STUDY

Our study began in 1992, with funding from the National Center for Medical Rehabilitation Research at the National Institute of Child Health and Human Development, National Institutes of Health (NIH). It was entitled "Psychosocial Behaviors of Women with Physical Disabilities" and focused on sexuality, relationships, health, and personal development. Results from the first phase of the study were compiled from qualitative open-ended interviews (Patton, 1990) with 31 women who had a variety of physical disabilities. Although a fair amount of literature exists on reproduction and disability, it is predominantly about men with spinal cord injury and deals with physiological issues much more than psychosocial issues. Because so little had been done in this area as it relates to women and because we did not presume to know the correct questions to ask (although several of us could draw on a wealth of personal experience with disability, we did not assume that our experience was universal), we began with an interview study to identify primary themes and issues about the sexuality of women with disabilities.

Thirty-one adult women with disabilities that resulted in functional impairments participated in the interviews. They were recruited through personal contact and by fliers distributed locally and nationally. Use of theoretical sampling (Glaser & Strauss, 1967) assured that the selection of individuals represented key variables hypothesized to affect sexual functioning, such as 1) type of disability, 2) age at onset of disability, 3) ethnicity, and 4) marital status.

The racial groups presented in the sample included Caucasian (18), Asian (4), Hispanic (3), and African American (6). Ages ranged from 22 to 69, with ages at onset of disability ranging from birth to 52. Disabilities included cerebral palsy, postpolio, spina bifida, amputation (bilateral upper limb, unilateral lower limb), rheumatic conditions (including rheumatoid arthritis and systemic lupus erythematosus), multiple sclerosis, spinal cord injury, traumatic brain injury, and stroke. Sexual orientation consisted of 29 heterosexuals and 2 lesbians. At the time of the interview, 15 of the participants were never married, 7 were divorced, and 9 were married; 14 had children. Level of education attained was unrepresentatively high: 10 had graduate degrees, 7 had bachelor's degrees, 10 had some college, and 4 had a high school education. Seventeen worked for pay, and thirteen were considered unemployed but productive—that is, involved in home-making, educational, or volunteer activities. Only one was considered inactive.

Our sample divided fairly neatly into two groups: those who had expressed problems in a more positive sense and those who expressed problems in a more negative sense. The latter were more overcome by these problems, which tended to dominate their lives. When we compared these two groups of women, we tried to determine what was common among the more positive women versus the more negative women. This is where our wellness study started.

A WELLNESS PERSPECTIVE OF SEXUALITY AMONG WOMEN WITH PHYSICAL DISABILITIES

After analyzing the interviews, five thematic domains related to sexuality emerged. Stated from a wellness perspective, they are

1. Having a positive sexual self-concept
2. Having information about sexuality
3. Having positive, productive relationships
4. Managing barriers
5. Maintaining optimal health and physical sexual functioning

After elaborating on the data from which the domains were derived, our analysis is compared with some of the models of wellness in the literature mentioned earlier.

Having a Positive Sexual Self-Concept

The most expansive and complex grouping of themes in this study fall under the label "Sense of Self." It includes a broad array of themes covering self-concept, self-esteem, body image, sexual identity, and perception of roles, as well as the influence of family, friends, sexual partners, and society on the development of all of these. In considering sexuality from a wellness perspective, the notion of "sense of self" cannot be given a value label; however, several of its components can, such as self-esteem and body image. The following characteristics are common among women with disabilities who have a positive sexual self-concept.

She appreciates her own value. Despite any negative influences during the development of her self-concept, she thinks of herself as a sexually attractive and potent individual. The majority of women with early-onset disabilities who participated in the study reported hearing negative statements about their worth from family members. They were told, for example, that they should never hope for much in life, they could never be attractive to a sexual partner because of their disability, and no one would ever marry them. Many were told outright that they were a burden to the family. For some, persistent but unsuccessful efforts by medical professionals and faith healers to cure them imposed the notion that they were failures. A few in the sample had rejected these negative influences and defined their sexuality and attractiveness for themselves. Without exception, those raised by families who encouraged exploration of both personal and professional potential exhibited a more positive sexual self-concept. For women with later-onset disabilities, the effects of injury or illness may have challenged their already-determined self-concept. Many participants cited the positive effect of spirituality on their self-concept, whether it was through involvement in religious organizations or individual spiritual quests. According to one participant, "It sort of helps me to identify myself, thinking I am a woman created by God and I am so precious and I am so loved and I have so much beauty inside of me."

She asserts her right to make a choice. Even when life options seem limited, she acknowledges that she deserves the best and makes choices that will improve her life. Many women interviewed reported being told to accept whatever they were given, especially by abusive family members and partners. As a result, some were promiscuous in their sexual activities, desperately accepting anyone who came along. Those who were raised to develop and commit to their own sense of value were more selective and more satisfied with their choices. The woman with a more positive sexual self-concept respects her right to say no in any situation.

She feels ownership of her body. As a result of experiencing more physical abuse and many more medical procedures than most people, some women with disabilities, particularly those with an early age at onset, often feel that they must allow physical contact with any part of their body and must cooperate with anything demanded by an authority. This manifests in a dissociation from the body, apathy toward its care, and often a lack of awareness of the right to set boundaries around personal space. The sexually healthy woman accepts responsibility for her body, sets and maintains appropriate boundaries, and defends against inappropriate touch.

She is able to restrict the limitations resulting from her disability to physical functioning only and does not impose those limitations on her sexual self. Beatrice Wright, in her classic analysis of the psychosocial approach to disability (Wright, 1983), discusses the concept of spread, or the power of a single characteristic to evoke inferences about a person. The sexually well woman is able to isolate functional impairment to the body function impaired, even if that function is related to sexual activity, without perceiving her entire sexual being as impaired.

She takes action to improve herself and her relationships. One behavior common to women interviewed who demonstrated a more positive sexual self-concept was the effort to improve themselves through various means, including pursuing educational interests and engaging in social and recreational activities that enhanced life quality. For some, this characteristic takes the form of ending an unsatisfying relationship, changing jobs, suspending a career to take on a primary role of mother, or getting involved in new social groups. The woman with a positive sexual self-concept is not afraid to initiate contact with others and engages in productive activities.

She is accepting, not ashamed, of her body. A common theme was covering up one's body during sexual activities and turning out the lights so the partner would not see scars or deformities. One Hispanic participant, who, as a child, had experienced numerous surgeries and unsuccessful encounters with faith healers, reported finally feeling comfortable with letting her partner see her body in full light when she engaged in sexual activity with a man who also had a disability. This is not to say that a woman must embrace her body and disregard its limitations. Rather, women with more positive body images accepted their bodies, limitations and all, as a given and not a negative and were successful in maintaining a perception of themselves as attractive.

She makes her own decisions about assistive devices. Dealing with assistive and orthotic devices is a major challenge to developing a positive self-concept for women with physical disabilities, especially during adolescence. There is often a push from family and medical professionals to use braces instead of wheelchairs or prosthetic limbs instead of going without. One participant who had a bilateral arm amputation at birth grew up using her feet like hands, but was humiliated for doing so by her sixth grade teacher because the teacher felt it was inappropriate. She used cumbersome artificial arms with hooks whenever she was away from home until this past year. She is currently in counseling and has recently been able to feel comfortable in public without her prostheses. Another participant with lupus did not use a three-wheeled scooter even though ambulating long distances was getting more and more difficult. She succumbed to pressure from her husband, who did not want that symbol of disability around him. Others had more positive attitudes toward the devices that compensated for their functional limitations, regarding them as means of liberation rather than confinement or stigma.

She takes action to enhance her attractiveness. This is expressed in many different ways according to taste and values. For some women, it means maintaining cleanliness and neatness. For others, it extends to using makeup and clothing appropriately and fashionably. One participant with a severe disability from polio commented that she likes to wear makeup and fashionable clothes so she will look "less disabled."

Having Information About Sexuality

Among the women interviewed, especially those with early-onset disabilities, there was a pervasive lack of information about their own sexuality.

They tended not to know about the sexual functioning of their bodies, were often uninformed about sexually transmitted diseases, and, mostly out of fear, did not receive gynecological care until later in life. We have found examples in our sample where this deficit resulted in failure to recognize sexual abuse and exploitation, unwanted pregnancies, and preventable postpartum complications for the mother. Here are the characteristics present in the women who were the best informed about their sexuality.

She has general information about sexuality and is able to apply it to herself. Some women who were in special education classes never had the opportunity to see the sex education films traditionally shown in elementary school or were excused from taking high school gym and health class and therefore never learned about such topics as sexually transmitted diseases or breast self-examination. More than a few reported receiving this information along with everyone else, but never thought it applied to them because of their disability. The sexually well woman has the information she needs to understand and care for her own body.

She actively seeks information about how her disability affects her sexuality. She has access to resources, be they books, medical professionals, or other women with or without disabilities, and consults them to obtain answers to questions about her own sexual functioning. Many women interviewed relayed encounters with physicians who either said they did not know how their disabilities affected sexual functioning, said nothing at all, or provided inaccurate information. Among those few who had received comprehensive medical rehabilitation, none reported receiving the information they needed or wanted during that time. One participant with cerebral palsy was afraid to even ask about whether or not she could have sex until she was in her mid-20s. She finally got up the nerve to ask if she could get pregnant when she found a sex partner in her late 20s, and, at the time of the interview, was still too afraid to ask if she could carry a child to term. Those who exhibited sexual wellness actively sought information when it was needed and persisted until their questions were answered.

Having Positive, Productive Relationships

In this holistic approach to sexuality, relationships play a primary role. For women whose disabilities severely restrict the amount and quality of sexual activity, the role of relationships is even more important. Several characteristics of the woman with positive, productive relationships follow.

She feels generally satisfied with her relationships. Interacting with others, be they family, friends, work colleagues, or assistants, is a source of fulfillment for those women who felt that they were an integral part of a group or community. The women interviewed who did not have spouses or close family are very active in organizations and spend considerable time with friends. The sexually well-adjusted woman strikes a satisfying balance among her relationships.

She is able to communicate effectively with others. The sexually well woman is able to express her thoughts, feelings, and needs and, reciprocally, is able to respond when others do the same. The participants who exhibit higher levels of sexual wellness know if they are pleasing their partners and are able to talk about any problems and limitations and arrive at solutions together. When disability affects the ability to speak, as often occurs with cerebral palsy or brain injury, there can be severe limitations on social development. The issue becomes not only communicating feelings and desires to potential sexual partners, but also finding assistants to interpret effectively without speaking for the individual, thereby opening doors for social integration.

She feels stability in her relationships. Although she often has a variety of relationships, some long-standing, some short-term, the woman with greater sexual wellness has a few strong, very stable relationships that serve as anchors in her life. This could be a long-term, satisfying marriage, living together in a committed relationship, or, for those who are single, a strong friendship, a strong tie to family, or even a long-term working relationship with a personal assistant.

She is able to control the amount and nature of contact with others. Women with traits of sexual wellness were able to say no when they did not wish to be with someone, even if the relationship was strong and satisfying. This issue was particularly problematic with families. Participants related numerous accounts of overprotectiveness and dominance by parents and siblings, even after leaving home and gaining independence. Every woman is challenged to nurture relationships, yet protect her needs for privacy and solitude, but the woman with a disability struggles even harder to maintain this balance in light of her greater need for assistance from others.

Some special considerations relevant to the broad range of people with whom women with disabilities relate follow:

1. Family: The sexually well woman is able to maintain a satisfactory relationship with parents, siblings, and others without compromising her autonomy.
2. Friends: She has effective social skills and is able to initiate and sustain friendships.
3. Dates: She is able to initiate contacts or respond to overtures with no more fear of rejection than anyone else normally experiences. Her choice of dates is not governed primarily by disability considerations, but by other factors, such as mutual attraction, interests, and goals. She is able to maintain healthy relationships and end unsatisfactory ones.

4. Spouse/partner: If the disability occurs or worsens after marriage, she and her spouse are able to adapt to her loss and redefine their relationship, roles, and sexual behavior patterns as needed. For women with early-onset disabilities, once the challenges of dating have been resolved, many marriage issues are the same as for anyone else.

5. Children: There is congruence between the sexually well woman's desire to be a mother and actually becoming a mother. She is able to appraise realistically and carry out or supervise child care duties, using support resources as needed. She is able to resolve problems that arise in trying to make a house accessible yet childproof. She is satisfied with her fulfillment in her role as a mother.

6. Personal assistants: She is able to garner the assistance resources needed to support her in fulfilling the roles she has chosen. The resulting arrangement for receiving personal assistance is satisfactory. She is comfortable asking her assistant to help with personal hygiene and preparation for sexual activity.

Managing Barriers

Women with physical disabilities face long-standing, substantial barriers to expressing their sexuality. Sources of these barriers include the physical environment, the attitudes of society, and the abusive behaviors of people close to them. The number of reported incidents of psychological, physical, and sexual abuse and exploitation in this sample is alarmingly high. Although further analysis and data collection are necessary before any conclusions can be drawn, there appears to be a strong tendency for physical disability to increase the vulnerability of women to abuse (Ammerman, Cassisi, Hersen, & Van Hasselt, 1986; Cole, 1986; Doucette, 1986; Mullan & Cole, 1991; Murphy, 1993; Sobsey & Doe, 1991; Waxman, 1991). In many cases the cause of the abuse or barriers cannot be removed, so the issue becomes one of management and minimizing the negative impact as much as possible. Here are the characteristics found in the woman who has experienced abuse and exploitation or who has encountered environmental and societal barriers yet has been able to develop a positive sense of her sexual self.

She is able to recognize psychological, physical, and sexual abuse and exploitation and take action to reduce or eliminate it or to neutralize its impact. Some of the women interviewed had been so poorly informed about sexuality and life in general that they did not recognize the abuse until much later. They reported considerable psychological abuse and some physical and sexual abuse by parents, grandparents, siblings, spouses, dates, medical professionals, and strangers. Many were solitary incidents, but a large number were long-term, some current. The national survey, which will be Phase II of this study, will yield data on whether the incidence and prevalence of such experiences is higher in women with disabilities than in the population as a whole. The women in this sample who took action to end the abuse did so through divorce, counseling, avoidance, and escape. It is a major life challenge for women who have had these experiences to come to terms with them and develop positive sexuality in spite of them. For those with very limited life options, denial becomes the least damaging means of coping available to them.

She has learned to reduce her vulnerability. She recognizes what type of situation to avoid, be it with a date or a relative, in order to protect her emotional and physical health. Some of the participants who experienced long-term childhood abuse reported learning survival skills, such as talking their way out of it, seeking emotional support outside the family, and learning how to have back-up support available if a situation ever became life threatening.

She understands her disability-related environmental needs and seeks information on how to meet those needs. One participant had difficulty rising from soft couches and made a point of announcing that to all her friends to avoid embarrassing situations. For women who have progressive or fluctuating disabilities, this represents a constant learning process. It requires the ability to know whom to ask (often a medical professional or another woman with a disability) and where to get resources to obtain the required devices or modifications.

She recognizes her right to live in a barrier-free environment and takes action to achieve it. There were very few women in this sample who tolerated inaccessibilities. While total access is sometimes unobtainable, especially for those with very severe disabilities, the woman with a positive self-concept strives toward that goal. If a barrier cannot be removed, she finds creative ways around it. She does not respond by constantly complaining or by manipulating others.

She confronts societal barriers by using good communication skills to educate her partner, friends, and family. The sexually well women we interviewed were unlikely to listen without protest to overt expressions of stereotypes about the sexuality of women with disabilities. As painful as those assaults may be, they did not internalize them and they took actions to refute them. Communication skills are also needed to explain to others about personal needs. Several women reported an awkwardness over the timing and method of explaining to their dates about their catheters, yet they did it; and, once done, it was not an issue of concern to either party.

Maintaining Optimal Health and Physical Sexual Functioning

Disability can impose significant limitations on a woman's ability to maintain general good health and satisfactory physical sexual functioning. The following are the characteristics of the woman who manages these limitations most effectively.

She participates in health maintenance activities and engages in health-promoting behaviors. Many women in our study expressed this desire, but they were frustrated by inaccessible exercise and health care facilities, lack of information on how they could stay fit (including losing weight, when many did not have accessible scales), inadequate support services (transportation, personal assistance) to enable them to participate in health maintenance activities, and lack of health insurance to cover preventive measures and, for some, even basic care. As a reflection of their sense of self-worth, they valued their health and took steps to preserve it.

She feels congruity between her values/desires and her sexual behaviors. Even though many of the women interviewed expressed unfulfilled desire and frustration, the ones with the strongest sexual self-concept were doing something about it by initiating social contacts, participating in informal or formal support groups, or seeking counseling. Conversely, women with strong self-concepts did not engage in undesired sexual behavior simply because someone asked. They were true to themselves and took action to bring about the sought-after harmony.

She manages her environment to optimize privacy for intimate activities. This was a particularly serious problem for women who live with their parents or require assistance of another person to prepare for sexual activity. Those who were in such situations, but were satisfied with their privacy, had achieved high levels of communication with their personal assistants and partners.

She is satisfied with the frequency and quality of sexual activity. Our study showed that the relationship between satisfaction and level of sexual activity by women with disabilities must be interpreted in light of several factors. Many have been raised to believe that they should not expect sexual satisfaction. Others who acquire disability later in life accept the social stereotype that disability means the end of sex life. Some of the women interviewed who had never had a sexual experience with another person gravitated toward fundamentalist religious groups that subordinate sexual desire and discourage sexual activity. Disability itself may interfere with fertility and the ability to perform various types of sexual activity. Women who are prone to urinary tract infections or who must make elaborate preparations before and after sexual activity (for example, those who use ventilators) expressed the desire for more spontaneous and more frequent activity, but made their best effort to maximize enjoyment of the activities available to them.

She is able to communicate freely with her partner about her limitations and devices and about what pleases her sexually. The ability to talk with their partners was a strong common theme among participants with positive sexual self-concepts. It was an effective means of resolving problems and dealing with fears. It was often accompanied by a willingness to experiment to identify resolutions to problems or just to discover techniques for mutual pleasure.

CONCLUSIONS

All of the elements discussed in wellness models surfaced in this qualitative study of sexuality among women with physical disabilities. One of the most salient components was, of course, physical, but in a much different way from anticipated in many of the models. Intact physical functioning seemed to have little relevance to determining the individual's sexual wellness in this sample; rather, it set the stage for the interaction of all the other components. In Antonovsky's terms, physical impairment is a stressor that must be counterbalanced by psychological and social resistance courses.

The developmental component was particularly important for women with early-onset disabilities. The social climate and integration opportunities available during childhood—especially in terms of education, technology, and social attitudes toward disability—strongly influenced the development of a positive sexual self-concept among these women. Parents and siblings displaying an attitude of positive acceptance of the disability rather than enduring the disability as a tragedy also fostered a positive sexual self-concept.

The sociocultural component, that is, social resources and the general attitude toward disability, probably has a more powerful influence on the wellness of women with disabilities than on the population at large. On the one hand, it is a barrier, a stressor, a force that can strengthen resilience or cause defeat. Constant exposure to negative feedback (women with disabilities are ugly, worthless, burdensome to society, and unable to ever fulfill their proper role as women); the absence and, in some cases, withholding of information about one's body; and environmental barriers compounded by a lack of appropriate assistive technology are not factors most people have to deal with in their daily lives. On the other hand, sociocultural elements such as encouraging, supportive family and friends have an inestimable value in counteracting these negative forces. Living in an accessible environment has become possible only recently thanks to design and construction standards legislated since the 1970s (most recently, the Americans with Disabilities Act). The effect of enhanced accessibility on the development of a positive self-concept deserves serious investigation. In this study, culture had a strong influence on family attitude toward disability and the availability of family for support. The presence of supportive social systems was highly variable in this sample, dependent largely on geographic location and socioeconomic status.

Of the psychological elements mentioned—coherence, self-regulation, competence, resilience, empowerment, and health awareness—resilience seems to be the most relevant to the results of this study. There is a whole body of literature on resilience, yet it is seldom applied to women with disabilities. The setting of boundaries, or in Neuman's terms, lines of resistance and defense, emerged as an important part of this resilience. These boundaries were constantly threatened by insensitive behaviors of medical professionals and overwhelming overprotectiveness by family for many participants. The unexpectedly high incidence of abuse was another factor causing the hardening of defense mechanisms in this sample. Participants who exhibited the most signs of wellness tended to be assertive, resourceful, and proactive in their search for information and solutions to the barriers life presented.

Only a few participants commented on spirituality. For some, involvement in a religious organization was a means for finding refuge and comfort in situations of unbearable isolation and despair. A few of these sought out fundamentalist groups that subordinated sexuality. Others cited a strong sense of values that may or may not have stemmed from a church as an influence on their attitudes and behaviors. Although the spirituality of women with disabilities has been discussed (Lane, 1992), spirituality in the context of wellness needs considerably more definition before its interaction with psychological, social, and physical elements can be understood.

In conclusion, the sexual wellness of women with disabilities is gaining more attention. Cowen's (1991) notion of social system modification as a component of wellness clearly relates to the sexuality of women with physical disabilities. As far as policy makers are concerned, the change in perspective—from person-centered to situation-centered—is of fundamental importance. The way a social problem is defined determines the way policies are written, strategies for change are selected, social delivery systems are designed and implemented, and criteria for evaluation are considered. As long as women with physical disabilities are viewed as deviating from the sexual norm solely on the basis of disability, they will continue to be ignored by the medical and social services emerging to promote women's health and sexual wellness. What we are asking for is not only the removal of physical requirements from concepts of sexual wellness, but a redefinition of womanhood in its proper holistic sense throughout all segments of society. Schorr (1989) emphasized that breaking the cycle of disadvantage cannot occur through piecemeal interventions typical of the "blaming the victim" mentality; instead, they can come about only through comprehensive programs addressing the needs of individuals within a family and community context. Ultimately, such programs would promote a rich knowledge base and practices capable of improving all aspects of physical and psychological wellness.

REFERENCES

Abood, D.A., & Burkhead, E.J. (1988). Wellness: A valuable resource for persons with disabilities. *Health Education, 19*(2), 21–25.

Abood, D.A., & Mundy, C.J. (1986). *Wellness lifestyle model.* Unpublished manuscript, Florida State University, Tallahassee.

Adcock, C., & Newbigging, K. (1990). Women in the shadows: Women, feminism, and clinical psychology. In E. Burman (Ed.), *Feminists and psychological practice* (pp. 132–188). London: Sage.

Americans with Disabilities Act of 1990 (ADA), PL 101-336. (July 26, 1990). Title 42, U.S.C. 12101 et seq.: *U.S. Statutes at Large, 104,* 327–378.

Ammerman, R.T., Cassisi, J.E., Hersen, M., & Van Hasselt, V.B. (1986). Consequences of physical abuse and neglect in children. *Clinical Psychology Review, 6*(4), 291–310.

Antonovsky, A. (1979). *Health, stress, and coping.* San Francisco: Jossey-Bass.

Antonovsky, A. (1987). *Unraveling the mystery of health.* San Francisco: Jossey-Bass.

Architectural Barriers Act of 1968, PL 90-480. (August 12, 1968). Title 42, U.S.C. 4151 et seq.: *U.S. Statutes at Large, 82,* 718–719.

Cole, S.S. (1986). Facing the challenges of sexual abuse in persons with disabilities. *Sexuality and Disability, 7,* 71–88.

Cowen, E.L. (1991). In pursuit of wellness. *American Psychologist, 46,* 404–408.

Danek, M.M. (1992). The status of women with disabilities revisited. *Journal of Applied Rehabilitation Counseling, 23*(4), 7–13.

DeJong, G. (1979). Independent living: From social movement to analytic paradigm. *Archives of Physical Medicine and Rehabilitation, 60,* 435–446.

Doucette, J. (1986). *Violent acts against disabled women.* Toronto: DAWN (DisAbled Women's Network).

Education for All Handicapped Children Act of 1975, PL 94-142. (August 23, 1977). Title 20, U.S.C. 1400 et seq.: *U.S. Statutes at Large, 89,* 773–796.

Glaser, B.G., & Strauss, A.L. (1967). *Discovery of grounded theory: Strategies for qualitative research.* Chicago: Aldine.

Hanna, W.J., & Rogovsky, E. (1991). Women with disabilities: Two handicaps plus. *Disability, Handicap & Society, 6*(1), 49–62.

Hanna, W.J., & Rogovsky, E. (1992). On the situation of African-American women with disabilities. *Journal of Applied Rehabilitation Counseling, 23*(4), 39–45.

Individuals with Disabilities Education Act of 1990 (IDEA), PL 101-476. (October 30, 1990). Title 20, U.S.C. 1400 et seq.: *U.S. Statutes at Large, 104,* 1103–1151.

Lane, N.J. (1992). A spirituality of being: Women with disabilities. *Journal of Applied Rehabilitation Counseling, 23*(4), 53–58.

Lesh, K., & Marshall, C. (1984). Rehabilitation: Focus on women with disabilities. *Journal of Applied Rehabilitation Counseling, 15*(1), 18–21.

Mullan, P.B., & Cole, S.S. (1991). Health care providers' perceptions of the vulnerability of persons with disabilities: Sociological frameworks and empirical analyses. *Sexuality and Disability, 93,* 221–241.

Murphy, P. (1993). *Making the connections: Women, work, and abuse.* Orlando, FL: Paul M. Deutsch Press, Inc.

Neuman, B. (1982). *The Neuman systems model: Application to nursing education and practice.* Norwalk, CT: Appleton-Century-Crofts.

Nosek, M.A., & Fuhrer, M.J. (1992). Independence among people with disabilities: I. A heuristic model. *Rehabilitation Counseling Bulletin, 36,* 6–20.

Patton, M.Q. (1990). *Qualitative evaluation and research methods* (2nd ed.). Newbury Park, CA: Sage Publications.

Rehabilitation Act of 1973, PL 93-112. (September 26, 1973). Title 29, U.S.C. 794 et seq.: *U.S. Statutes at Large, 87,* 355–394.

Schorr, L.B. (1989). *Within our reach: Breaking the cycle of disadvantage.* New York: Doubleday/Anchor Books.

Sobsey, D., & Doe, T. (1991). Patterns of sexual abuse and assault. *Sexuality and Disability, 9,* 243–259.

Waxman, B.F. (1991). Hatred: The unacknowledged dimension in violence against disabled people. *Sexuality and Disability, 9*(3), 185–199.

Witmer, J.M., & Sweeney, T.J. (1992). A holistic model for wellness and prevention over the life span. *Journal of Counseling and Development, 71*(2), 140–148.

Wright, B.A. (1983). *Physical disability: A psychosocial approach* (2nd ed.). New York: Harper & Row.

chapter 3

Causes, Risks, and Consequences of Disability Among Women

Barbara M. Altman

Since the 1970s, various issues regarding persons with disabilities have gained wider recognition. Among these issues are employment, benefit programs, and health plans. Men with disabilities who serve as "bread-winners" for their families have long been eligible for federal and state supplemental income programs. More recently, other segments of the population with disabilities have received special attention, particularly education and benefits for children and long-term care issues for the increasing elderly population. However, despite the fact that one fifth of women in the United States have disabilities (McNeil, 1993), efforts to address the problems of women with disabilities are just beginning to gain interest.

In the early 1980s, there was an awakening to the general lack of research on women's health care problems (Moore, 1980; Public Health Service Task Force on Women's Issues, 1985). At the same time, the neglect of women with disabilities in the ongoing research on disability was also recognized (Altman, 1982, 1985; Barnartt, 1982; Deegan & Brooks, 1985; Fine & Asch, 1985). In the early 1990s, these two parallel streams began to address their one common concern, the relationship of disability to women's health problems. Because the risk of disability is generally associated with a woman's physical and mental health, the merging of these two research streams is an important step in understanding the causes and consequences of disability among women.

Except for one specific statistical data publication on demographics about women with disabilities (Bowe, 1984) and a few on access to benefits by women with disabilities (Johnson, 1979; Kutza, 1981; Mudrick, 1988), descriptive, statistical information about risks, causes, and consequences of disability among women at the national level is limited. When available at all, such information is buried within larger, more general publications (Collins, 1993; Haber, 1971; LaPlante, 1988, 1991; McNeil, 1993).[1] This chapter brings together published statistical information about women with disabilities in order to examine the causes and risks of impairment or disability for women in the United States and the social and economic outcomes associated with disability for that population.

DATA SOURCES

The primary sources of data for this chapter consist of other published work that used nationally representative data sets. Information on health conditions associated with disability is taken from analyses of the Health Interview Survey (HIS), sponsored by the National Center for Health Statistics. Two publications by LaPlante (1988, 1991) are the sources for the data from the HIS and the material on social epidemiology.

It is necessary to cumulate information from the HIS over several years in order to have a population with disability large enough to examine the less prevalent conditions. In one publication, data are cumulated from 1983–1985 (LaPlante, 1988). The second publication (1991) cumulates the data over a period of 4 years, instead of 3, from 1983 to 1986. Data from the tables in these publications were either excerpted or used in calculations to create the tables appearing here. Limitations were experienced because of what was available in the published material. Although it would have been preferable to use the data cumulated over 4 years alone, the content of that publication did not provide all the data necessary to calculate all the information presented here.

Information on the population estimates of women with disabilities and their sociodemographic characteristics is taken from published data based on a combined sample of the 1990 and 1991 panels of the Survey of Income and Program participation (SIPP), collected by the census (McNeil, 1993). These data supplied the information on socioeconomic characteristics that can be considered related to the consequences of disability as well. In addition, data on access to and utilization of health care among women with disabilities are reported from the National Medical

---

[1]This is just a recent sample of material that contains such information. Social Security data from the 1972, 1974, and 1978 surveys, for example, provided information on people with disabilities who received Social Security benefits. Other sources that could provide possible information would be ones that used data from the National Health Interview Survey sponsored annually by the National Center for Health Statistics or data from the 1977 and 1987 household surveys on Medical Expenditures sponsored by the Agency for Health Care Policy and Research (formerly the National Center for Health Services Research).

Expenditure Survey (NMES). NMES took place from January 1 to December 31, 1987, and collected data on health care utilization and expenditures from a nationally representative sample of households. The NMES material discussed on here is the result of an analysis done specifically for this chapter and has not been published previously. Further information on the National Medical Expenditure Survey can be found in Edwards and Berlin (1989).

Definitions of disability in this report are based on three commonly accepted measures: activity limitations, major activity limitations, and basic activity limitations (ADLs & IADLs); however, the exact questions may differ slightly between data sources. *Activity limitations* reflect limitations in role or role-related activities associated with one's age and gender. They can include but are not limited to major activities such as work, school, or housework. The measure is based on a question that generally asks the following: Are you limited in any way in any activities because of an impairment or health problem?

Major activity limitations focus on limitation of the person's major role activities, primarily those associated with work, school, or housework. The data also refer to *need for help in basic activities*. These are measures of ability to perform tasks associated with daily life. With this information, it is possible to identify those with more severe limitations; however, although this information is commonly used, it tends to provide limited sample sizes when used to analyze the wide range of conditions that can cause disability. Therefore, interpretation of information using this measure is limited at times because of estimates with relative standard errors greater than 30%.

ABOUT THE POPULATION

According to a recent census publication, as many as 26 million women in the United States are estimated to have some level of disability (McNeil, 1993). That is more than half (53%) of the estimated 49 million persons with a disability in the United States. Although disability is most often a correlate of increasing age, more than 1.4 million women under age 18 are estimated to have a disability (Table 1), and the largest proportion of the total population of women with a disability are ages 18–44 (28.4%). However, they represent only 13.7% of all women in that age group. As with men, the presence of disability is more common among the female population as it ages. Estimates from the census data indicate that, among women 85 years and over, approximately 86% have some type of activity limitation or disability.

Table 1. Women with a disability, as a percent of all women by sociodemographic characteristics

	Total number (1,000s)	Number with a disability	Percent of all women	Percent distribution among those with a disability
Total	129,104	26,020	20.2	100.0
Age				
Less than 18	32,256	1,412	4.4	5.4
18–44 years	54,112	7,400	13.7	28.4
45–64 years	24,880	7,203	29.0	27.7
65–74 years	10,156	4,608	45.4	17.7
75–84 years	6,002	3,939	65.6	15.1
85 years and over	1,699	1,458	85.8	5.6
Race / ethnicity				
White	98,322	20,326	20.7	78.1
Black	16,656	3,622	21.7	13.9
Hispanic	10,948	1,775	16.2	6.8
American, Eskimo, or Aleut	797	174	21.8	0.7
Asian or Pacific Islander	4,066	434	10.7	1.7
Years of school completed				
Persons 25 years old and over	84,338	23,342	27.7	
Less than 12	18,900	9,275	49.1	39.8
12	32,931	8,42	25.6	36.0
13–15	16,602	3,440	20.7	14.7
16 and over	15,905	2,206	13.9	9.5

Adapted from McNeil (1993).

Census data also indicate some racial/ethnic differences in rates of disability among women. Caucasian, African American, and Native American women are more likely to have a disability than are women of Hispanic or Asian descent (Table 1). Only 10.7% of the Asian and Pacific Islander population and 16.2% of the Hispanic population have a disability compared with 20.7% of Caucasian women, 21.7% of African American women, and 21.8% of Native American women.

Of women ages 25 and over, those with higher levels of education are less likely to have a disability. Only 13.9% of those with 16 or more years of education have a disability, while almost half of those who have less that 12 full years of education have disabilities, according to the estimates reported by McNeil (1993) (Table 1).

From this descriptive material, it is clear that some ascribed and achieved characteristics of these individuals are associated with creating more risk for disability during their lifetime. Older age, race, and even level of education or combinations of the three can contribute to the potential for acquiring a disability. However, to truly understand the factors that contribute to the risk for a woman to acquire a disability, a social epidemiological approach is best.

SOCIAL EPIDEMIOLOGY

Generally, disabilities result from some chronic physical or mental health condition that limits one's ability to perform activities associated with his or her social roles or with tasks associated with maintaining life. The chronic physical or mental health problem can be caused by either a birth defect, an accident, or disease. Although chronic conditions or impairments are precursors to disability, they vary widely in their risk of causing disability. To understand the risk of disability as a result of various diseases and impairments, several factors must be taken into account. These factors form two classes: "those intrinsic to health conditions and those related to the characteristics of the individual and the social and physical environment" (LaPlante, 1991, p. 1).

The differences noted in Table 1 are associated with the demographic and social characteristics of the individual. For example, education is an element usually associated with social class because persons with higher levels of education generally have better jobs, which result in higher incomes. In this case, persons with higher levels of education show a lower proportion with disability. This is consistent with the literature, which has shown that chronic physical and mental health conditions are found more frequently among people of lower income (Dutton, 1986). This is an example of social class (as represented by education) becoming a social risk factor associated with disability.

The factors intrinsic to health conditions include the clinical aspects of the disease or impairment, such as prognosis, course of treatment, degree of functional limitation, and rehabilitation potential (LaPlante, 1991). An accurate comparison of the risks of disability associated with chronic diseases would require knowledge of the natural history of the disease. However, this is a difficult task in the individual case and next to impossible to achieve on a national level. In addition, social and environmental factors discussed earlier contribute to effects of diseases and could not be controlled adequately to effectively isolate the intrinsic factors.

To arrive at a crude estimate of risk, an alternative is to use our knowledge of the prevalence of chronic physical and mental conditions and the prevalence of disability as attributed by the individual to that condition, within each type of chronic condition or impairment. If we look only at the proportion of persons with a specific chronic condition among those who have a disability, we can overstate the disability risks of less severe conditions. That is because the assessment of risks is often complicated by the presence of multiple chronic conditions, only one of which is primarily responsible for the disability. Some conditions, such as hypertension and arthritis, are quite common, especially as people age. If we calculate the number of persons with hypertension who have a disability, some disability caused by other conditions will be misattributed to hypertension.

The commonly accepted alternative to the problem of estimating disability risk, which avoids the complications of multiple conditions, is to identify only the condition considered to be the main cause of disability. This method, called *direct causal attribution*, accepts the affected individual's judgment (or a professional's) of which condition is the primary cause of his or her disability (LaPlante, 1991). When one condition alone is specified, it is simpler to obtain an estimate of the number of cases in which a particular condition causes a disability. An estimate of risk can then be calculated by dividing the estimated number of cases in which a condition causes a disability by the estimated total number of cases of that condition. This correction for the total number of cases with a condition controls for the actual prevalence of the condition in the total population. Using such a technique, we find that conditions with a high prevalence in the population have relatively low risks of disability, while conditions that occur less frequently can have a much greater risk of causing disability.

Using the main cause of disability reported by respondents in the Health Interview Survey (Table 2), we note conditions with the highest prevalence of activity limitation for the total population, for men only, and for women only. In the total population, three types of conditions account for more than one third of all conditions identified as the main cause of disability: orthopedic impairments, arthritis, and heart disease. The same three types of conditions are the leading main causes of disability among men and women separately; however, the rankings differ. Arthritis is the leading condition among women (16.3% compared to 7.6%), while orthopedic impairments are the leading condition associated with disability among men.

When genders are separated, we also see that the remaining rankings vary both between men and women and among men, women, and the total population. For example, among women, hypertension is ranked as the fourth cause of disability, while it is ranked twelfth among men and eighth in the total population. Another example of information gained by looking at women separately is that the types of conditions most prevalent are not consistent within each group. Prevalence of emphysema and other respiratory diseases are among the top 15 main causes of disability for men, but not for women. Rather, osteomyelitis/bone disorders and phlebitis/varicose veins are more prevalent main causes of disability for women. Gender differences, then, are masked by viewing the main causes of disability in the total population.

As indicated earlier, prevalence of conditions associated with disability does not accurately reflect the relative risk of disability for an individual

Table 2. Prevalence of activity limitation due to chronic conditions by main cause of limitation and gender: U.S. civilian noninstitutionalized population, 1983–1985 (3-year average)

Main cause of limitation	Both genders			Males			Females		
	Prevalence (1,000s)	%	Rank	Prevalence	%	Rank	Prevalence	%	Rank
All conditions	32,540	100.0		15,178	100.0		17,362	100	
Orthopedic impairments	5,220	16.0	1	2,607	17.2	1	2,612	15.0	2
Arthritis	4,000	12.3	2	1,161	7.6	3	2,839	16.3	1
Heart disease	3,736	11.4	3	1,971	13.0	2	1,765	10.2	3
Visual impairment	1,438	4.4	4	704	4.6	6	736	4.3	6
Intervertebral disk disorder	1,424	4.4	5	741	4.9	5	683	3.9	7
Mental disorders[a]	1,425	4.3	6	748	5.0	4	680	3.8	8
Asthma	1,411	4.3	7	657	4.3	7	754	4.3	5
Hypertension	1,239	3.8	8	406	2.7	12	834	4.8	4
Nervous system disorders[b]	1,148	3.6	9	529	3.4	9	622	3.6	9
Mental retardation	947	2.9	10	583	3.8	8	364	2.1	12
Diabetes	885	2.7	11	346	2.3	13	539	3.1	10
Hearing impairments	813	2.5	12	443	2.9	11	370	2.1	11
Emphysema	649	2.0	13	416	3.1	10	183	1.1	—
Cerebrovascular disease	610	1.9	14	340	2.2	14	270	1.6	13
Osteomyelitis/bone disorders	360	1.1	15	109	0.7	—	251	1.4	14
Other respiratory disease	321	1.0	—	209	1.4	15	112	0.6	—
Phlebitis/varicose veins	271	0.8	—	68	0.4	—	203	1.2	15

Adapted from LaPlante (1988).

[a] Combines schizophrenia/other psychoses, neuroses/personality disorders, other mental illness, alcohol or drug dependency and senility from Table 6A, LaPlante (1988).

[b] Combines epilepsy, multiple sclerosis, Parkinson's disease, other nervous disorders from Table 6A, LaPlante (1988).

with a specific condition. Crude estimates of risks of disability for women are shown in Table 3. Conditions in this table are not grouped to the extent they are in Table 2. For example, the condition *arthritis*, which appeared in Table 2, is represented by two forms of arthritis in the original risk tables (LaPlante, 1991). Only one type of arthritis, rheumatoid arthritis, is among the 15 conditions with the highest risk of disability for women. Those 15 conditions are ranked in Table 3 for each type of disability, any activity limitation, major activity limitation, or need for help with basic life activities. In some instances, the condition is so rare that the relative standard errors of the estimates are large, which precludes us from making a dependable estimate of risk. This is the case for the first condition in the table, absence of leg(s). However, all the other estimates of risk of disability are not subject to precision problems.

Of the 15 conditions with the highest risks of activity limitation for women, only six are diseases. The remaining conditions are impairments. Setting absence of leg(s) aside, multiple sclerosis and mental retardation are clearly the conditions with the greatest risk of any activity limitation or major activity limitations for women of all ages. Risks of activity limitation from other diseases such as heart disease, emphysema, or diabetes are about 50% less than for the leading high-risk conditions. However, it is important to note that even the 15th-ranked condition, emphysema, causes some activity limitation in about 43% of those with the condition. Of the three high prevalence conditions, only orthopedic impairments and one form of arthritis, rheumatoid arthritis, fall into the top 10 conditions associated with higher risks of disability. When compared to conditions with the highest risks for disability among men (see LaPlante, 1991), the most notable differences are that, for men, multiple sclerosis, epilepsy, and rheumatoid arthritis are not among the top 15 conditions associated with risk.

Rankings of the conditions causing risks of major activity limitation are very similar to those causing activity limitation, although epilepsy and emphysema fall out of the top 15. Cardiovascular disease and diabetes are included in their place. Overall a larger proportion of conditions cause activity limitations for women than cause major activity limitations (11.2% compared with 7.9%).

The need for assistance in basic life activities is associated with more severe limitations and occurs less frequently than activity limitation. Among women, it is caused by only 3.1% of conditions. Conditions with the highest risk of causing need for assistance in basic life activities are ranked somewhat differently. While multiple sclerosis still ranks as the highest risk factor, lung or bronchial cancer and complete paralysis rank second and fourth, once again excluding absence of leg(s). At this level of disability particularly, we can see that the most prevalent conditions are

Table 3. Conditions with highest risk of disability for women, by type of disability: United States 1983–1986 (4-year average)

Chronic conditions	Number of conditions (1,000s)	Percentage causing any activity limitation	Rank	Percentage causing major activity limitation	Rank	Percentage causing need for help in basic life activities	Rank
All selected chronic conditions	230,096	11.2		7.9		3.1	
Absence of leg(s)	56[a]	86.3[a]	1	81.2[a]	1	55.8[a]	3
Multiple sclerosis	123	84.0	2	73.8	2	48.9	1
Mental retardation	440	79.0	3	73.2	3	22.0	9
Lung or bronchial cancer	90	68.7	4	61.4	4	37.1	2
Cerebral palsy	85	68.3	5	61.1	5	28.2	6
Other orthopedic impairments	161	60.8	6	50.3	6	18.1[a]	12
Complete paralysis in extremity	277	55.3	7	43.3	8	28.9	4
Blind in both eyes	205	54.9	8	47.8	7	28.8	5
Rheumatoid arthritis	902	53.6	9	41.5	10	18.7	11
Partial paralysis in extremity	259	50.8	10	40.1	11	27.7	7
Intervertebral disk disorders	1,775	46.6	11	36.8	12	7.4	—
Epilepsy	584	45.5	12	28.7	—	10.5	—
Other heart disease / disorders[b]	2,633	45.4	13	33.1	13	15.0	13
Cancer of digestive sites	121	45.4	14	42.8	9	20.6	10
Emphysema	675	42.8	15	26.8	—	12.2	14
Cardiovascular disease	1,331	36.8	—	30.4	14	25.3	8
Diabetes	3,487	37.8	—	30.1	15	12.0	15

Adapted from LaPlante (1991).

[a] Relative standard error exceeds 30%; number has low statistical reliability or precision.

[b] Heart failure, valve disorders, congenital disorders, all other, and ill-defined heart conditions.

43

not necessarily the ones with the greatest risk for causing limitation. The most prevalent conditions on the table—diabetes, other heart disease/disorders, and intervertebral disk disorders—are at the lower ends of the ranking or are not ranked in the first 15 at all. However, the rarer conditions (such as multiple sclerosis [MS], lung or bronchial cancer, complete paralysis, and blindness in both eyes) have the highest risks of causing the most serious limitations.

Because some chronic conditions become more prevalent with age, it is not always useful to look at prevalence and risk across the total age range exclusively. Conditions associated with aging, such as heart disease and arthritis, although present in younger age groups, are quite rare at younger ages. Considering conditions with the greatest prevalence among persons with disabilities of all ages may mask conditions, such as asthma, more prevalent during a particular age range. In the same way, considerations of risk of limitations caused by such conditions over the complete age range may misrepresent the actual risk during the age range when the condition is more prevalent or less prevalent. The next two tables introduce age into the discussion of prevalence and risks of conditions associated with disability among women.

Focusing on the main cause of limitation reported by different age cohorts in Table 4, we observe the prevalence of the 15 conditions reported in Table 2 as the leading conditions associated with activity limitations. Clearly, the most prevalent conditions for those under age 18 are very dissimilar for those in the other age groups. Asthma and mental retardation account for one third of conditions associated with activity limitations among women under 18. Orthopedic impairments account for another 8.8%. Hearing impairments and mental disorders complete the top five. For women ages 18–44, orthopedic conditions alone are associated with activity limitations three times as frequently as among those under 18 and more than twice as frequently as in the next oldest age cohort, 45–69. In fact, among those ages 18–44, orthopedic impairments are four times more prevalent than the next most prevalent condition, asthma. In addition, nervous system disorders, which include the condition (MS) associated with the greatest risk of limitation for women, are most prevalent between the ages 18 and 44.

Arthritis becomes the most prevalent condition associated with activity limitation for women ages 45–69 and continues as the most prevalent after age 70. Heart disease is second in both age cohorts, followed by orthopedic impairments. Hypertension reaches its peak of prevalence in association with activity limitations between the ages 45 and 69 (7.4%); it is more than twice as prevalent during that age range than in any other age range. Among women age 70 or over, visual impairment is ranked fourth, the highest prevalence for that condition compared with the other age categories.

Table 4. Prevalence of activity limitation due to chronic conditions among women by main cause of limitation and age: U.S. civilian noninstitutionalized population, 1983–1985 (3-year average)

Main cause of limitation[b]	Under 18		18–44		45–69		70+	
	1,293	100.0	4,144	100.0	7,675	100.0	4,250	100.0
Arthritis	13[a]	1.1[a]	276	6.7	1,538	20.1	717	16.8
Orthopedic impairment	146	8.8	1090	26.2	960	12.5	286	6.7
Heart disease	34	2.6	171	4.1	912	11.8	466	11.0
Hypertension	2[a]	0.1	114	2.8	567	7.4	113	2.7
Asthma	225	17.4	284	6.8	198	2.6	36	0.8
Visual impairment	37	2.9	103	2.5	223	3.0	233	5.5
Intervertebral disk disorder	—	—	274	6.6	358	4.7	38	0.9
Mental disorders[c]	77	6.0	154	3.7	192	2.4	130	3.0
Nervous system disorder[d]	48	3.7	238	5.7	236	3.0	74	1.7
Diabetes	10[a]	0.8[a]	79	1.9	304	4.0	111	2.6
Hearing impairments	99	7.7	89	2.2	100	1.3	54	1.3
Mental retardation	205	15.9	123	3.0	31	0.4	3	0.1
Cerebrovascular disease	3[a]	0.2[a]	14[a]	0.3[a]	97	1.3	107	2.5
Osteomyelitis/bone disorders	12[a]	0.9[a]	35	0.9	124	1.6	57	1.3
Phlebitis/varicose veins	2[a]	0.2[a]	51	1.2	125	1.6	19	0.4

Number of conditions in thousands and percent distribution

Adapted from LaPlante (1988).

[a]Relative standard error exceeds 30%; number has low statistical reliability or precision.

[b]Uses order of prevalence ranking conditions for all women, as calculated in Table 2.

[c]Combines schizophrenia / other psychoses, neuroses / personality disorders, other mental illness, alcohol or drug dependency and senility from Table 6A, LaPlante (1988).

[d]Combined epilepsy, multiple sclerosis, Parkinson's disease, other nervous disorders from Table 6A, LaPlante (1988).

Examining the risk of conditions causing disability among women in the various age categories is difficult for a number of reasons. First, the less prevalent conditions become even rarer occurrences when we focus on a single age group that is a subportion of the population. The low sample sizes that are used to represent the less frequently occurring conditions translate into estimates with relative standard errors greater than 30%, which in turn lowers the reliability of the estimate. Second, the NHIS data used for this analysis include many conditions that have low prevalence among children under age 18 and do not include some conditions specific to that population. This limits our ability to make estimates for that group. Finally, this report is based on published data and is limited by the classifications and the form of analysis chosen by the original authors. Within those constrictions, Table 5 presents the conditions with the highest risks of causing work limitations for two groups of women ages 18–69.

The top 15 conditions with the highest risk associated with work limitations for women ages 18–44 and 45–69 are ranked in Table 5, regardless of their relative standard errors. Because of the unreliability of those estimates (with relative standard errors over 30%), which occurs in approximately 50% of the cells of this table, these results are discussed in very general terms. Among women ages 18–44, there are some conditions unambiguously associated with risk of work limitation, including mental retardation, epilepsy, intervertebral disk disorders, rheumatoid arthritis, and orthopedic impairment in the upper extremities. When age is considered along with gender, some new conditions are introduced into the top 15 high-risk conditions. Among this group (ages 18–44), orthopedic impairment in the upper extremities and cancer of the breast are conditions with more than a 20% risk of causing work limitations and rank 14th and 15th. Less than 1% of conditions are associated with a high risk of need for help in basic life activities in this younger group, and the risk estimate for only one condition, mental retardation, can be considered precise.

Among older women, ages 45–69, several conditions show greater risk of causing a work limitation than among the younger group. Conditions with the highest risk of work limitations that can be discussed with some precision include mental retardation, epilepsy, intervertebral disk disorders, and rheumatoid arthritis. All four conditions were noted among the younger women as well. In addition, older women risk work limitations if they have complete paralysis in the extremities. Although orthopedic impairments in upper extremities and cancer of the breast are also associated with over 20% risk of work limitations, other heart disease/disorders and cancer of the genitourinary sites demonstrate higher risks not evident among the younger group. As with the younger group, few of the estimates of risk associated with the need for help in basic activities can be considered precise. However, rheumatoid arthritis and intervertebral disk disorders can be interpreted as reliable estimates of risk.

Table 5. Conditions with highest risk of disability for women by age and type of disability: United States 1983–1986 (4-year average)

Chronic condition	Ages 18–44				Ages 45–69			
	Number of conditions (1,000s)	Percent causing any work limitation	Rank	Percent causing need for help in basic life activities	Number of conditions (1,000s)	Percent causing any work limitation	Rank	Percent causing need for help in basic life activities
All selected chronic conditions	82,431	4.0		0.5	83,803	11.2		2.3
Absence of leg(s)	3[a]	100.0[a]	1	0.0	24[a]	84.7[a]	1	38.3[a]
Lung or bronchial cancer	3[a]	100.0[a]	2	0.0	39[a]	67.6[a]	6	28.0[a]
Mental retardation	132	65.0	3	43.8	65	74.5	3	26.7[a]
Blind in both eyes	42[a]	62.9[a]	4	10.2[a]	48[a]	78.1[a]	2	38.1[a]
Complete paralysis in extremity	36[a]	62.5[a]	5	21.8[a]	115	42.9	12	19.5[a]
Multiple sclerosis	52[a]	61.8[a]	6	34.9[a]	59[a]	69.9[a]	5	51.1[a]
Cerebral palsy	32[a]	54.7[a]	7	55.3[a]	13[a]	73.2[a]	4	0.0
Cancer of digestive sites	6[a]	49.0[a]	8	0.0	77	39.3[a]	15	14.1[a]
Epilepsy	276	40.7	9	10.7[a]	106	47.1	7	7.4[a]
Intervertebral disk disorder	671	36.7	10	6.2[a]	908	43.8	10	8.1
Rheumatoid arthritis	164	36.5	11	2.3[a]	550	42.3	13	14.5
Other orthopedic impairments	60[a]	32.7[a]	12	0.0	74	43.0[a]	11	19.5[a]
Partial paralysis in extremity	38[a]	27.1[a]	13	0.0	99	45.9	8	27.5[a]
Orthopedic impairment in upper extremity	467	22.9	14	1.9[a]	525	27.0	—	4.4[a]
Cancer of female breast	59[a]	21.4[a]	15	0.0	247	22.3	—	3.4[a]
Other heart disease/disorders[b]	520	16.6	—	1.9[a]	988	44.8	9	5.8[a]
Cancer of genitourinary sites	109	7.1[a]	—	3.5[a]	75	40.9[a]	14	0.0

Adapted from LaPlante (1991).

Note that the definition of disability is limited in this table to two types, Work Limitations (or what in early tables had been defined as "Major Activity" limitations) and Need for Help in Basic Life Activities. Any Work Limitations rather than Any Activity limitations are used in this table because that is the only published data readily available.

[a] Relative standard error exceeds 30%; number has low statistical reliability or precision.

[b] Heart failure, valve disorder, congenital disorder, all other ill-defined heart conditions.

As can be seen from this examination of risks of disability among women of different ages, crude estimates subsume differences in many characteristics of populations with specific conditions. However, populations with specific conditions vary not only by age and gender, but also by many other sociodemographic variables such as race, marital status, educational attainment, duration of the condition, and other factors associated with disability risk. For this reason, it is appropriate to provide estimates of the risks of chronic conditions causing disability *adjusted* for all of those population characteristics. Classic adjustments are made by the method of direct standardization: Risks are estimated for various categories of one compositional variable and weighted according to a standard population distribution to obtain a summary adjusted risk factor. When the populations differ with respect to many variables, multivariate adjustment is more appropriate. Such a multivariate analysis for women is not available in published data at this point, but would contribute further to our understanding the combined effects of disease, impairment, and environment on risks of disability for women. LaPlante (1991), our main resource for this portion of the chapter, does use two multivariate analyses of risk of chronic conditions and impairments causing activity and work limitations for the total population. Gender is a variable included in that analysis. The reader is referred to LaPlante (1991) for an interesting discussion of the methodology and results.

OUTCOMES ASSOCIATED WITH DISABILITY STATUS

It cannot be unequivocally stated that disability is the cause of many of the social outcomes experienced by women with various levels of limitations, but there are some associations that are noteworthy. Economic status of women with disabilities, ages 15–64, is displayed in Table 6 in terms of income and use of means-tested assistance. Although women with disabilities make up 17.9% of all women ages 15–64, they account for 28.2% of women below the poverty level, 25.1% of women near the poverty level, and only 11.1% of women at the highest income level. The situation among women with severe disabilities, about half of the women ages 15–64 with a disabilities, is more economically limited. Only 3.8% of that group have incomes in the highest range, whereas twice their actual proportion in the population (17.6%) are below the poverty level.

The economic difficulties of this population are further elaborated by the information on the use of means-tested assistance. These data show that women with disabilities are a very large proportion of those covered by Medicaid, those receiving cash assistance, and those receiving housing assistance (44.0%, 49.8%, and 34.1%, respectively). A majority of those with disabilities receiving these benefits have severe disabilities (77% of

Table 6.   Income, benefits, for women 15–64 with disability, by level of disability: 1991–1992

	Total (1,000s)	With a disability		With a severe disability	
		N	%	N	%
	83,886	14,978	17.9	7,309	8.7
Ratio of income to two-income threshold					
Less than 1.00	13,931	3,935	28.2	2,455	17.6
1.00 to 1.49	7,713	1,939	25.1	1,146	14.9
1.50 to 1.99	8,180	1,675	20.5	841	10.3
2.00 to 2.99	16,068	2,774	17.3	1,189	7.4
3.00 to 3.99	12,794	1,853	14.5	730	5.7
4.00 and over	25,183	2,798	11.1	944	3.8
Means-tested assistance					
Covered by Medicaid	7,309	3,215	44.0	2,497	34.2
Received cash assistance	5,203	2,590	49.8	2,108	40.5
Received food stamps	5,405	2,127	29.4	1,488	27.5
Received housing assistance	3,579	1,221	34.1	845	23.6
Received both cash assistance and food stamps	3,764	1,569	41.7	1,166	31.0
Received all those benefits	1,332	581	43.7	432	32.5
Did not receive assistance	75,275	11,452	15.2	4,662	6.2

Adapted from McNeil (1993).

those covered by Medicaid and 81% of those receiving cash benefits—calculations not shown on Table 6). However, overall, about 36% of those with severe disabilities receive means-tested assistance, while 49% are below or close to the poverty threshold.

The economic status of women with disabilities can be explained in part by their employment and earnings. Indications of those associations are shown in Table 7, which contains information on the employment status of all women, and Table 8, which compares the mean earnings of men and women.

When compared with women without disabilities, women with disabilities are less likely to be employed (Table 7). According to the census data for women age 21–64, 72.6% of women without a disability were employed, while only 45.2% of women with a disability had any employment. The employment rate for women with a severe disability was half of that for all women with a disability, only 22.7%. Examining women with severe disability more closely reveals the extent of the disadvantage. Women with a severe disability make up 9.5% of the total population of women ages 21–64, but only 3.2% of all employed women. Instead they account for more than twice their proportion in the population among all women who are not employed (22.5%).

Table 7. Work outcomes for women with and without a disability, age 21–64 by level of disability

	Total (1,000s)	Without a disability			With a disability			With a severe disability		
		N	%	Percent distribution[a]	N	%	Percent distribution[a]	N	%	Percent distribution[a]
	73,855	59,688	80.8	100.0	14,167	19.2	100.0	7,019	9.5	100.0
Employment status										
Employed	49,709	43,301	87.1	72.6	6,408	12.9	45.2	1,594	3.2	22.7
Not employed	24,146	16,387	67.9	27.4	7,759	32.1	54.8	5,425	22.5	77.3

Adapted from McNeil (1993).
[a]Percent distribution among those without a disability, those with a disability, and those with a severe disability, as appropriate.

Table 8. Mean monthly earnings by sex and type of disability

	Men			Women		
	With earnings (1,000s)	Value	Standard error	With earnings (1,000s)	Value	Standard error
Total	66,298	$2,367	$23	56,070	$1,406	$10
Disability status						
with no disability	57,311	2,405	23	48,842	1,441	11
With a disability	8,986	2,122	90	7,228	1,171	24
Severe	1,544	1,890	368	1,831	1,028	42
Not severe	7,443	2,170	77	5,397	1,220	29

Adapted from McNeil (1993).

Table 8 shows the mean monthly earnings of employed men and women with and without disability. Even when women with disabilities are employed, their mean earnings are the lowest as compared with men with and without a disability and women without a disability (Table 8). Using the salary of men without a disability as the standard, we find that men with disabilities have mean monthly earnings 88% of the standard (calculation not shown). The mean monthly earnings of women without a disability is 60% of the standard, and women with a disability have mean monthly earnings that is only 49% of the standard.

The discrepancy also exists when earnings of women without a disability are used as the standard. In that case, mean monthly earnings of women with a disability are 81% of that of women without a disability. For women with a severe disability, the comparison with women without a disability indicates they earn only 71% of what is earned by women without a disability and 84% of what is earned by women with less severe disabilities. Gender, disability, and severity of disability are characteristics that combine to create a clear-cut hierarchy of earnings that demonstrates a disadvantage to women with disability. Unfortunately, these data verify that earnings outcomes for women with a disability have changed little since the 1970s (Altman, 1982, 1985).

The economic status of women with disabilities probably accounts for their health insurance status and access to health care. An analysis of the National Medical Expenditure Survey data for women age 18 and over shows that, although there is no significant difference between women with and without disabilities in terms of having health insurance, the sources of that insurance are very different (Table 9). Women with disabilities are significantly less likely to have private insurance and more likely to have public insurance or some combination of public and private insurance. This combination reflects the larger proportion of elderly women among those with disabilities. There is a relatively small proportion of women with disabilities who are uninsured, similar to women without disabilities.

In spite of the reliance on public insurance, women with disabilities are more likely to have a general practitioner as their source of care and less likely than women without disabilities to have no source of care at all. However, their insurance status is an important factor in the nature of their source of care (Table 10). Women with disabilities who are uninsured are likely to have no source of care or to have no regular doctor at their source of care. In contrast, women with both private and public insurance are the least likely to be without a source of care or a regular doctor.

Table 11 displays data regarding the volume of medical care use among women. In 1987, women without disabilities reported an average of 7 ambulatory visits, while women with a disability had an average of 13.6 visits, almost twice as many as women without disabilities. Of those

Table 9. Health insurance and source of health care among women ages 18 and over by disability status, 1987

	Women with a disability[a]	Women without a disability
Total (1,000s)	17,910	74,120
Any insurance	93.1	91.5
Type of insurance		
Private	34.7	73.0
Public	22.2	7.0
Both private and public	36.2	11.4
Uninsured	6.9	8.6
Source of care		
No source	9.9	19.2
Source / No doctor[b]	7.6	12.4
General practitioner	71.2	58.3
Specialist	11.3	10.1

Data from Agency for Health Care Policy and Research: National Medical Expenditure Survey, 1987.

[a] Disability is measured by limitations in kind or amount of work or inability to work.

[b] Respondents indicated they had a source of care but did not see a specific doctor regularly at that source of care.

13.6 visits, an average of 8.3 are doctor visits, about 61% of the ambulatory visits. For women without disabilities, the average number of doctor visits per year is 4.8, about 68% of ambulatory visits. Women with disabilities have approximately 73% more doctor visits than do women without disabilities, but have only about 33% more hospital stays during the year, an average of 1.6 compared to an average of 1.2 for women without disabilities. The data indicate that in the face of lower incomes and different types of insurance coverage, women with disabilities are receiving greater

Table 10. Sources of health care among women with disabilities ages 18 and over by type of health insurance, 1987

	Type of insurance			
	Private insurance	Public insurance	Both private and public	Uninsured
Total (1,000s)	6,214	3,979	6,477	1,235
Source of care				
No source	12.7	8.0	5.4	25.7
Source / No doctor[a]	6.4	13.0	3.4	18.2
General practitioner	69.6	68.8	79.0	45.6
Specialist	11.3	10.2	12.2	10.5

Data from Agency for Health Care Policy and Research: National Medical Expenditure Survey, 1987.

Note. Disability is measured by limitations in kind or amount of work or inability to work.

[a] Respondents indicated they had a source of care but did not see a specific doctor regularly at that source of care.

Table 11. Mean number of visits to health care providers and hosptial stays among women age 18 and over with and without disabilities, 1987

	Mean number ambulatory visits[a]	Mean number doctor visits	Mean number hospital stays
Women with disabilities	13.6	8.3	1.6
Women without disabilities	7.0	4.8	1.2

Data from Agency for Health Care Policy and Research: National Medical Expenditure Survey (1987).
[a]Ambulatory visits include all doctor visits and outpatient and emergency room visits.

amounts of health care services. In light of the greater need for care associated with disabling conditions, this is not unexpected. The data, however, do not indicate whether the level of services is sufficient to meet the needs. A mean or average number of visits indicates that some persons in the sample may be receiving substantially more service then the average, while others are receiving less. Those who are uninsured and without a source of health care or regular doctor at their health care centers are certainly not receiving the mean level of care. Further research on health care access and utilization by women with disabilities is necessary to understand the effects of low income and the varieties of insurance.

CONCLUSIONS

This chapter has examined the factors associated with disability among women, with an emphasis on the types of chronic conditions and impairments that have the greatest risks of causing disability for this population. Arthritis is the most prevalent condition associated with disability among women, followed by orthopedic impairment and heart disease. These are the same top three conditions that are found among men, but in a slightly different order. When the 15 most prevalent conditions are considered, however, some conditions not so prevalent among women are replaced by others, so the list changes in content as well as ranking from that of men. Apparently, the conditions that have the greatest risk for causing disability among women (as with the general population) are the least prevalent conditions. These include MS, mental retardation, lung and bronchial cancer, and cerebral palsy.

Further elaboration on the prevalence of conditions and risks of disability for women indicate that age is an important cofactor to be considered. Younger women are more likely to have limitations associated with asthma, mental retardation, orthopedic impairments, and hearing impairments. However, the risk of having a work limitation is greater for the younger group, ages 18–44, if they have mental retardation, epilepsy, intervertebral disk disorders, and rheumatoid arthritis. We have not mentioned those conditions whose relative standard errors were greater than 30%, because such estimates must be considered less precise. Other chronic conditions and impairments increase in prevalence at later stages in life. By ages 45–69, arthritis, orthopedic impairments, and heart disease have become the most prevalent conditions associated with disability for women. The ranking of risks of work limitations for the older group differs as well and incorporates heart disease/disorders in the top 15 in place of cancer of the breast for younger women.

Meanwhile, published data on the socioeconomic status of women with disabilities show that having a disability is associated with low income and receipt of means-tested assistance. Women of working age with disabilities are less likely than women without disabilities to be employed, particularly if they have severe disabilities. They have the lowest earnings when they are employed when compared with all men and women without disabilities. Health care access appears to be closely related to the availability and type of health care insurance. Although the average use of health care services in this population is greater among women with disabilities, the full impact of low incomes and type of health insurance has yet to be determined.

The information reported here is based primarily on previously published survey material. Viewing it here together, however, gives a clear picture of the risks and consequences of disability among women. At the same time, such a survey stresses the importance of studying the problem of disability separately for women and men side-by-side with the study of disability issues in the population as a whole.

REFERENCES

Altman, B.M. (1982, September). *Disabled women: Doubly disadvantaged members of the social structure.* Paper presented at the meetings of the American Sociological Association, San Francisco, CA.

Altman, B.M. (1985). Disabled women in the social structure. In S.E. Browne, D. Connors, & N. Stern (Eds.), *With the power of each breath* (pp. 69–76). Pittsburgh, PA: Cleis Press.

Barnartt, S. (1982). The socio-economic status of deaf women: Are they doubly disadvantaged? In J. Christiansen & K. Egelston-Dodd (Eds.), *Socioeconomic status of the deaf population* (pp. 1–31). Washington, DC: Gallaudet College.

Bowe, F. (1984). *Disabled women in America.* Washington, DC: President's Committee on Employment of the Handicapped.

Collins, J.G. (1993). Prevalence of selected chronic conditions, United States, 1986–1988. National Center for Health Statistics. *Vital Health Statistics, 10*(182).

Deegan, M.J., & Brooks, N.A. (Eds.). (1985). *Women and disability.* New Brunswick, NJ: Transaction Books.

Dutton, D.B. (1986). Social class, health and illness. In L.H. Aiken & D. Mechanic (Eds.), *Applications of social science to clinical medicine and health policy* (31–62). New Brunswick, NJ: Rutgers University Press.

Edwards, W.S., & Berlin, M. (1989). *Questionnaires and data collection methods for the household survey and the survey of American Indians and Alaska Natives.*

Department of Health and Human Services, Public Health Service, National Center for Health Services Research and Health Care Technology. DHHS Publication No. (PHS) 89-3450.

Fine, M., & Asch, A. (Eds.). (1988). *Women with disabilities: Essays in psychology, culture, and politics.* Philadelphia: Temple University Press.

Haber, L.D. (1971). Disabling effects of chronic disease and impairment. *Journal of Chronic Disease, 24,* 469–487.

Johnson, W.G. (1979). Disability, income support, and social insurance. In E.D. Berkowitz (Ed.), *Disability policies and government programs* (pp. 87–132). New York: Praeger Publishers.

Kutza, E. (1981). Benefits for the disabled: How beneficial for women? *Journal of Sociology and Social Welfare, 8*(2), 298–319.

LaPlante, M.P. (1988). *Data on disability from the National Health Interview Survey, 1983–1985.* National Institute on Disability and Rehabilitation Research. U.S. Department of Education, Washington, DC.

LaPlante, M.P. (1991). *Disability risks of chronic illnesses and impairments.* National Institute on Disability and Rehabilitation Research. U.S. Department of Education, Office of Special Education and Rehabilitative Services, Washington, DC.

McNeil, J.M. (1993). *Americans with disabilities: 1991–92.* U.S. Bureau of the Census. Current population reports, P70-33. U.S. Government Printing Office, Washington, DC.

Moore, E.C. (1980, September–October). Women and health: United States 1980. *Public Health Reports, Supplement,* 9–84.

Mudrick, N.R. (1988). Disabled women and public policies for income support. In M. Fine & A. Asch (Eds.), *Women with disabilities: Essays in psychology, culture and politics.* Philadelphia: Temple University Press.

Public Health Service Task Force on Women's Health Issues. (1985). Women's health: Report of the Public Health Service task force on women's health issues. *Public Health Reports, 100,* 74–106.

chapter 4

The Perspective of Ethnicity on Women's Health and Disability

More Questions than Answers

Deborah L. Bernal

> The oppression of a majority is detestable and odious; the oppression of a minority is only by one degree less detestable and odious. (William Ewart Gladstone [1809–1898], from a speech)

This chapter examines the circumstance of women minorities with disabilities. Women currently represent a 51% majority of the work force. Demographic projections for the work force in the year 2000 suggest that new entrants will be principally women of ethnic origin (U.S. Department of Health and Human Services, 1990). The neglect of concerns of women with disabilities is compounded for minority women with disabilities. This neglect is reflected by the paucity of demographic data and research information vital to this underserved population.

What do we know of minorities with disabilities? We get some information on this subject from 1988 census data prepared by Bowe (1993) for the President's Committee on Employment of Persons with Disabilities:

> The "typical" adult with a work disability as of March, 1988 is a high school graduate about 48 years old whose disability is so severe that he or she believes that work, at least full-time work, is not possible. The individual is equally as likely to be male as to be female. A former blue collar worker, in a factory or service occupation, he or she did not work last year. He or she is married, lives in a metropolitan area, and had a mean income from all sources in 1987 of $9,379 a year. (p. 11)

The trend in the 1980s was toward an increasing percentage of women with disabilities. The shift appears related to the aging of disabled World War II Veterans. African Americans are more likely to have disabilities

(13.7%) than are Hispanics (8.2%) and whites (7.9%). The Hispanic population is growing at five times the rate of all ethnic and minority groups (Bowe, 1988b). Of working-age adults with severe disabilities, 24% or nearly one fourth are African American, while 12.6% are Hispanic. Therefore, over one third of all working-age adults with severe disabilities are from minority groups (Bowe, 1993). The typical Hispanic adult with a work disability is described as follows:

> The "typical" adult of Hispanic origin who has a work disability as of March, 1988 is a high school graduate about 43 years old whose disability is so severe that he or she believes that work, at least full-time work, is not possible. The individual is slightly more likely to be male (51.8%) than female (48.2%). A former blue-collar worker, in a factory or service occupation, he or she did not work last year. He or she is married, lives in a metropolitan area, and had a mean income from all sources in 1987 of about $11,000 a year. (Bowe, 1988b; p. 7)

Among Hispanic adults without disabilities, the population is 50% male and 50% female (Bowe, 1988b).

The typical African American adult with a work disability is also described by Bowe (1988a):

> The "typical" black adult with a work disability as of March, 1988 is a non–high school graduate about 47 years old whose disability is so severe that he or she believes that work, at least full-time work, is not possible. The individual is more likely to be female (54.5%) than male (45.5%), largely because women outnumber men among Blacks in the working-age range. A former blue-collar worker, in a factory or service occupation, he or she did not work last year. He or she is not married, lives in a metropolitan area, and had a mean income from all sources in 1987 of under $9,000 a year. (p. 10)

African American males have a markedly lower life expectancy than either white men or African American women (U.S. Department of Health and Human Services, 1985). The working age population of African American women is 54.2% of all African Americans; therefore, their percentage of African Americans with disabilities approximates their population.

Bowe (1988c) describes women with a work disability as follows:

> The "typical" woman with a work disability as of March, 1988 is a high school graduate about 47 years old whose disability is so severe she believes that work, at least full-time work, is not possible. A former blue or pink-collar service worker, she did not work the previous year. She is married, lives in a metropolitan area, and had a mean income from all sources in 1987 of $6,355 a year. (p. 11)

A total of 13.8% of all African American women have work disabilities, compared with 7.9% for Hispanic women and 7.7% for white women. Further, 9.5% of all African American women have severe disabilities, compared with 5.2% of Hispanic women and 3.9% of white women. Bowe

(1988c) provides the following information regarding women with disabilities: In terms of the total population of women with severe disabilities, 26% are African American and 8.8% are Hispanic. Thus, over one third of all women with severe disabilities are minorities. One half of these women are single heads of households (i.e., they have children but no husband), one quarter of them are married, and one quarter are single with no children. Three quarters live in metropolitan areas, while a quarter live in rural areas. A quarter receive Supplemental Security Income (SSI) or Social Security Disability Insurance (SSDI), and a quarter are looking for work. They are four times more likely than white women to have less than an eighth grade education, and, as you might guess, a high percentage live in poverty. And unfortunately, 46% of African American and Hispanic women with disabilities are not covered by any health insurance or pension plan.

The report of the Secretary's Task Force on Black and Minority Health (U.S. Department of Health and Human Services, 1985) contained a review of mortality and morbidity indicators of minority health. The task force found that though minority and nonminority women have a longer life expectancy than men, minority women still experience similar disparities in health status as compared to nonminority women. Asian females, however, have the highest life expectancy of any group.

The data reviewed by the task force (U.S. Department of Health and Human Services, 1985) clearly show that African Americans have the greatest disparity in mortality and morbidity among minorities compared with whites. Data for Hispanics cover only a limited segment of this minority; however, they do indicate disparities in mortality. Major areas of disparity exist between Native Americans and the white majority (perhaps most prominently due to several causes related to alcohol abuse). The Asian and Pacific Island minority, in aggregate, is healthier than all racial or ethnic groups in the United States, including whites.

Disabilities are disproportionately high within the minority, elderly, lower socioeconomic, and rural populations. Native Americans have the highest rate of activity limitations, followed by African Americans, Hispanics, and whites; Asians and Pacific Islanders have the least.

So what is the solution to this dilemma? As the problem is multifaceted, the solution must take on a comparable level of complexity. There are no easy answers. Currently we are laying the groundwork to ask the right questions. This will take

- Painstaking culturally sensitive research on minority women with disabilities
- A network of minority female health professionals and researchers
- Empowerment of minority females with disabilities to act as advocates

One facet of this problem is the lack of research data about this important population. Research must be directed at female minorities related to demographics, etiology of disability, and impact of the disability on the quality of life. Prevention of secondary disabilities, as well as health and social service delivery provided to persons with disabilities, must be considered. All aspects of disability should be taken into account, including those related to developmental disabilities, injuries, and chronic conditions.

From the general data reviewed here, several factors clearly emerge that may account for disparities between the sexes and among different racial groups. Behavioral, social, economic, cultural, and ethnic variables can be very hard to determine. Existing studies suggest that health professionals who are from the same cultural background as their patients may be able to communicate better with these populations (U.S. Department of Health and Human Services, 1985).

For this research to be culturally sensitive, it must include care providers and an infrastructure that targets underserved minority female populations for the research and collection of data. Only in this way can we assure that we are able to obtain the appropriate information from these sources. In order to gather reliable data, we have to target women and underserved minority populations in training programs for research and health care delivery.

"Females are under-represented in the population of physicians in this country. They were 18.1% of physicians in 1992 and are projected to be 30% by 2010" (American Medical Association, 1993, p. 1). Of all medical students admitted in 1993, 42% were women. However, "women constitute 61% of black and 45% of other under-represented minority entrants in the class" (Association of American Medical Colleges, 1993).

African Americans, while 11.7% of the U.S. population, represent only 3.7% of the population of physicians. Hispanics are 9% of the general population and 4.7% of the physician population, while Native Americans are only 0.7% of the population and only 0.1% of physicians. These groups together represent 21.4% of the general population, but only 8.5% of physicians. The only minority group that is not underrepresented is that of Asians and Pacific Islanders. While only 1.8% of the population, they are 11.8% of physicians in the United States. The Association of American Medical Colleges (AAMC) "Project 3000 by 2000" targets underrepresented minorities for 3,000 entrants to medical school by the year 2000 (Association of American Medical Colleges, 1994). We should applaud this effort and similar efforts to increase women's participation in medicine.

The last, and one of the most important, aspects is advocacy for minority women with disabilities. We need their input to design programs for prevention of disability based on the data that we collect. We need their insight to improve our current service and delivery infrastructure and co-ordination of services based on the information that we are able to collect. And we need their cooperation to improve the reentry of minority females with disabilities into the work force. Unless we change the tide of poverty within this population, we are not going to see an improvement in their health, health care delivery, or their abilities to afford a decent lifestyle.

In my years of working with the National Medical Association and with my own patients, it has become obvious to me that there are many minorities with disabilities—many females with disabilities—that are feeling alone, feeling that no one has an interest in their well-being, and feeling no one is assisting them or addressing their needs. If we focus on gaining access to these groups so that they can discuss their issues, and be advocates for themselves, then the quality of research, delivery of services, and their reentry into the work force will be pushed forward.

> With malice toward none, with charity for all, with firmness in the right, as God gives us to see the right, let us strive on to finish the work we are in. (Abraham Lincoln, [1809–1865], second Inaugural Address)

REFERENCES

American Medical Association. (1993). *Women in medical services.* Chicago: Author.

Association of American Medical Colleges. (1993). *Minority students in medical education: Facts and figures VII.* Washington, DC: Author.

Association of American Medical Colleges. (1994). *Medical school admission requirements 1994–95* (44th ed.). Washington, DC: Author.

Bowe, F. (1988a). *Black adults with disabilities: A portrait.* Washington, DC: President's Committee on Employment of People with Disabilities.

Bowe, F. (1988b). *Disabled adults of Hispanic origin: A portrait.* Washington, DC: President's Committee on Employment of People with Disabilities.

Bowe, F. (1988c). *Women with disabilities: A portrait.* Washington, DC: President's Committee on Employment of People with Disabilities.

Bowe, F. (1993). *Adults with disabilities: A portrait.* Washington, DC: President's Committee on Employment of People with Disabilities.

U.S. Department of Health and Human Services. (1985). *Report of the Secretary's Task Force on Black and Minority Health* (Vol. 1). Washington, DC: Author.

U.S. Department of Health and Human Services. (1990). *Healthy people 2000: National health promotion and disease prevention objectives.* Washington, DC: Author.

SEXUALITY AND REPRODUCTIVE HEALTH

Margaret A. Nosek

Women with physical disabilities have the same sexual feelings and desires and the same basic reproductive health care needs as women in general, yet these feelings, desires, and health care needs have been fundamentally ignored by service providers, health care professionals, families, and even many women with disabilities themselves. The awareness of this inequity is increasing, thanks to the pioneering leadership of advocates such as Carol Gill in Chicago, Marsha Saxton in Boston, Barbara Waxman in Los Angeles, and many other women with disabilities throughout the United States who are working to dispel stereotypes and create new models of service delivery that will be inclusive and well informed. As the network of advocates for women with disabilities grows and strengthens, its impact can be felt in many sectors, including the National Institutes of Health (NIH).

Justice cannot be done to the subject of sexuality and reproductive health without addressing its psychological, social, and environmental aspects, as well as its physical or clinical aspects. The following chapters reflect the intention to present what is known (and not known) about sexual response, reproductive health, pregnancy, and delivery, as well as the psychosocial issues of sense of self, relationships, parenting, sexual orientation, abuse, gaining access to health care systems, and the politics surrounding the sexuality of women with disabilities. The purpose of compiling this information is to enable clinicians, service providers, researchers, and advocates to expand their knowledge in these areas and identify the issues that demand more information and systems change.

The first question in many people's minds is whether women with disabilities are able to respond sexually. In Chapter 5, Beverly Whipple and her colleagues discuss the physiological aspects of sexual response in women with spinal cord injuries (SCI). Their research examined the effect of self-stimulation by women with complete SCI on activating sexual response, suppressing neurogenic or experimental pain, and suppressing spasticity. In qualitative interviews with women who have SCI, they identified the common pattern of cognitive dissociation, sexual disenfranchisement, and sexual rediscovery after injury.

Sandra Welner (Chapter 6) examines gynecological issues facing women with a variety of disabilities. There are many fears on the part of both physicians and consumers about possible dangers in taking oral contraceptives, particularly the risk of thrombosis. Welner presents various tests that can be administered to determine the seriousness of various risk factors, and she reviews the scant literature on the negative effects of taking estrogen and progesterone for certain disabilities. She concludes by looking at two seriously neglected areas: the effect of disability on the detection and treatment of sexually transmitted diseases and the experience of menopause by women with physical disabilities.

Historically, there has been a tendency for physicians to discourage women with physical disabilities from having children. Consequently, very little is known about some of their unique needs. Amie Jackson (Chapter 7) conducted a study of 472 women with SCI, asking about their experiences with pregnancy and delivery pre- and post-injury. She paid special attention to complications, including exacerbation of disability-related problems, such as urinary tract infections and autonomic dysreflexia, and catalogued types of anesthesia used. She raises the question of whether the high rate of cesarean sections reflects medical necessity or comfort of the physician. She found increased rates of low birth weight babies and other neonatal health problems.

Judy Rogers (Chapter 8) looks at pregnancy from a qualitative perspective. Her interviews with women who had a variety of disabilities revealed problems in the attitude of physicians, quality of communication, and a lack of information about the effect of disability on pregnancy. She outlines recommendations for research on various common problems experienced by pregnant women with physical disabilities.

The psychological, social, and relationship aspects of sexuality are often viewed as more important than the physical aspect by women with disabilities. Harilyn Rousso (Chapter 9) masterfully discusses the critical effect disability can have on the development of a positive sense of self in adolescent girls. Her interview studies showed that negative social and parental attitudes are often internalized by girls who acquire a disability before adolescence. They tend to feel excluded, rejected, and regarded as asexual. It is very common for parents to have low expectations for them socially and very high expectations academically and vocationally. Rousso identifies the need to address their needs as girls first as a key to successful social and sexual development.

Carol Gill dives deeper into theories of romantic disadvantage for women with disabilities in Chapter 10. The need to demonstrate and prove their womanhood often pressures them into accepting abusive relationships and staying in them. She analyzes some of the strong negative social influences on able-bodied men against marrying women with disabilities, and the many familial, social, and physical barriers that work against women with disabilities establishing successful relationships with men with disabilities. Later in this book (Chapter 22) Sonya Perduta-Fulginiti looks at how a woman's sexuality, self-esteem, and ability to enter into intimate relationships may be compromised by bladder and bowel management problems.

Megan Kirshbaum (Chapter 11) has conducted numerous studies of parents with disabilities. She discusses some of the inappropriate conclusions that have been reached about the capabilities of mothers with disabilities to parent and the impact of the mother's disability on the children. Abuse surfaces once again as a significant barrier to successful fulfillment of the role of mother. She outlines topics that demand further research and emphasizes the need to choose research methodologies carefully so that problems associated with disability are distinguishable from psychological and social problems that are common among women in general. She issues a strong call for observational studies and research on service and equipment needs of mothers with disabilities.

Corbett O'Toole discusses sexuality among disabled lesbians in Chapter 12. This population is culturally invisible to both women with disabilities and women in general. She cites the lack of role models within families and the compounded effect of shame instilled by families because of having a disability and being a lesbian. The stereotype of asexuality affects them in some different ways, and puts them at an even greater disadvantage in receiving appropriate reproductive care and general health care.

All of the authors addressing the psychosocial aspects of sexuality in this section have observed the high prevalence and devastating effects of abuse on women with disabilities. Margaret Nosek (Chapter 13) examines this problem in considerable detail. After discussing the definitional and methodological challenges inherent in conducting abuse research, she critically reviews the literature on the sexual abuse of girls and women with disabilities. She then describes the results of her qualitative interview study of 31 women with a variety of physical disabilities and summarizes the sexual abuse experiences reported by 11 of the participants. In trying to isolate the effect of disability on the occurrence of sexual abuse, she describes several ways in which disability increases a woman's vulnerability and reduces her options for escape. She concludes with recommendations on how to identify and prevent the sexual abuse of women with disabilities.

Marsha Saxton (Chapter 14) discusses interactions between women with disabilities and health care systems. She analyzes the ways in which health care providers regard women with disabilities and describes methods she has used successfully to raise their awareness of disability issues and basic legal and community resources. Levels of anger are very high among women who feel they have been damaged and marginalized by health care systems. Saxton encourages galvanizing this anger by promoting compliance with the Americans with Disabilities Act of 1990. She encourages interactions that reflect a true partnership between health care providers and women with disabilities.

This section concludes with a commentary by Barbara Waxman (Chapter 15) on various sexuality and reproductive issues. She describes four facts that underlie the historical scientific indifference to the reproductive health needs of women with disabilities: 1) research on disability has been gender-nonspecific; 2) sexuality and reproductive research have been predominantly on the needs of men with spinal cord injury; 3) research has been pathologically oriented, focusing not on the whole woman, but on the defective woman; and 4) the eugenic underpinnings of efforts to control the fertility of women with disabilities.

At the conclusion of the segment on sexuality and reproductive health at the NIH conference on the health of women with physical disabilities, participants brainstormed about topics requiring further research. The extensive lists of ideas are roughly summarized as follows:

1. What are the characteristics shared by women with disabilities who are satisfied with their sexuality? What disability-related physical, emotional, and social benefits are there to being sexually active?
2. What factors contribute to the development of a positive sexual sense of self among adolescent girls with disabilities?
3. Describe the gynecologic and obstetric problems that are faced disproportionately by women with disabilities, as related to such areas as menstruation, infertility, contraception, pregnancy and delivery, sexually transmitted diseases, menopause, and access to cancer screening.
4. What is the effect of various systems of health care delivery on the reproductive health of women with disabilities?
5. What is the impact of some of the unique aspects of intimate relationships that are experienced by women with disabilities, such as the dual role of partner and attendant, privacy and boundaries, and attitudes toward the use of assistive technology?
6. Identify factors that contribute to violence and abuse against women with disabilities and develop effective strategies for prevention and treatment.
7. What are the characteristics of women who are successful in the role of mother, including personal traits, family dynamics, support services, and availability of accessible equipment?

8. Identify the most crucial training needs of medical and allied health professionals to expand their understanding of the needs of women with physical disabilities.

9. Develop and implement effective strategies for the dissemination of information about sexuality and reproductive health to girls and women with disabilities.

Participants stressed the need for greater use of qualitative and observational methods of research, as well as longitudinal research. Studies should also consider the effects of minority status, economic level, sexual orientation, age at onset of disability, type of disability, and program access issues in examining all of the topics listed above. There was a strong call for special efforts in encouraging and assisting women with disabilities to pursue careers in health care delivery and research, and to serve on grant review panels.

chapter 5

Sexual Response in Women with Complete Spinal Cord Injury

Beverly Whipple, Eleanor Richards,
Mitchell Tepper, and Barry R. Komisaruk

Sexual response in women with complete spinal cord injury cannot be understood without first defining sexuality. In the past, sexuality was viewed as having one purpose—reproduction. Today it is seen as an important aspect of health and personality functioning; it enhances the quality of life, fosters personal growth, and contributes to human fulfillment (Whipple & Gick, 1980). When the term *sexuality* is viewed holistically, it refers to the totality of a being. It encompasses human qualities, not just the genitals and their functions. It includes all of the qualities—biological, psychological, emotional, social, cultural, and spiritual—that make people who they are. People have the capacity to express their sexuality in any of these areas without necessarily involving the genitalia.

What the person and/or the couple view as their goal of sexual expression must also be considered. According to Timmers (1976), there are two commonly held views. The most common view is goal directed, which is analogous to climbing a flight of stairs. The first step is touching, the next step kissing, followed by caressing, vagina/penis contact, intercourse, and orgasm. The goal of both partners or one partner is orgasm. If the sexual experience does not lead to the achievement of that goal, then the partners do not feel satisfied with what they have experienced (Whipple, 1987).

The alternative view is pleasure directed, which can be conceptualized as a circle, with each expression on the circle considered an end in itself.

This work was supported in part by the National Institute of Child Health and Human Development, Grant HD 30156.

Whether the experience involves kissing, oral sex, holding, or other physical contact, each is an end in itself and each is satisfying to the couple. There is no need to have this form of expression lead to anything else (Whipple, 1987). If one person in a couple is goal directed and one is pleasure directed, problems may occur if they do not realize their goals or do not communicate their goals to each other.

SEXUAL RESPONSE IN WOMEN

Little was known about the physiology of sexual response before Masters and Johnson published their pioneering research in 1966 (Masters & Johnson, 1966). They found that two principal physiological changes take place—vasocongestion (e.g., blood engorgement) and myotonia (e.g., muscle tension). Reporting their findings using arbitrarily chosen phases of excitement, plateau, orgasm, and resolution, Masters and Johnson stated that these phases correspond to the level of sexual arousal and describe typical responses.

Not all researchers or women agreed with Masters and Johnson's monolithic pattern and their report of one reflexive pathway in sexual response. Some women reported that they had orgasm from vaginal stimulation and some women reported an expulsion of fluid with orgasm, which Masters and Johnson said did not occur (Masters & Johnson, 1966). After listening to the reports of these women, Perry and Whipple designed research studies that led to their naming the Grafenberg spot and their documenting the phenomenon of female ejaculation (Addiego et al., 1981; Perry & Whipple, 1981). Perry and Whipple (1981) hypothesized that there were two different nerve pathways involved in sexual response. One pathway, via the pudendal nerve, is the major sensory pathway from clitoral stimulation as identified by Masters and Johnson (1966). Perry and Whipple (1981) identified the hypogastric plexus and the pelvic nerve as the sensory pathways in sexual response in women when there is vaginal stimulation.

In a later study that was also designed to validate the reported experiences of women, Whipple, Ogden, and Komisaruk (1992) documented in the laboratory that women could achieve orgasm from fantasy alone, without touching their bodies. During this study, orgasm from both self-induced imagery and genital self-stimulation was associated with significant increases in blood pressure, heart rate, pupil diameter, and pain thresholds over resting control conditions. These two orgasm conditions did not differ significantly from each other on any of the physiological measures (Whipple, Ogden, & Komisaruk, 1992). On the basis of these findings, it is evident that physical genital stimulation is not necessary to produce a state that is reported to be an orgasm.

SEXUALITY AND WOMEN WITH
SPINAL CORD INJURY: LITERATURE REVIEW

There is a paucity of literature concerning female sexual response after spinal cord injury (SCI). Perhaps the reason for this is that the ratio of males to females with SCI is 4:1 and that it is much easier to study sexual response in males, because they have external genitalia (Sipski, 1991). Based on the literature concerning female sexual function after SCI, it is clear that women with spinal cord injuries are capable of menstruating, conceiving, and giving birth (Whipple, 1990). Most of the current literature is not concerned with whether women with SCI have any sexual desire or response. For example, Billings and Stokes (1982) report that women with SCI, because their role can be *passive*, may enjoy intercourse and be perfectly capable of satisfying the male. Billings and Stokes (1982) also state that little is known about their capacity for orgasm.

Sandowski (1976) reported the following:

> Far less has been written about the female paraplegic, probably because her ability to participate in sexual activities is less affected than the male's. The female paraplegic can have intercourse in the usual position of the female lying on her back with the male facing her on top. . . . With the help of an understanding husband, it is quite possible for the female paraplegic to satisfy his needs and for the couple to achieve a fairly normal sex life. (p. 323)

As late as 1992, Szasz stated that in women with complete spinal cord injuries, "although vaginal lubrication may still occur in response to either touch or mental stimuli, there can be no orgasmic response arising from or detected in the genitalia" (Szasz, 1992, p. 178). He further stated that "whenever the injury is complete, genital signals cannot get to the brain to generate neuromuscular tensions" (Szasz, 1992, p. 180). Perduta-Fulginiti (1992) agrees that orgasm cannot be physiologically achieved. She further reports that "in all complete spinal cord injuries at the Sacral 4 segment and above, total vaginal and anal sensation are lost" (p. 109). Although Money (1960) acknowledged that orgasm was reported by people with SCI, he labeled these orgasms "phantom," a label that is still used today. As late as 1992, Perduta-Fulginiti reports that some women with complete SCI report orgasm of a nongenital nature, which have been labeled as "phantom," although they are described as having intense psychological pleasure and similar subjective physical sensations as detailed during the orgasm phase of the sexual response pattern. She suggests that visceral motor and sensory components of the autonomic nervous system may relay information between the cortex, the hypothalamus, and the genitalia (Perduta-Fulginiti, 1992). However, she does not identify the sensory pathways.

As early as 1976, Bregman and Hadley interviewed 31 women with SCI and reported that most of the women's descriptions of orgasm since their injury were very similar to those of women without disabilities. Three of the women reported orgasms that were not different from the orgasms they experienced before their injuries (Bregman & Hadley, 1976). Berard (1989) discusses physiological responses based on interviews of 15 women with SCI and reports a correlation between richness of fantasy and fulfillment of sexual life. Berard (1989) does address orgasm and states that pleasure may be heightened by concomitant stimulation of an erogenous zone either above or at the level of injury.

Charlifue, Gerhart, Menter, and Whiteneck (1992) surveyed 231 women and noted that half of their subjects reported they had experienced orgasms since their injuries. The stimulus was generally genital or a combination of genital and breast stimulation. They do not specify if these women had complete or incomplete injuries.

Kettl et al. (1991) surveyed 74 women, and 52% of their sample reported orgasm after SCI; however, half of these women stated that it was different after their injuries. They do not state if these women had complete or incomplete injuries.

Although it is claimed that women with complete SCI cannot achieve orgasm or that their orgasms are labeled as "phantom" orgasms, subjective reports of women do not support these contentions. Indeed, some women with complete SCI report that they can experience the psychological and even physical sensation of orgasm. In addition, Axel (1982) found that 56% of her sample experienced the same discomfort with their menstrual period as before their SCI, 22% had less discomfort, and 22% had more discomfort. Again, she does not state if these women have a complete or an incomplete injury. Having a spinal cord injury does not necessarily prevent a woman from being orgasmic or from having menstrual discomfort.

These psychosexual data are generally based on anecdotal evidence or information from questionnaires and interviews. This type of data collection and dissemination has inherent biases because it is based on subjective reports (Whipple & Komisaruk, 1993). Laboratory data documenting these subjective reports are lacking.

CURRENT STUDIES

In 1992, the National Center for Medical Rehabilitation Research funded two studies that are addressing some of these psychosexual issues. Using a population of women with complete and incomplete injuries above the level of T6, Dr. Marca Sipski and colleagues are investigating "The Physiological Effects of SCI on Females" (M. Sipski, personal communication,

September 1, 1992). In another study, Komisaruk, Whipple, and Richards are investigating the effects of vaginal and cervical self-stimulation on pain, spasticity, and sexual response in women with complete spinal cord injury at or below T6. In addition to these physiological studies, supplemental funding was received by the latter researchers for qualitative research to investigate additional understudied areas of sexuality in women with complete SCI. This part of the study is addressing the psychosocial, emotional, and relationship components, using a phenomenological approach and is described in the qualitative section.

QUANTITATIVE STUDY

Methods

The basic premise of this study is that after SCI, the sensory, sensorimotor, and perceptual capabilities of the nervous system may be underestimated. The specific aims are to identify sensory, sensorimotor, and perceptual responses to vaginal and cervical self-stimulation (such as effect on pain, spasticity, and sexual responses) that are intact and potentially functional in women with complete SCI. The long-term objective of this study is to identify the actual capabilities of the nervous system after SCI so that they can be utilized to the fullest extent and thereby enrich the quality of life of women with complete SCI.

This study is designed to ask the following research questions. In women with complete SCI, are vaginal, cervical, and/or hypersensitive zone self-stimulation effective in 1) activating sexual response, 2) suppressing neurogenic or experimental pain, and 3) suppressing spasticity?

This study is also determining if there are differential responses depending on the level of SCI. Two of the nerves that carry sensory input from the vagina and cervix are the pelvic and hypogastric nerves. Because these nerves enter the spinal cord at different levels, their relative contribution is being determined by studying women whose levels of complete SCI are expected to either block these pathways or leave them intact.

This study uses the same methodology used in previous studies from this laboratory (Whipple & Komisaruk, 1985, 1988; Whipple, Ogden, & Komisaruk, 1992), with the addition of a disposable tampon stimulator used for vaginal self-stimulation and cervical self-stimulation. There is a pressure transducer embedded in the holder for the stimulator so that the amount of pressure the subject is self-applying can be monitored. A tampon is attached to a diaphragm with Velcro discs when the stimulator is used for cervical self-stimulation.

Results

The following are *preliminary* results of the sexuality data from the first 13 subjects. Five are controls without disabilities, four have a complete

SCI between the levels of T6 and T10, and four have a complete SCI between the levels of T11 and L2.

The mean age of the women with SCI is 39 years (range: 32–47 years). Seven of the women are Caucasian; one is African American. Five are married; one is living with a partner, and two are separated. The mean length of time since injury is 11.7 years (range: 2–21 years).

The preliminary physiological data are summarized in terms of pain thresholds, cervical and vaginal sensibility, level of arousal, blood pressure, and heart rate.

Pain Thresholds   The subjects in each group showed a significant increase in pain detection threshold (as measured with a Ugo Basile Analgesia meter [Stoelting, Chicago] on the fingers) from prestimulation to during the stimulation condition, in response to vaginal, cervical, or hypersensitive area self-stimulation. There were no significant differences among the groups within each stimulus condition by analysis of variance (ANOVA) (see Figure 1).

This is a major preliminary finding of the study; that is, evidence that genital self-stimulation exerts a perceptual effect after complete SCI at these levels. To our knowledge, this is also the first demonstration that cervical self-stimulation produces analgesia. (There was no increase in tactile thresholds.) The pain tolerance thresholds were also significantly increased, and there were no significant differences between any pairs of groups in response to each form of self-stimulation.

Based on this evidence in our sample to date, the existence of SCI did not significantly reduce the magnitude of the pain-blocking effect of vaginal or cervical self-stimulation.

Cervical and Vaginal Sensibility   All of the women tested in the control group perceived cervical and vaginal pressure. In the SCI groups, two of four women in each of the T6–T10 and T11–L2 groups perceived cervical and vaginal pressure to self-stimulation.

Of the women with complete SCI, seven of the eight reported that they experienced menstrual cramps. Three of these seven women said they experienced menstrual cramps as lower back pain, which was below the level of their injury.

One woman with complete SCI at T11–T12 experienced multiple orgasms from vaginal self-stimulation and from cervical self-stimulation during the testing, but reported that she did not feel the stimuli.

Arousal   There were no significant differences in arousal between any pairs of groups for any stimulus type (i.e., vaginal, cervical, or hypersensitive area self-stimulation) as reported on the visual analog scale (see Figure 2).

Thus, under other conditions in which group differences were observed, it is unlikely that elevated levels of arousal could account for these

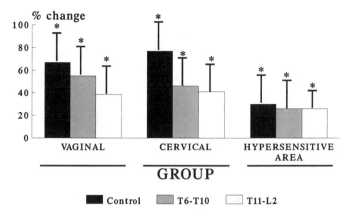

Figure 1. *Pain-detection threshold.* Each of the three modalities of self-stimulation (vaginal, cervical, and hypersensitive area) induced a significant increase in pain detection threshold over the corresponding prestimulation baseline levels (*asterisks*). There were no significant differences among the control, T6–T10, and T11–T12 groups under any of the stimulus conditions (*solid line* under each stimulus condition).

effects. For example, pain thresholds during vaginal, cervical, or hypersensitive area self-stimulation were not significantly correlated with the magnitude of arousal reported during the corresponding type of self-stimulation.

Heart Rate and Blood Pressure Heart rate and blood pressure increased significantly in the control group in response to vaginal and cervical, but not hypersensitive area, self-stimulation. These findings confirm

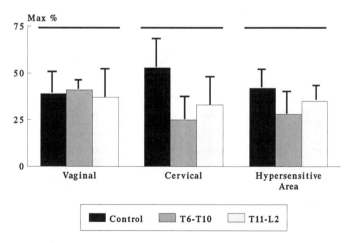

Figure 2. *Arousal.* Each stimulus condition produced a significant increase in arousal, and there were no significant differences in level of arousal among the control, T6–T10, or T11–T12 groups on any of the stimulus conditions.

our earlier findings (Whipple, Ogden, & Komisaruk, 1992). In addition, this is the first demonstration of which we are aware that cervical self-stimulation in women increases heart rate and blood pressure (see Figure 3).

Cervical self-stimulation increased heart rate significantly in the T11–L2 group, but not in the T6–T10 group. By contrast, cervical self-stimulation increased blood pressure significantly in the T6–T10, but not in the T11–L2 group.

These findings, taken together, suggest that a mechanism related to that underlying autonomic dysreflexia may be responsible, although the levels of SCI in this study were too low for the women to experience any crisis of autonomic dysreflexia.

There was no significant correlation between blood pressure, heart rate, or pain thresholds. Consequently, heart rate, blood pressure, arousal, and pain thresholds may be controlled by mechanisms that function independently of each other under the conditions of the present study.

Discussion

There are a number of possible mechanisms suggested by these data:

1. The spinal cord near the central canal could be undamaged but integrity untested.
2. The sensory input could bypass the level of injury ascending via the sympathetic chain and enter at a higher level, or an extramedullary

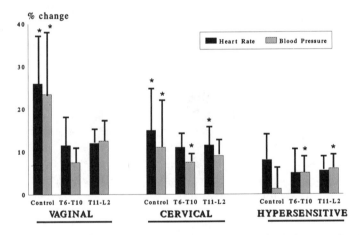

Figure 3. *Heart rate and blood pressure.* Vaginal and cervical self-stimulation produced a significant increase in heart rate and blood pressure in the control group. Cervical self-stimulation produced a significant increase in blood pressure in the T6–T10 group and a significant increase in heart rate in the T11–T12 group. See text for interpretation.

pathway via a cranial nerve, such as the sensory vagus, which enters the brain directly. This hypothesis is currently being tested in laboratory animals.

3. There could be humoral effects; however, the response is too fast, and some subjects could perceive vaginal and cervical pressure.

4. There could be a cognitive effect, similar to our imagery-induced orgasm results. However, some of these women report menstrual cramps and vaginal and cervical pressure in response to sensory stimulation.

Based on the present findings and the recent study on imagery-induced orgasms, the current concepts of orgasm and sexual response need reformulation. In the present study, two women with complete SCI reported orgasm induced by cervical and vaginal self-stimulation in the absence of perception of these stimuli as sensory stimuli per se. Previous studies documented increases in autonomic response and pain thresholds in response to imagery with no stimulation of any body region (Whipple, Ogden, & Komisaruk, 1992) and in response to hypersensitive area stimulation in the absence of physical genital stimulation (Sipski, Komisaruk, Whipple, & Alexander, 1993).

Further research into the nature and mechanism of orgasm is warranted to advance our understanding of this significant physical and cognitive process. One ultimate benefit could be to improve the quality of life of people with SCI by making them aware of responses that have been underestimated in the past.

QUALITATIVE STUDY

The qualitative component of this study provides additional information about the subjects and their sexuality. Preliminary data from interviews with the eight women with complete SCI are summarized in the following sections.

Methods

Phenomenology, a qualitative research approach, permits emerging data to be described through the uniqueness of the experience of participants. This methodology was used to expand the depth of understanding of sexuality and relationship experiences. An Ethnograph (Qualis Research Associates, Corvallis, OR) computer program was used to analyze the content of tape-recorded semistructured interviews with the subjects. This analysis identified a trajectory of sexuality in women with complete SCI. For interview purposes, data were clustered in phases according to sexuality and relationship experiences: 1) prior to injury, 2) immediately postinjury, and 3) during the rehabilitation process until the present.

Results

Prior to injury, there were no clear commonalities in subjects' perceptions of sexuality or relationship experiences. All participants reported that they experienced coitus prior to their injury.

Immediately postinjury, participants reported a "shutting down and closing up" of their sexuality, or a shelving of sexual interest. On the basis of observed or assumed absence of genital sensation, women believed that physical sexual pleasure was no longer possible for them. Familiar sexual responses were perceived as unattainable. A cognitive awareness and conscious decision not to deal with their sexuality emerged from the data. We labeled this phenomenon "cognitive genital dissociation."

Energies were focused on maintaining or regaining salient physiological functions (mobility, bowel, and bladder). Sexuality was not perceived as being of high priority, although some concerns were expressed. Between 3 months and 3 years postinjury, participants experienced coitus. There was a stated curiosity of what the experience "would be like." The experience generally resulted in sexual dissonance, a comparison between pleasure (what was) and disappointment (what is). This experience activated for most women a lengthy sexual readjustment and reevaluation of the nature of sexual pleasure.

Beginning with the immediate postinjury period and continuing with the rehabilitative process, participants described a loss of their sexuality or a "sexual disenfranchisement." More graphically, they felt "robbed" of their sexuality, including sexual desirability.

A period of "sexual rediscovery" emerged following sexual disenfranchisement. For some women, significant life events (such as a 40th birthday), or situational events (such as a new sexual partner) were turning points. Postinjury (in some cases 7, 8, or 15 years), women who were engaged in unaffirming and destructive relationships tended to move toward relationships that were affirming or constructive. Affirming relationships characterized by open communication, creativity, and resourcefulness played a key role in positive sexual self-concept. In the period of sexual rediscovery, reciprocity in relationships (partner meeting needs) was critical in the shift from negatively to positively perceived sexual readjustment.

There was also a reevaluation of the meaning of sexual pleasure. Exploration resulted in a self-awareness of alternative approaches to sexual arousal and, in some instances, orgasm. Four women reported experiencing orgasm, one with a T6–T7 injury, one with a T10–T11 injury, and two with T11–T12 injuries. Participants reported arousal or orgasm through breast, cervical/vaginal, and/or hypersensitive area stimulation. There were no consistently preferred sexual positions.

Participants were asked to comment on the extent and quality of their postinjury sexuality education by health professionals. The overall quality was considered poor. Generally included with information on bowel and bladder functioning, the materials that were distributed were of poor quality, outdated, and usually targeted for men. The focus of female sexuality education was on giving, rather than receiving, sexual pleasure and on reproductive issues, such as fertility and conception. All women reported a clear preference for the formation of female groups to discuss issues of sexuality.

Discussion

A sexual trajectory emerged from our study, the major phases of which were, in sequence, cognitive dissociation, sexual disenfranchisement, and sexual rediscovery. The preliminary results of this qualitative study indicate the need for further sexuality research in these identified phases. Research is also needed to identify critical points for sexuality education and counseling in women with SCI with the goal of shortening the sexual adjustment process.

CONCLUSIONS

There is still much we do not know about sexuality and women with SCI. Nevertheless, positive steps are being taken to learn more about the physiological and interpersonal aspects of sexuality. Ultimately, these efforts will enhance the quality of life for women with SCI.

REFERENCES

Addiego, F., Belzer, E.G., Comolli, J., Moger, W., Perry, J.D., & Whipple, B. (1981). Female ejaculation: A case study. *Journal of Sex Research, 17*, 99–100.

Axel, S.J. (1982). Spinal cord injured women's concerns: Menstruation and pregnancy. *Rehabilitation Nursing, 7*, 10–15.

Berard, E.J.J. (1989). The sexuality of spinal cord injured women: Physiology and pathophysiology: A review. *Paraplegia, 27*, 99–112.

Billings, D.M., & Stokes, L.G. (1982). *Medical surgical nursing.* St. Louis: C.V. Mosby.

Bregman, S, & Hadley, R.G. (1976). Sexual adjustment and feminine attractiveness among spinal cord injured women. *Archives of Physical Medicine, 57*, 448–450.

Charlifue, S.W., Gerhart, K.A., Menter, R.R., & Whiteneck, G.G. (1992). Sexual issues of women with spinal cord injuries. *Paraplegia, 30*, 192–199.

Kettl, P., Zarefoss, S., Jacoby, K., Garman, C., Hulse, C., Rowley, F., Corey, R., Sredy, M., Bixler, E., & Tyson, K. (1991). Female sexuality after spinal cord injury. *Sexuality and Disability, 9*(4), 287–295.

Masters, W., & Johnson, V. (1966). *Human sexual response.* Boston: Little, Brown & Co.

Money, J. (1960). Phantom orgasm in the dreams of paraplegic men and women. *Archives of General Psychiatry, 3*, 373–382.

Perduta-Fulginiti, P.S. (1992). Sexual functioning of women with complete spinal cord injury: Nursing implications. *Sexuality and Disability, 10*(2), 103–118.

Perry, J.D., & Whipple, B. (1981). Pelvic muscle strength of female ejaculators: Evidence in support of a new theory of orgasm. *Journal of Sex Research, 17,* 22–39.

Sandowski, C. (1976). Sexuality and the paraplegic. *Rehabilitation Literature, 37*(11–12), 322–327.

Sipski, M.L. (1991). Spinal cord injury: What is the effect on sexual response? *Journal of the American Paraplegia Society, 14*(2), 40–43.

Sipski, M.L., Komisaruk, B.R., Whipple, B., & Alexander, C.J. (1993). Physiological responses associated with orgasm in the spinal cord injured female. *Proceedings of the American Academy of Physiological Medicine and Rehabilitation, 74,* 1270.

Szasz, G. (1992). Sexual health care. In C.P. Zejdlik (Ed.), *Management of spinal cord injury* (pp. 175–201). Boston: Jones and Bartlett Publishers.

Timmers, P.O. (1976). Treating goal-directed intimacy. *Social Work,* 401–402.

Whipple, B. (1987). Sexual counseling of couples after a mastectomy or a myocardial infarction. *Nursing Forum, 23*(3), 85–91.

Whipple, B. (1990). Female sexuality. In J.F.J. Leyson (Ed.), *Sexual rehabilitation of the spinal-cord-injured patient* (pp. 19–38). Clifton, NJ: Humana Press.

Whipple, B., & Gick, R. (1980). A holistic view of sexuality: Education for the health professional. *Topics in Clinical Nursing, 1,* 91–98.

Whipple, B., & Komisaruk, B.R. (1985). Elevation of pain threshold by vaginal stimulation in women. *Pain, 21,* 357–367.

Whipple, B., & Komisaruk, B.R. (1988). Analgesia produced in women by genital self-stimulation. *Journal of Sex Research, 24,* 130–140.

Whipple, B., & Komisaruk, B.R. (1993). Current research trends in spinal cord injuries. In F.B. Haseltine, S.S. Cole, & D.B. Gray (Eds.), *Reproductive issues for persons with physical disabilities* (pp. 197–207). Baltimore: Paul H. Brookes Publishing Co.

Whipple, B., Ogden, G., & Komisaruk, B.R. (1992). Relative analgesic effect of imagery compared to genital self-stimulation. *Archives of Sexual Behavior, 21,* 121–133.

chapter **6**

Contraception, Sexually Transmitted Diseases, and Menopause

Sandra Welner

The gynecological needs of women with disabilities have not received adequate attention. This chapter highlights that which is already known and identifies areas about which more information is needed. It discusses contraceptive choices for women with disabilities and the diagnosis of sexually transmitted diseases in these women. Possible alterations in symptoms and signs as well as in medical therapy for sexually transmitted diseases in women with disabilities are also reviewed. Important issues regarding the impact of disabilities on menopausal women are examined.

CONTRACEPTION

Women with disabilities are sexual and have the need to be able to control their fertility. The myth that women with disabilities are asexual may produce a barrier for physical access as well as for accurate information about contraceptive options. It is standard practice in a gynecologist's office to ask any woman of reproductive age, "Are there any contraceptive needs or issues that we need to discuss?" This is often not an automatic question for women with disabilities. Perhaps this omission results from a lack of information regarding the most appropriate way to manage contraception in women with disabilities. Nevertheless, it is critical to identify accurate birth control information both for women with disabilities and for health care providers.

Published data regarding contraception for women with disabilities are limited and are primarily reported in the neurological, rehabilitation, and nursing literature rather than in the mainstream gynecological literature. Two studies have described oral contraceptive use in women with multiple sclerosis (MS). A case study published in *The American Journal of Physical Medicine and Rehabilitation* reported that one woman experienced a cerebrovascular accident while taking oral contraceptives (Malanga & Gangemi, 1994). The study did not discuss baseline disability levels, dosage of estrogen, birth control pills, or cofactors such as age or smoking. An earlier study concluded that the birth control pill, most likely at a dosage of over 100 micrograms (mcg) of ethinyl estradiol, caused women with MS to have significant exacerbation of symptoms and an increase in the risk of thrombosis. With this high dosage, women without disabilities are also at risk for thrombosis (Speroff, Glass, & Kase, 1989). In an article reviewing women with spinal cord injury (SCI), 4 of 70 women developed thrombosis after using high-dose oral contraceptives (Sipski & Alexander, 1992).

Women experience a variety of disabling conditions with a wide range of considerations that cannot be comprehensively discussed in one text. To define more clearly the population's contraceptive needs, impairments are categorized into three main groups. The three categories include mobility impairments, chronic diseases, and cognitive impairments with other mental dysfunctions. It is important to remember that overlaps will occur within these groups.

Women with Mobility Impairments

Women with mobility impairments constitute a substantial population of women with disabilities. The etiologies of mobility impairments can vary significantly. The most common of these include SCI, MS, cerebral palsy (CP), spina bifida, and amputations. Despite the inherent differences in the underlying pathophysiology, certain generalizations about contraceptive risks in women with mobility impairments can be made. The most significant concern in this population is the theoretical risk of thrombotic predisposition. Measurement of thrombotic tendencies can be accomplished using a number of sensitive coagulation markers. The usefulness of these markers in the decision-making process regarding oral contraceptives has never been evaluated comprehensively. This issue has furthermore not been evaluated in women with mobility impairments. The most commonly used coagulation markers are antithrombin III, protein S, protein C, and anticardiolipin antibody. One clinician has measured antithrombin III levels as a screening tool in determining whether it is advisable to prescribe oral contraceptives in women with SCI (McCarren, 1993). Antithrombin III was measured at baseline and again 3 weeks later in women with severe spasticity. No increase in levels of antithrombin III were observed. Other factors have not been measured, and these women have not been followed beyond 3 months. In patients with severe leg spasticity, muscle contractions may make thrombosis less likely. In some Scandinavian countries, as well as some centers in the United States, birth control pills are being administered to spinal cord–injured women with marked leg spasticity, because this spasticity is felt to prevent venous pooling and thus to limit thrombosis risk. The safety of this approach has yet to be verified (McCarren, 1993). As a consequence, it is important to include in any study women with flaccid lower extremities as well as with other disability etiologies where thrombosis may be more of a concern.

Gynecological research on women without disabilities supports the assumption that oral contraceptives provide some beneficial effects, such as prevention of ovarian and endometrial cancer, decreases in blood cholesterol levels, and enhancing bone mass (Speroff, Glass, & Kase, 1994). These benefits are seen in the low-dose estrogen pills currently used (Speroff et al., 1994). It would be helpful to ascertain whether this method of contraception is safe in women with mobility impairments so that these women might derive the same benefits from this contraceptive method.

Contraceptive methods most commonly offered to the woman with mobility impairments include nonestrogenic formulations such as Depo-Provera and Norplant. There is some concern about long-term use of Depo-Provera because it can be associated with decreased circulating estradiol levels in some women. Prolonged amenorrhea has been reported in 2%–5% of women using Depo-Provera, even 1 year after stopping the injections (Speroff et al., 1994). This amenorrhea is usually welcomed by women in whom menstrual periods present hygiene problems. Decreased estradiol levels have also been reported, which may result in vaginal dryness. A very serious concern for the woman with a mobility impairment is the impact of decreased estradiol levels on bone mass. There have been a few reported cases of Depo-Provera leading to decreased bone mineral density even in women without disabilities (Speroff et al., 1994). It has been hypothesized that the drop in estradiol levels seen with this method of contraception can predispose women to osteoporosis. Thus far, data have not been conclusive and have not been studied with regard to women with disabilities. Since this is a significant issue to women with mobility impairments, more studies are needed (Ettinger, Genant, Steiger, & Maduig, 1989). Studies should be performed that evaluate bone mass in women with disabilities using Depo-Provera, Depo-Provera with calcium supplementation, and also possibly Depo-Provera with estrogen supplemental therapy in the form of a low-dose transdermal estrogen patch.

Norplant is a convenient method of birth control. However, because of the high incidence of erratic bleeding, it may be a less desirable alternative. Additionally, some women with disabilities have altered upper arm positioning, which may compromise the access for Norplant insertion and removal. Data regarding the behavior of sex steroids on the vascular system have demonstrated that estrogen can be thrombogenic and that progesterone may lead to vasospasm (Speroff et al., 1994). How much hormone is needed for these effects to develop is not known, because the information is so limited.

Currently, intrauterine devices (IUDs) can be safely recommended if the woman does not have sensory impairments and if the woman is monogamous and multiparous. Barrier methods require the contribution of the partner's assistance.

Women with Chronic Diseases

Women with disabilities are subject to the same chronic diseases as the rest of the population. Numerous women who are diabetic also have disabilities. What are the appropriate choices for contraception in the diabetic population? What do we know about the way hormones act on diabetes? There have been few studies that have examined the effects of estrogen and progesterone on glucose metabolism. There are data to suggest that estrogen possibly impairs glucose tolerance and that progesterone possibly causes insulin resistance (Speroff et al., 1994). It is still very unclear at what doses these side effects develop. Dose response by components of the oral contraceptive (i.e., progesterone used and the stability of the diabetes) can be a factor that may affect the safety of oral contraception in the diabetic woman.

Central nervous system disorders such as strokes, aneurysms, and head trauma also pose significant problems for contraceptive choice. With their newly acquired limitations, these women's sexual feelings, needs, and desires may be overlooked, minimized, and negated even by themselves, as discussed for women with SCI by Whipple in Chapter 5. Their needs for contraception are more challenging but still deserve attention. Barrier methods, IUDs, and possibly Depo-Provera and Norplant could be acceptable. The impact of these hormonal agents on the underlying disabilities has not been well studied. According to some researchers, estrogen reduces the threshold in seizure disorders, whereas progesterone raises the seizure threshold (Neinstein & Katz, 1986). This observation requires more confirmatory studies prior to establishing birth control protocols for women prone to seizures.

Lupus erythematosus affects many women in the reproductive age group. This disease may have a benign course or may be very debilitating. Patients with lupus are predisposed to thrombosis and other related complications such as strokes and deep vein thrombosis. Thus, they may develop further disabilities. Estrogen-containing oral contraceptives have a tendency to provoke thrombosis in patients with lupus erythematosus (Sipski & Alexander, 1992). It is not known whether there are specific markers that identify women at risk for this complication. Progesterone is not known to be thrombogenic, and therefore, theoretically, progesterone-only contraception such as Depo-Provera and Norplant may be safer options than the combination oral contraceptives. The Progestasert® and Pera-guard® IUDs have not been evaluated in relation to effects on lupus erythematosus, but their use is probably a safe option in monogamous, multiparous women.

For women with rheumatoid arthritis, oral contraceptives appear to improve the condition or have no effect (Leavesley & Porter, 1982). The improvement may result from the steroid effects of estrogen.

Women with cystic fibrosis are living longer because of improved medical management that has reduced the incidence of pneumonia or bowel complications. Contraceptive options for this population have not been examined. It is known that progesterone increases cervical mucus viscosity and may have similar effects on bronchial secretions (Dooley, Braustein, & Osher, 1979), which may be of concern to women with this condition.

SEXUALLY TRANSMITTED DISEASES

Sexually transmitted diseases (STDs) are occurring in epidemic proportions in the general population. This concern is not exclusive to nondisabled women. Women with disabilities who are sexually active should have routine testing for STDs. Tests for syphilis, gonorrhea, chlamydia, hepatitis, and human immunodeficiency virus (HIV) should be included in the workup. If an ulcer is present, herpes should also be tested for. Two issues that are of particular concern for this population include sensory impairments in the pelvic area that limit self-diagnosis, as well as physical access issues that prevent prompt intervention. Sometimes these infections may be the only indicators of an abusive relationship to which a woman with a disability is being subjected. Thus, this evaluation is very important. Gentle questioning to raise these potentially difficult issues and supportive intervention should be offered.

What are some complicating factors about STDs in women with disabilities? Women with disabilities may or may not have complete motor and sensory capacities, especially if they have high spinal cord lesions. Women with multiple sclerosis and other disabling conditions affecting the spinal cord may have sensory deficits in their pelvis that could result in an inability to detect a STD. Health care providers who treat women with disabilities or debilitating diseases that affect neurologic sensations must be trained to understand and recognize the so-called "sneaky" signs. Spasms or sensations of pressure, sweating, and flushing may imply full bladder, constipation, urinary tract infection, STDs, ectopic pregnancy, appendicitis, or a decubitus ulcer in the woman with an SCI (Welner, 1993). Other factors, such as vaginal discharge and odor, may be helpful to differentiate these conditions. Women with disabilities need to be taught to distinguish these signs to help identify circumstances that require intervention (Welner, 1993).

Besides diagnostic dilemmas, various barrier issues affect a woman's ability to obtain prompt, appropriate treatment for sexually transmitted diseases. Many women with mobility impairments depend on paratransit services, which may not be easy to arrange. Services may require assistance from a family member whom the woman may rather not involve. In addition, accessible examination rooms and tables are not universally available, and this may cause the woman to delay seeking care.

Just as symptoms may be masked, findings may be equally puzzling. For example, differentiating ulcer lesions in a woman with decubitus ulcer propensity may be challenging. A decubitus ulcer could appear similar to a herpetic ulcer, especially from primary herpes. Human immune deficiency dermatosis may be deceptive, and the differentiation of these lesions may be somewhat difficult. The important take-home lesson for the health care team caring for the woman with a disability is this: Think about sexually transmitted diseases, and test for them.

When treating any infections in women with disabilities, including sexually transmitted diseases, it is important to ensure that the woman is able to take her medication. For women with dysphagia, liquid forms are preferable to large pills. Physicians should be certain to designate packages for easy opening to prevent frustration and encourage compliance. Simplified dosing, when at all possible, should be considered. For example, a single-dose formulation of Azithromycin (Xithromox®), taken for 1 day, would be simpler than 7 days of Doxycycline, to treat chlamydia (Welner, 1992). Additionally, safe-sex messages are as important for the disabled patient as they are for the patient without a disability. Communicating the importance of this behavior may be even more important for the woman who has compromised sensation or is subject to situations where her disability may make her vulnerable to exploitation.

MENOPAUSAL ISSUES

Women with disabilities are living longer, continuing to be productive, and remaining in better health. Therefore, research on menopausal issues is gaining in importance. Estrogen replacement therapy has become well accepted as a useful intervention to help decrease cardiovascular morbidity as well as to impede progression of osteoporosis in the able-bodied menopausal population. Women with long-term disabilities enter menopause with many years of decreased weight bearing and limited participation in aerobic activities (Collins et al., 1993; Lufkin, Wahner, & O'Fallun, 1992). Little is known regarding the quantitative impact of disabilities on the menopausal state. It is important to determine whether, and to what degree, hormonal intervention will be beneficial to this vulnerable population.

A number of organ systems are affected by the reduced estrogen levels that occur as a consequence of menopause. Decreased estrogen levels result in a reduction in bone mineral density. For women with mobility limitations who may already have secondary osteoporosis, this potential acceleration of bone loss has not yet been quantified.

Data exist on the impact of osteoporosis in the general community, but not regarding women with disabilities (Ryon, Harrison, Blake, & Fogelman, 1992). Because this population is in part immobile, the impact of osteoporosis is theoretically much more significant. Studies should be undertaken to examine the effect of disabilities on osteoporosis by measuring bone metabolism in women with SCI and other immobilizing disabilities. There are simple, noninvasive assays to measure bone metabolism and bone turnover. Serum calcium, 24-hour calcium excretion, creatine clearance, bone-specific alkaline phosphatase, 25-hydroxy vitamin D, and parathyroid hormone (PTH) were previously used as common markers for assessing bone loss (Delmas, 1990). Currently, serum osteocalcin and urine hydroxyproline are available and are much more sensitive markers for detecting bone turnover (Ferrandez, Martin, & Fernandez, 1990). Superior markers are being developed that have the potential for enhancing our understanding of bone mineral metabolism. These include collagen cross-linkers and deoxypyridinoline, and plasma bone Gla protein (Garnero, Vassy, Bertholin, Riou, & Delmas, 1994; Munk et al., 1994).

It would be helpful to assemble data regarding the bone-mineral density status and quantitative measurements using the dual X-ray absorptiometry (DEXA) (Munk et al., 1994). Acquisition of data for women with disabilities regarding DEXA measurements would be very helpful. Unfortunately, the impact of the variance in disabilities on bone mineral density is quite complex and therefore does not easily lend itself to clear and standardized information. An intricate assembly of data that includes type of disability, age at onset of disability, and many other factors contributing to bone loss needs to be examined to develop such standardization, if this is achievable. Thus, bone loss could be quantified in this population and could provide a guide to corrective interventions. By comparing bone-mineral density measurements in the lower body skeletal structures, such as in the hips and femurs of women with and without disabilities, the differences between bone mass measurements in these two groups could be compared.

Decreased tissue turgor and strength, loss of skin elasticity, and reduced blood supply to the skin and soft tissues occur as a result of menopause (Speroff et al., 1989). These issues can be of great significance in a person with a disability. Vasomotor instability may be more pronounced in patients with MS because of sensitivity to temperature changes and also in SCI patients with high (above T6) lesions (Colachis, 1990; Duquette et al., 1992).

An additional benefit of estrogen replacement therapy that is in the process of being confirmed, but is currently fairly well accepted, is enhancement of cardiovascular health. This includes improved perfusion of coronary and peripheral vasculature as well as improvement in lipid profiles (Nabulsi et al., 1993; Writing Group for PEPI Trial, 1995). Cardiovascular health is often compromised in women with disabilities because of decreased ability to engage in protective aerobic activity.

The benefit of estrogen replacement therapy needs to be investigated. There has been fear of widely prescribing estrogen replacement therapy in the population of women with disabilities. Some clinicians are concerned about inducing thrombotic complications, but there has been little to support and document these concerns. To verify the safety of this important intervention, sensitive hypercoagulability markers need to be studied in this population to discern their baseline risks of thrombosis, as discussed earlier in this chapter. If there are no abnormalities in these markers, hesitation to use this therapy more widely may be put to rest. Clotting studies to ascertain risk of thrombotic predisposition are not using sensitive enough markers (Bick & Pegram, 1994). The less sensitive, previously used markers may be abnormal only when there is an actively propagating thrombus. More sensitive markers are being developed, and they should be able to detect the thrombogenic condition before the acute danger has been realized. These very sensitive assays will enable the researcher, and in the future the clinician, to identify those women with disabilities who can safely take estrogen replacement therapy and those for whom this therapy will be contraindicated. As of 1995, these markers are not commercially available. These markers include deficiencies of protein C, protein S, antithrombin III activity, and resistance to activated C (Baur & Rosenburg, 1991; Baur, 1994). Additional markers include plasminogen activator inhibitor, fibrinogen, and prothrombin fragment 1.2 (Ginsberg, Hirsh, & Morder, 1994; Greer, 1994).

CONCLUSIONS

In summary, the preceding pages address research concerns regarding contraception, sexually transmitted diseases, and menopause in disabled women. Although it is known that women with disabilities need safe and effective contraception, appropriate options are still unclear and require more study. Women with disabilities who are sexually active are at risk of developing STDs. Still, there has been some difficulty in identifying the best methods to educate women and their health care providers about identifying these infections, given the paucity of traditional symptoms and findings. Menopausal women without disabilities can develop osteoporosis and cardiac disease due to estrogen deficiency. It is unknown what impact the woman's disability has on the progression of these conditions. Each of these areas has great potential for research innovation.

REFERENCES

Baur, K.A. (1994). Inherited hypercoagulable states. *Thrombosis and Hemorrhage,* 809–834.

Baur, K.A., & Rosenburg, R.D. (1991). The hypercoagulable state. *Disorders of Hemostasis,* 267–291.

Bick, R.L., & Pegram, M. (1994). Syndromes of hypercoagulability and thrombosis. *Seminars in Thrombosis and Hemostasis, 20,* 109–131.

Colachis, S.C. (1990). Autonomic hyperflexia with spinal cord injury. *Journal of the American Paraplegia Society, 15,* 171–186.

Collins, P., Rosano, G.M., Jiang, C., Lindsay, D., Sarrel, P., & Poole-Wilson, P. (1993). Cardiovascular protection by oestrogen. *Lancet, 341,* 1264–1265.

Delmas, P.D. (1990). Biochemical markers of bone turnover for the clinical assessment of metabolic bone disease. *Endocrinology and Metabolism Clinics of North America, 19,* 1–18.

Dooley, R., Braustein, H., & Osher, A.B. (1979). Polypoid cervicitis in cystic fibrosis patients receiving oral contraceptives. *American Journal of Obstetrical Gynecology, 118,* 971–974.

Duquette, P., Pleines, J., Girard, M., Charest, L., Senecal-Quevileon, M., & Masse, C. (1992). The increased susceptibility of women with multiple sclerosis. *Canadian Journal of Neurological Sciences, 19,* 466–471.

Ettinger, B., Genant, H., Steiger, P., & Maduig, P. (1989). Low-dosage micronized B-estradiol prevents bone loss in post-menopausal women. *American Journal of Obstetrics and Gynecology, 166*(2), 479–488.

Ferrandez, L., Martin, M., & Fernandez, M. (1990). Calcitonin, estradiol, and hydroxyproline as parameters in the early diagnosis of involutional osteoporosis. *Archives of Orthopedic Trauma Surgery, 109,* 181–185.

Garnero, P., Vassy, V., Bertholin, A., Riou, J., & Delmas, P. (1994). Markers of bone turnover in hyperthyroidism and the effect of treatment. *Journal of Endocrinology and Metabolism, 78,* 955–958.

Ginsberg, J.S., Hirsh, J., & Morder, V.J. (1994). Thrombotic and hemorrhagic complications in the obstetric patient. *Hemostasis and Thrombosis,* 981–988.

Greer, I.A. (1994). Haemostasis and thrombosis in pregnancy. *Hemostasis and Thrombosis,* 989–1015.

Leavesley, G., & Porter, J. (1982). Sexuality, fertility, and contraception. *Contraception, 26,* 417–441.

Lufkin, E.G., Wahner, H.W., & O'Fallun, W.M. (1992). Treatment of post-menopausal osteoporosis with transdermal estrogen. *Annual Internal Medicine, 117,* 1–9.

Malanga, G.A., & Gangemi, E. (1994). Intracranial venous thrombosis in a patient with multiple sclerosis. *American Journal of Physical Medicine & Rehabilitation,* 283–285.

McCarren, M. (1993). Birth control. In S. Maddox (Ed.), *Spinal network* (pp. 360–361). Philadelphia: J.B. Lippincott.

Munk, N., Nielsen, P., von der Decke, M., Hansen, K., Overgaard, K., & Christianson, C. (1994). Estimation of the effect of salmon calcitonin in established osteoporosis by biochemical bone markers. *Calcif Tissue International, 55,* 8–11.

Nabulsi, A.A., Folsom, A.R., White, A., Wolfgang, P., Heiss, G., & Wu, K. (1993). Association of hormone replacement therapy with various cardiovascular risk factors. *New England Journal of Medicine, 328,* 1070–1117.

Neinstein, L.S., & Katz, B. (1986). Contraceptive use in the chronically ill adolescent female: Part I. *Journal of Adolescent Health Care, 7,* 123–133.

Ryon, P.J., Harrison, R., Blake, G.M., & Fogelman, I. (1992). Compliance with hormone replacement therapy (HRT) after screening for post menopausal osteoporosis. *British Journal of Obstetrics and Gynaecology, 99,* 325–328.

Sipski, M.L., & Alexander, C.J. (1992). Sexual function and dysfunction after spinal cord injury. *Traumatic Spinal Cord Injury, 3,* 811–828.

Speroff, L., Glass, R.H., & Kase, N.G. (1989). *Clinical gynecologic endocrinology and infertility* (4th ed.) Baltimore: Williams & Wilkins.

Speroff, L., Glass, R.H., & Kase, N.G. (1994). *Clinical gynecologic endocrinology and infertility* (5th ed.). Baltimore: Williams & Wilkins.

Welner, S. (1992). Evaluation of azithromycin as a one day treatment for *chlamydia trachomatous.* Research Project, Yale University, New Haven, CT.

Welner, S. (1993). Treatment of sexually transmitted diseases in the physically disabled woman. In F.B. Haseltine, S.S. Cole, & D.B. Gray (Eds.), *Reproductive issues for persons with physical disabilities* (pp. 275–290). Baltimore: Paul H. Brookes Publishing Co.

Writing Group for PEPI Trial. (1995). Effects of estrogen or estrogen/progestin regimens on heart disease risk factors in postmenopausal women. *Journal of the American Medical Association, 273,* 199–208.

chapter 7

Pregnancy and Delivery

Amie B. Jackson

In 1988, the University of Alabama at Birmingham founded the nation's first clinic for women with disabilities. The focus of the clinic was on reproductive health. Since its establishment, women with many different disabilities, including spinal cord injury, multiple sclerosis, cerebral palsy, stroke, head injury, arthritis, and spina bifida, have been seen at the clinic. One of the first observations was that women with newly acquired disabilities presented with a unique set of problems compared with women who had had their disabilities for many years or from birth. For example, women with a newly acquired spinal cord injury (SCI) had unique complications, such as prolactinemia, breast enlargement, galactorrhea, and amenorrhea (Jackson & Varner, 1990). Women who had had chronic disabilities, such as SCI for longer than a year, came to the clinic with questions regarding sexual function, birth control, urological issues, and obstetrical issues. The physical accessibility of the clinic was reported by most of the women as being a major reason for their visit. Many had neglected getting routine primary health care for years because of physical barriers and ignorance in their communities.

When the clinic first opened, the women who came to receive care asked many questions, but answers and data were limited. Because of the medical problems faced by these women and the lack of health information available, a large study was initiated in 1992 in collaboration with 10 regional model SCI systems. The study involved the development of an extensive questionnaire that explored gynecological problems, menstrual history, Pap smear results, gynecological examinations, sexual activity, birth control, menopause issues, and obstetrical histories in women with SCI. Comparison information related to their experiences prior to their injury was also obtained.

QUESTIONNAIRE DISTRIBUTION AND RESULTS

To date, information has been collected on 472 women with SCI across the country. In these results, many important issues stand out and lead the way for future research directives. It is important to note that these data were collected only on women who have had an SCI, which underscores the absence of data on the sexual, gynecological, and obstetrical issues for women with other types of disabilities.

The questionnaire was sent to 10 regional SCI centers located in Birmingham, Seattle, New York, Chicago, Houston, Denver, Philadelphia, Ann Arbor, West Orange (New Jersey), and Detroit. Women who had had an SCI at least 1 year prior to the study were included. All 472 women were interviewed by a woman trained both in information collection and with regard to the sensitivity of the subject matter. The questionnaire was divided into gynecological histories and obstetrical histories. The results showed that the average age at injury was 32 years, with a mean age of 26. The degree of neurological impairment was evenly divided, with approximately half of the women having quadriplegia and half having neurologically complete injuries. A total of 54 women (11.4%) were injured 1 year prior to answering the questionnaire. A total of 249 women (52.7%) were injured 2–10 years prior to the study, and 169 (35.8%) were injured 11 or more years prior to the study.

Prior to their SCI, 246 of the women, or 52.1%, had had at least one pregnancy. There were a total of 665 pregnancies experienced by the participants of this study prior to injury, which represented approximately 2.7 pregnancies per woman. There was a significant decrease in the number of women having babies following their injury. Of the 472 women questioned, 66 (13.9%) had had at least one pregnancy postinjury. There was a total of 101 postinjury pregnancies, which represented 1.53 pregnancies per woman, or 2.14 pregnancies for all of the women in the study. Essentially no differences were reported regarding the incidence of problems with intercourse, ovulation requiring medication, or infertility before and after injury.

Of the 66 women who became pregnant following their injury, 24 had had at least one pregnancy prior to their injury, which represented 36.4% of the women who became pregnant postinjury. However, there were 42 women who became pregnant for the first time after an injury. Thus, approximately two thirds of the pregnancies that occurred postinjury were first-time pregnancies. Upon examination of the pregnancy outcomes, several interesting trends are evident (Table 1). Although women had the same percentage of live births (78%) prior to their injury as they did postinjury, a greater percentage of women reported miscarriages before injury (12.7%) than after injury (6.0%). However, the abortion frequency was higher in

Table 1. Pregnancy outcomes

	Preinjury	Postinjury
Live births	521 (78.8%)	78 (78.0%)
Miscarriage	84 (12.7%)	6 (6.0%)
Abortion	43 (6.5%)	14 (14.0%)
Multiple births	9 (1.4%)	1 (2.0%)
Stillbirth	2 (0.03%)	0
Unknown	46 (6.9%)	2 (2.0%)

postinjury pregnancies (14%) compared with that of women prior to injury (6.5%). The reasons for this trend may have far-reaching psychosocial implications that have not been examined.

Tables 2 and 3 provide information on women who had more than one pregnancy. Of the 46 women who became pregnant following SCI, 40 women (60.6%) had only one pregnancy. Approximately 30% had two pregnancies. One woman reported five pregnancies, the highest number reported in this group. There were also considerable differences in the number of pregnancies that occurred prior to injury. For example, 72 of the 246 women in this category (29.3%) reported a single pregnancy prior to their injury. The range in number of pregnancies varied, with one woman reporting 12 pregnancies. These statistics provide an initial glimpse of the population and should be viewed with caution to avoid overgeneralization.

REPORTED COMPLICATIONS

Complications were seen in pregnancies both before and after injury (Table 4). Pregnancy experiences were similar for both groups with the exception of the frequency of symptomatic urinary tract infections (UTIs). Some 8% of the women reported UTIs before injury and 45.5% after injury. This difference was statistically significant. For other complications, such as persistent high blood pressure, vaginal bleeding, toxemia, diabetes, severe morning sickness, and anemia, however, there were no significant differences between the two groups. Some 26% of women complained of other types of postinjury pregnancy complications that may have fetal health

Table 2. Postinjury pregnancies

	Number of women	Number of pregnancies
	40 (60.6%)	1
	20 (30.3%)	2
	4 (6.1%)	3
	1 (1.5%)	4
	1 (1.5%)	5
Total	66	101

Table 3. Preinjury pregnancies

Number of women	Number of pregnancies
72 (29.3%)	1
63 (25.6%)	2
42 (17.1%)	3
37 (15.0%)	4
14 (5.7%)	5
5 (2.0%)	6
2 (0.8%)	7
2 (0.8%)	8
2 (0.8%)	9
1 (0.4%)	12
6 (2.4%)	Unknown
Total 246	665

consequences. Thus, aggressive medical management may need to be advocated for these women.

Many women with SCI reported exacerbation of disability-related difficulties during their pregnancy (Table 5). For example, 12% reported frequent autonomic dysreflexia; 6% developed pressure sores; and 12% reported worsening of their spasticity. Independence was also affected because approximately 11% of the women reported a new inability to transfer at the end of their pregnancy, and 4.5% were no longer able to propel their wheelchairs. The study also addressed urological problems seen in postinjury pregnancies. Fifteen percent of women with disabilities reported an increase in leakage around their indwelling urinary catheter, and 9.1% reported more frequent bladder spasms that expelled the catheter. Of women on intermittent catheterization for bladder management, 27.3% had to catheterize more frequently during the day. Many (25.8%) women re-

Table 4. Pregnancy complications

Complication	Women pregnant preinjury	Women pregnant postinjury
Persistent high blood pressure	18 (7.4%)	7 (10.6%)
Vaginal bleeding	14 (5.8%)	2 (3.0%)
Toxemia	16 (6.6%)	2 (3.0%)
Diabetes of pregnancy	5 (2.1%)	6 (9.1%)
Urinary tract infections[a]	20 (8.2%)	30 (45.5%)
Severe morning sickness with nausea, vomiting, and weight loss	89 (36.6%)	24 (36.4%)
Anemia requiring treatment	21 (8.6%)	4 (6.1%)
Other	15 (6.2%)	17 (25.8%)

[a]Statistically significant, $p < .05$.

Table 5. Pregnancy complications (spinal cord injury related)

Frequent autonomic dysreflexia	8 (12.1%)
Developed pressure sore(s)	4 (6.1%)
Unable to transfer at end of pregnancy	7 (10.6%)
Could no longer propel wheelchair	3 (4.5%)
Spasticity worsened	8 (12.1%)

ported that they had to change their usual bladder management method during their pregnancy. Finally, a staggering ($p < .05$) complication rate for women with disabilities was found in this study. Of the women who had postinjury pregnancies, 75% complained of at least one or more pregnancy complications. In comparison, 49.8% of the pregnancies prior to the injuries had one or more complication.

The questionnaire results also provided information on labor symptoms. The majority (62%) of women experienced conventional uterine contraction labor pains and/or rupture of membranes to signify the onset of labor prior to their injury. Postinjury, however, a wider variety of labor symptomatology was observed. These included pains above the level of injury (41%), abnormal pains (29%), ruptured membranes (53%), significantly increased spasticity (15%), increased frequency of autonomic dysreflexia (18%), and increased bladder spasms (17%). Some women did not experience any type of labor sensations, and some reported normal labor symptomatology.

Results concerning method of delivery showed an increased incidence of cesarean sections in postinjury pregnancies, (Table 6). In addition, there was a higher frequency of vacuum or forceps delivery in postinjury pregnancies and fewer spontaneous vaginal deliveries. This information raises questions as to whether these practices result from difficulties with progression of the delivery or whether factors such as habits and comfort of the obstetrician play a role.

Table 7 provides information on delivery complications experienced by the respondents. After SCI, women developed significantly higher incidence of problems with blood pressure instability than prior to injury.

Table 6. Method of delivery

	Preinjury	Postinjury
Spontaneous vaginal	418 (62%)	48 (48%)
Forceps or vacuum	46 (7%)	14 (14%)
Cesarean section	55 (8%)	18 (18%)
Unknown (including abortion or miscarriage)	146 (22%)	21 (21%)

Table 7. Labor and delivery complications

Complication	Women pregnant preinjury	Women pregnant postinjury
Problems with blood pressure instability[a]	13 (5.3%)	15 (22.7%)
Excessive bleeding requiring transfusion	5 (2.1%)	2 (3.0%)
Abnormal bleeding prior to delivery	11 (4.5%)	2 (3.0%)
Prolonged postpartum bleeding (greater than 1 month)	10 (4.1%)	3 (4.5%)
Prolonged labor requiring cesarean section	11 (4.5%)	4 (6.1%)
Premature labor and delivery[b]	31 (12.8%)	14 (21.2%)
Fetal distress requiring cesarean section	10 (4.1%)	3 (4.5%)
Other	16 (6.6%)	3 (4.5%)

[a]Statistically significant, $p < .05$.
[b]Approaches statistical significance, $p = .07$.

Premature (prior to 36 weeks gestation) labor and delivery were seen more frequently in individuals with SCI. Although this did not quite reach statistical significance, it was very close. Other complications that were seen infrequently in both groups included excessive bleeding requiring transfusion, abnormal bleeding prior to delivery, prolonged postpartum bleeding, prolonged labor requiring cesarean section, and fetal distress requiring cesarean section.

The type of anesthesia utilized is described in Table 8 and is similar in all groups except for the "none" category. These data indicate that women with SCI require less anesthesia for delivery because of apparent reduction in pain sensation. Complications from anesthesia were low, and no statistical differences were noted in the two patient groups (Table 9).

Table 8. Anesthesia used in labor and delivery

	Women pregnant preinjury	Women pregnant postinjury
Epidural	32 (13.2%)	15 (22.7%)
General	64 (26.3%)	9 (13.6%)
Local	19 (7.8%)	3 (4.5%)
Spinal	53 (21.8%)	2 (3.0%)
Other	19 (7.8%)	4 (6.1%)
None[a]	59 (23.9%)	33 (50.0%)

[a]Statistically significant, $p < .05$.

Table 9.   Complications from anesthesia

Complication	Women pregnant preinjury	Women pregnant postinjury
High blood pressure	0	0
Low blood pressure	1 (0.4%)	1 (1.5%)
Too high of a block with epidural or spinal	0	1 (1.5%)
Electrolyte abnormality	0	0
Hyperthermia	1 (0.4%)	1 (1.5%)
Other	18 (7.4%)	4 (6.1%)

POSTPARTUM ISSUES

Of great concern to women with SCI contemplating pregnancy is the possibility of congenital disabilities in their children. There was no statistical difference in the frequency of the most common congenital disabilities in both groups (Table 10). That is not to say that problems with the infant at the time of birth did not arise (Table 11). Quite surprisingly, there was a statistically greater incidence of low birth weight infants (less than 5 lbs., 6 oz., but not born prematurely) born to women with SCI. In addition, there was a trend for women with SCI to have an infant who had difficulties breathing at birth. This finding has never been described; thus, the implications are powerful and warrant further study. Furthermore, there appeared to be a trend for all problems with the baby to be more frequent in the postinjury pregnancies. These included the baby having a fever and requiring antibiotics, requiring a blood transfusion, or being jaundiced.

The final section of this study dealt with breast-feeding habits of women following injury. A total of 28% of women breast-fed their babies born prior to their SCI for an average of 4.1 months. However, only about 11% of women breast-fed their babies born following SCI, and this period averaged 6.2 months. This difference was statistically significant. The study did not examine the reasons why fewer women chose to breast-feed their infants following the onset of their disability. This opens the door for future

Table 10.   Birth with congenital disabilities

	Preinjury pregnancies	Postinjury pregnancies
Cerebral palsy	1 (0.4%)	0
Down syndrome	1 (0.4%)	0
Cleft palate	0	0
Spina bifida	1 (0.4%)	0
Birth injury	3 (1.2%)	0
Other	10 (4.1%)	4 (6.1%)

Table 11. Birth with problems other than congenital disabilities

	Preinjury pregnancies	Postinjury pregnancies
Low birth weight[a] (less than 5 lbs. 6 oz. but not born prematurely)	11 (4.5%)	9 (13.6%)
Baby had problems breathing	18 (7.4%)	10 (15.2%)
Baby had fever and required antibiotics	7 (2.9%)	3 (4.5%)
Baby required a blood transfusion	6 (2.5%)	4 (6.1%)
Baby was jaundiced	42 (17.3%)	16 (24.2%)
Other	20 (8.2%)	5 (7.6%)

[a]Statistically significant, $p < .05$.
[b]Approaches statistical significance, $p = .1$.

investigations of psychosocial and physiological inhibitions to breast-feeding.

CONCLUSIONS

This study has provided much-needed information regarding obstetrical outcomes for women who have SCI. Unfortunately, however, it leaves researchers with many more questions than answers. For example, do women with SCI experience difficulties becoming pregnant? If so, for what reasons? We saw significantly fewer women having babies following their injuries. The reasons for this are unclear. Questions regarding psychosocial versus physiological reasons are raised. The literature, to date, reports that there is no reason why a woman cannot conceive after SCI. No studies, however, have really explored if this is true. There have been studies (DeVivo & Fine, 1985) that report a decrease in marriage rates, an increase in divorce rates, and an older age of pregnancy for women who have babies following injury. Factors such as infertility associated with aging in women should be considered.

Another question focuses on identifying the neuroendocrine consequences following SCI. It is known that immediately after SCI, women develop hormonal imbalances that can affect the reproductive endocrine system (Comarr, 1966; Terbizan & Schneeweiss, 1983). Normal menstruation does resume, at least by the end of the first year following an injury; but normal menstrual cycles, as well as the contribution of the endocrine system for normal ovulation, have not been established in this patient population.

Other important questions concern the long- and short-term complications that may arise during pregnancy, labor, and delivery. For example, does the increased frequency of symptomatic UTIs and autonomic dysreflexia have a relationship to the outcome of pregnancy, labor, and delivery?

More important, regarding fetal health, what are the neonatal risks of a pregnancy in women with SCI? Although congenital anomalies do not appear to be greater in the offspring of these women, there appear to be some definite risks to the infant, either in utero or at the time of delivery. The pathogenesis of these risks needs to be explored so that appropriate interventional practices can be initiated to ensure the arrival of healthy infants. Undoubtedly, the most obvious outcome of this study is the need for more effective education of women, physicians, and society to the special obstetrical needs of women with disabilities.

REFERENCES

Comarr, A.E. (1966, July/August). Interesting observations on females with spinal cord injury. *Medical Services Journal*, 651–661.

DeVivo, M.J., & Fine, P.R. (1985). Spinal cord injury: Its short-term impact on marital status. *Archives of Physical Medicine & Rehabilitation, 66*, 501–504.

Jackson, A.B., & Varner, R.E. (1990). Gynecological problems encountered in women with acute and chronic spinal cord disabilities. *Journal of the American Paraplegia Society, 13*(1), 54.

Terbizan, A.T., & Schneeweiss, W.D. (1983). The value of gynecological examinations in spinal cord injured women. *Paraplegia, 21*, 266–269.

chapter 8

Pregnancy and Physical Disabilities

Judith G. Rogers

In 1980 I started writing *Mother to Be: A Guide to Pregnancy and Birth for Women with Disabilities* (Rogers & Matsumura, 1991). Of the 36 women I interviewed, 14 had physical disabilities. The group was composed of women whose disabilities were fairly common, such as spinal cord injuries, and others whose disabilities were uncommon, such as Friedreich's ataxia. Altogether, the women had experienced 62 pregnancies. Collecting the material for the book reinforced my observation that society holds a long-standing bias against parenthood among people with disabilities. This attitude continues to be disturbingly prevalent, and I believe that education can help to overcome this bias.

It is important to analyze biases about women with disabilities in order to enhance health care management. Despite the fact that the number of women with disabilities becoming pregnant is increasing, the specific health problems associated with their pregnancy and childbirth are not receiving the attention they deserve either from researchers or from health care providers. In addition, studying pregnancy, labor, and delivery as they relate to women with disabilities may help with labor and delivery for all women.

This chapter 1) reviews the effects of long-standing bias against parenting by people with disabilities and 2) outlines a research agenda to help improve service delivery to pregnant women with disabilities.

NEGATIVE BIAS AND WELL-BEING

It is important to remember that pregnancy issues are not only physical in nature; they include psychological concerns as well. Expectant mothers

This chapter was made possible by NIDRR, Rehabilitation and Research Training Center, Grant H133B30076. Its contents do not necessarily represent the policy of that agency. The reader should not assume endorsement by the federal government.

often worry about body image, the effect the discomforts of pregnancy may have on their disabilities, and, like most women, their ability to be good mothers. The other issues may be more complex. For example, some women who are disabled and are also able to walk have increased mobility problems during pregnancy. At first they seem to struggle with the idea of needing a wheelchair. This is not surprising, because professionals, society, and families have given them the message that it is important to walk. This may be one of the factors that causes women with decreasing mobility to use a chair later in their pregnancy than would have been comfortable for them. Many of the women I interviewed used a chair earlier in their second pregnancy. After having experienced one pregnancy, these women felt more secure in their role as a parent and were not as concerned with conforming to society's standards.

The natural insecurities that first-time mothers experience may be intensified by the attitudes of health professionals. For example, some women with inherited disabilities may feel that bringing another child into this world with their own disability is a good thing because the family can share the culture that goes with that particular disability (e.g., in the deaf community). However, genetic counselors, health professionals, and society at large may express that it is not acceptable to reproduce a child with that disability because they are unaware of the positive psychological and social aspects of a disability culture (again, as seen in deaf culture). Because many professionals question the decision of a woman with a disability to become pregnant, consultation with her on approaches to making her pregnancy, labor, and parenting easier may be infrequent, minimal, or completely absent. Responding to the insensitivity of these professionals, the pregnant woman with a disability may become angry or anxious or both, depending on her temperament. This emotional reaction may result in poor self-esteem, which in turn may cause her not to seek help for resolving various pregnancy and/or parenting issues. In addition, the negative feedback from professionals can make it harder to succeed as a parent and thus become a self-fulfilling prophecy.

The majority of the women interviewed reported that their physicians' attitudes were not negative, although some did have problems with the attitudes of their doctors' on-call partners. For example, one interviewee described an incident that occurred years earlier, in the 1970s, with the doctor on call during her labor. The physician had such a negative reaction to his new patient and her disability that he pressured her into a tubal ligation. Even though this incident happened many years ago, similar biases may still exist today. A client from the agency in which I work, Through the Looking Glass, located in Berkeley, California, was pressured into a tubal ligation prior to an emergency cesarean section that resulted from eclampsia. The woman is still in conflict with the decision to have the tubal ligation and wishes she could have another baby. The law is clear that the physician should have waited 48 hours to see if she still agreed to the procedure. The physician probably had a caring point of view. He could have been worried about the possibility of a stroke compounding her original disability. Yet, in the long run, the decision was devastating to the woman, and it did not matter that the medical procedure was recommended as a result of concern or biases—the outcome was the same. This woman will probably never be able to give birth again, because she does not have the resources to have tubal ligation reversal. In addition, she does not want to pursue the litigation process.

A paternalistic view by the medical professionals, such as the one illustrated above, does not give the responsibility of the decision to the woman and, therefore, compounds the problem. I believe it would be beneficial to hold a team meeting with all the woman's specialists involved, not only to exchange information but also to work on attitudes and expectations. Doctors who share call should also be involved because, as the previous example illustrates, they can have a strong impact on treatment, both medically and psychologically.

Improving the attitudes of health providers will help to establish more appropriate services for pregnant women with disabilities. However, many unanswered questions remain regarding reproductive issues facing women with physical disabilities. The following sections highlight a number of areas in which more knowledge is needed.

THE NEED FOR BETTER COMMUNICATION AND EDUCATION

To what extent do physicians talk to women about how their disability may affect their pregnancy and to what extent do women with disabilities talk to their physicians? It is important for the doctor to feel comfortable directing questions to the pregnant woman about her disability and also to her disability specialist. Verduyn (1994) noted that physicians may not know how to treat dysreflexia in labor, which could result in disastrous consequences to the woman: death or stroke. The following examples (Rogers & Matsumura, 1991) illustrate the importance of communication between the woman and her health care providers. One woman felt that her doctor did not appreciate the important effect her disability could have on her pregnancy until, at her insistence, he conferred with her disability specialist. Following the consultation, she felt that her care improved. A second woman who had an autoimmune disability required a cesarean section. The anesthesiologist attending her was unsure whether spinal anesthesia would be safe for her, so he used a general anesthetic without consulting her or her specialist.

The Effects of Anesthesia

Medical staff monitor recovery from spinal anesthesia by assessing the return of functioning below the level of anesthesia. For women with physical disabilities, the baseline is different from that of women without disabilities, and physicians should be aware of these differences in order to assess the return of normal functioning. Anesthesiologists should avail themselves of consultants who are well versed in assessing levels of physical functioning in women with various disabilities. Furthermore, better understanding is needed regarding effects of anesthesia, and documentation of results should be thorough and accessible. For example, a woman with Friedreich's ataxia reports that she was given a general anesthetic because the anesthesiologist was uncomfortable using regional anesthesia. He did not use regional anesthesia in part because he did not know what effect it would have on her disability. This mother was very disappointed because she was unconscious when the baby was born. Had more information been available on this topic, both he and the woman might have been better served.

It is also important to study the effects of anesthesia on the body and possible complications to the respiratory system and the musculoskeletal system. Some women with disabilities have respiratory problems secondary to their disability. Because general anesthesia can compromise respiration, physicians need to know the risk associated with specific disabilities.

Access to Information

It is important to examine ways to help physicians be more comfortable about consulting with other specialists. Clearly, one physician cannot be expected to know about every disability. Obstetricians serving women with disabilities should have access to information that consultants can provide, such as advice on treating or preventing dysreflexia during labor. A national database or network could be established to allow greater depth of research and understanding of pregnancy, labor, and delivery as they relate to disability. The information highway should be used to collect data to study the interaction of pregnancy and disability and possible treatments that could minimize the negative effects for women with different disabilities. Most likely, overall satisfaction and outcomes for women with disabilities would improve if more physicians were better informed.

Circulatory Problems

Increased blood volume may have negative as well as positive effects on the woman's well-being and functioning. One negative effect that occurs in women with and without disabilities is edema. Edema in pregnancy is currently being investigated, but is not being studied in women with disabilities. Medical professionals have anticipated that pregnancy-related thrombophlebitis would be more of a problem among women with disabilities because the biggest predisposition to thrombophlebitis is stasis or pooling of blood in the lower extremities. Of the women I interviewed, only one woman with a spinal cord injury developed thrombophlebitis (Rogers & Matsumura, 1991). She had this problem both before and during pregnancy. It is important to know what other factors contribute to thrombophlebitis.

Hormonal Changes

There are many side effects that are related to hormonal shifts during pregnancy that all women experience. Studies are needed that will characterize hormonal effects in pregnant women within disability groups. Women I interviewed who have either multiple sclerosis or rheumatoid arthritis reported both remissions and exacerbations of their symptoms.

Respiratory Problems

Respiratory problems are not necessarily inevitable in pregnant women with physical disabilities. In fact, one interviewee who had post polio syndrome found that her breathing improved because her baby acted like a corset (Rogers & Matsumura, 1991). Many women, however, reported shortness of breath. Research should be undertaken that will predict which women may have significant change in respiratory function. This could result in better treatment of women with and without disabilities.

Urinary Problems

Bladder problems seem to affect many pregnant women, regardless of whether they have a disability. Increased hormone levels during pregnancy have an effect on the urinary system by reducing bladder tone and creating urine stasis. In addition, pressure from the uterus may make it difficult for the bladder to empty completely, thereby increasing the likelihood of bacterial growth. All of the women with spinal cord dysfunction whom I interviewed reported increased bladder complications (Rogers & Matsumura, 1991). Research should document these changes in bladder function that occur in pregnant women with disabilities.

Neuromuscular Problems

Some women experience increased spasticity during labor and delivery. As a woman with cerebral palsy, I found this topic of particular interest because I experienced severe clonus (a strong muscle spasm that caused my leg to jerk) during delivery. The experience was very disconcerting because it not only was painful but also made me feel out of control. Although my husband was able to control my clonus by bracing my leg, it required a lot of physical strength and effort to hold my leg. I not only delivered beautiful children but also gave birth to a bruise on my husband's chest. Some possible interventions should be evaluated for effectiveness that can help control significant spasticity during delivery.

Working with a woman with cerebral palsy at Through the Looking Glass, I found that both range of motion and stretching exercises were helpful in reducing leg cramps during her pregnancy; however, during labor her symptoms reappeared. Range of motion exercises during labor resulted in minimal improvement.

Cesarean Section

Physicians sometimes think that a cesarean section is physically easier for the woman than going through labor and delivery. One woman I interviewed for my book, who has spinal muscular atrophy, reported having a cesarean section instead of experiencing labor because her doctors thought the surgery would be less stressful on her body; however, they seemed to ignore the question of the interaction between anesthesia and respiratory problems. This was also the case for a woman mentioned previously, who had a similar progressive disability. She delivered her first child by cesarean section. Six years later, because of her determination, she gave birth to her second child vaginally. In spite of the years between the births, she was able to recover faster from the vaginal birth. This is significant, not only because she was several years older, but also because she has a progressive disability that by then had reduced her physical strength. It is important to examine the attitudes of obstetricians regarding cesarean section. If it is found that doctors believe cesarean sections are inherently safer and easier than vaginal births for women with disabilities, research should test this belief.

Postpartum Recovery

Postpartum recovery is difficult for many women with disabilities. I have spoken with a woman with cerebral palsy who was seeking information about postpartum recovery for women with disabilities. A year after delivering her daughter, during which epidural anesthesia was used, she felt she still had not recovered. Her legs continued to feel weak and uncoordinated. Other women reported that they continue to have backaches after pregnancy and delivery. Some of the women with cerebral palsy have lost some of their ability to walk after giving birth. Did the extra strain of pregnancy and giving birth cause permanent problems? What are the dangers of epidural anesthesia? A comparison of the physical symptoms during the postpartum period of women with and without disabilities could help distinguish between postpartum symptoms and disability exacerbations. Results from such a study could establish different methods of treatment for recovery from the effects of pregnancy, labor, and delivery.

The effect of cesarean sections on postpartum recovery should also be evaluated for women with disabilities. Comparison studies between women who had a cesarean section and those who had vaginal birth with regional anesthesia should provide important information on differences associated with postpartum recovery. Studies should group women by type of disability, degree of disability, type of anesthesia, and type of delivery.

Accessibility

Equipment present in health providers' offices may also provide a series of problems for women with disabilities. Some women reported finding it difficult to have office visits where practitioners do not have examining tables that are accessible. Hydraulic tables are available that make transfers easier, not only for the pregnant woman but also for the medical support staff and the woman's support person. Equipment is also needed that allows a woman to communicate with the medical staff if she is left alone in the examining room. One of the women I interviewed was left alone in the examining room, making her feel very vulnerable because she was unable to get to her wheelchair (Rogers & Matsumura, 1991). This incident left her with a strong sense of distrust. A buzzer or intercom system placed in an accessible location, for instance, can alleviate anxiety as well as provide access to help if necessary. This should be viewed also as a safety consideration.

An accessible scale is also a necessary piece of equipment because the woman can be weighed while she is in her wheelchair. Such scales are available and are able to weigh up to 580 pounds. These scales are listed now in many catalogs, but few professionals or consumers are aware of this fact, making them an uncommon piece of equipment in most medical offices and clinics. Women have had to invent ways of being weighed. One woman I interviewed needed to go to a rehabilitation unit. Some women did not get weighed at all, because it was inconvenient. This is risky to both the mother's and her baby's health. Another equipment need is redesigned birthing stools and birthing tables for pregnant women with and without disabilities. Some existing models are not comfortable for the mother or birthing personnel.

A needs assessment of the importance of accessible medical equipment for pregnant women with disabilities must be conducted. Also, resources are needed for the intervention, development, and purchase of equipment, not only in hospitals but also for practitioners in private practice. It is also important to know where and how to locate medical equipment. The dissemination of this information and possible acquisition of the equipment may help to alleviate stress.

CONCLUSIONS

Clearly, women with disabilities may have more problems getting information, because there has not been much information available or collected. There is a need for greater sensitivity on the part of health care providers, better communication between doctors and patients, increased data exchange among providers, and better equipment and facilities to accommodate women with disabilities.

Specific areas of research should include the effect that the attitudes of professionals have on the care they give to pregnant women with disabilities and the influences on positive and negative attitudes in professionals toward people with a disability. Studies should be undertaken to examine the care received by women whose health care providers have been educated about the needs and issues of women with disabilities, versus the care received from health providers who have not.

Studying women with disabilities and pregnancy may help our understanding not only of disability but also of pregnancy, labor, and delivery in general. This is still an area in which we have little knowledge, despite its obvious importance. We in the disability community can be instrumental in effecting change in the treatment of women during pregnancy, delivery, and postpartum recovery by raising these questions and doing more research.

REFERENCES

Rogers, J., & Matsumura, M. (1991). *Mother to be: A guide to pregnancy and birth for women with disabilities.* New York: Demos Publishing.

Verduyn, W. (1994, May). *Obstetrical issues for women with disabilities.* Paper presented at the conference on The Health of Women with Physical Disabilities: Setting a Research Agenda for the 90s, Bethesda, MD.

chapter 9

Sexuality and a Positive Sense of Self

Harilyn Rousso

When I was growing up, I assumed that because I had a disability, cerebral palsy, I could not date, have sex, or get married. I believed the myth that people with disabilities, particularly women, were asexual. Of course I had my share of sexual fantasies. There was desire but little hope for fulfillment. I did not begin dating until my late 20s, when the mystique of able-bodied sexuality had begun to break down. I remember that awkward first kiss, when my date stopped in the middle and said, "My God, you don't even know how to kiss. How is that possible?" How indeed.

Entering the social scene later than my peers without disabilities had its consequences. I had missed opportunities for exploration, pleasure, and probably heartache. Also, I had disregarded a whole part of myself, the part longing for intimacy. In addition, my social isolation and inexperience became one more reason to feel different, out of the mainstream. I later discovered that my experiences were typical of many other young women with disabilities, particularly those with visible physical disabilities.

The few existing studies on the sexual development of women with disabilities—for example, those by Welbourne, Lifschitz, Selvin, and Green on blind women (1983); by Duffy on women with orthopedic disabilities (1981); and by Landis and Bolles on women with epilepsy, rheumatic heart disease, cerebral palsy, and a range of orthopedic disabilities (1942)—indicate that they fare less well socially and sexually during adolescence and that they have their first kiss, date, and sexual encounter later than their nondisabled peers. Their more limited social and sexual involvement results not from lack of interest, but rather, lack of opportunity. Architectural and transportation barriers as well as attitudinal barriers, such as low expectations by parents and other significant adults and rejection by potential partners, keep these young women out of the social arena.

Yet parents, professionals, and the community at large show little concern about the social exclusion of girls with disabilities. At a time when our society is preoccupied with adolescent pregnancy, sexually transmitted disease, and human immunodeficiency virus (HIV) and acquired immunodefeciency syndrome (AIDS), the sexual inactivity of any group of girls may seem more like an advantage than a problem. In fact, their lack of access to the social arena can have significant negative effects. For all young people, involvement in social and sexual activities fosters the development of crucial social skills, helps loosen family ties, and paves the way to adulthood (Blos, 1962). In addition, for adolescent women, specifically heterosexual encounters such as dating, kissing, sexual encounters, and going steady may be an important component of gender-role identity, fostering a sense of adequacy as women. The traditional measure of a woman's success in our culture is her capacity to attract and keep a man and bear his children. Adolescence is the training ground for adult roles. For young women, the flurry of heterosexual activities is perceived as a confirmation of womanhood, whereas the absence of such activities is seen as a sign of failure (Bardwick, 1971; Malmquist, 1985). Access to heterosexual activities may be significant for young lesbians as well as heterosexual women, although further research is needed. Most young women regardless of sexual orientation are likely to be influenced and limited by the narrow definitions of womanhood that prevail.

Although heterosexual interaction may be important for the gender identity of young women, there is little information on the factors that help or hinder social success during adolescence. There has been far more research on factors contributing to academic or vocational success and on strategies to reduce heterosexual involvement. The assumption that social success is the norm for most teens, as well as the view of teenage sexuality as a danger rather than as an essential component in healthy development, may contribute to the limited scientific curiosity in this area.

Some young women with disabilities are socially successful despite the barriers. Exclusion from the social scene is not an inevitable consequence of disability. What contributes to their resilience? Parental attitudes and expectations may be an important influence. Studies have documented the role of parental expectations in academic success (Malmquist, 1985) and in the development of gender role identity (Katz, 1979). Also, research on children with disabilities has demonstrated the importance of parental attitudes in the development of body image and self-esteem (Darling, 1979; Kris Study Group, Beres/Caldor Section, 1971; Lussier, 1980; Rousso, 1984).

In 1988, I conducted a pilot study to explore the impact of parental attitudes on social success for girls with disabilities (Rousso, 1988). The underlying hypothesis was that adolescent girls with disabilities would fare better in the heterosexual arena when their parents expected them to do well socially. In particular, I assumed that girls would be more socially and sexually active if parents expected them to date, marry, and have children. I also assumed that the greater their parents' ability to view them as whole women, capable of meeting traditional female role expectations of wife and mother, rather than viewing them as "defective" women, the more satisfying were their daughters' social lives. This was a retrospective study, in which 43 adult women with physical and sensory disabilities were asked to reflect on their social and sexual expectations, interests, and activities during adolescence and their parents' expectations for them at that time. A majority of these women were white, heterosexual, and single, in their 20s and 30s, with some college education. Of the 43 women, 12 acquired disabilities after adolescence. These served as a control group for the 31 women who went through adolescence with a disability.

Confirming the results of previous research, one key finding of this study was that women with preadolescence disabilities had their first date, kiss, sexual contact, experience with intercourse, and steady relationship later than those with postadolescence disabilities. Yet the two groups showed no difference in the age that they began to masturbate, suggesting that girls with preadolescence disabilities were interested in sex but had few opportunities to explore their interests beyond their own bodies. A majority of these women perceived themselves as less socially active than their peers without disabilities. Most attributed their more limited involvement in the social arena to barriers stemming from their disabilities, such as greater difficulties circulating because of architectural or transportation barriers, negative attitudes on the part of peers, or their own doubts about their desirability. Almost all of those women who experienced themselves as less socially active felt they paid a price in terms of lost opportunities and damage to their self-esteem as women. These findings suggest that for women with disabilities, as for women without disabilities, heterosexual activities may be linked to feelings of adequacy as women. In a society that devalues women with disabilities because of their disabilities, the lack of social success becomes another reason to feel unwomanly.

Although parental attitudes and expectations for the women who had disabilities during adolescence and for the control group were not significantly different, there were some important trends. Parents of girls disabled before adolescence had lower expectations for their daughters in the social and sexual arena (i.e., the capacity for dating, marriage, and childbearing) and higher expectations in the educational and vocational arena (i.e., the capacity to go to college and get a good job) compared to the control group. Although some of the women with preadolescence disabilities appreciated their parents' high career aspirations for them, enabling them to reach significant levels of academic and professional achievement, most felt that such support for their work lives was based on their parents' lack of faith in their social potential.

A related finding was that women with preadolescence disabilities were less likely to have conversations with their mothers about dating, marriage, and children than the control group, as though mothers were fearful of raising unrequitable longings or did not consider these relevant topics for their daughters. Both groups were equally likely to talk with their mothers about female anatomy and the physiology of sex, topics that might be less emotionally charged and imbued with expectations. Research suggests that mother–daughter communications about sexual issues can raise a daughter's awareness of her sexuality and help her make responsible choices (Fox, 1980). For girls with disabilities, such conversations can serve as a counterforce to the societal view that she is asexual, whereas parental silence can reinforce the stereotype (Rousso, 1981, 1984).

An in-depth study of the 31 women with preadolescence disabilities revealed further information about the link between parental expectations and social achievement. The findings suggested that this link might be more complex than originally envisioned. Positive parental expectations did facilitate heterosexual activities, but negative expectations resulted in a range of responses, depending on a variety of factors. Parents who had high social and sexual expectations for their daughters often assisted their daughters to take on the social scene; for example, by moving to a neighborhood that was accessible and hospitable to diversity, by helping the daughter develop strategies to overcome barriers, or by directly expressing confidence in the daughter's social capacity, which the young woman then internalized. Most of these daughters achieved a considerable degree of social success. One woman stated: "I was a social success in part because my mother expected me to succeed. In fact, she gave me no choice."

However, the vast majority of parents had limited social and sexual expectations for their daughters, and for many of the young women these low expectations contributed to their lack of social success. A few parents were not only pessimistic about their daughters' social future, but they viewed sexuality as potentially dangerous for them, fearful (e.g., men might abuse and abandon them). Women with such parents had not only limited social involvement but also a particularly traumatic time during adolescence, experiencing, for example, severe isolation, depression, or alcoholism.

Yet some of the women were able to succeed socially during adolescence despite their parents' pessimism. They were able to rebel against rather than to internalize negative expectations. Often these women had access to a positive counterforce, such as a supportive friend or relative who believed in them socially or a particularly accessible or nonjudgmental community that was receptive to difference among its members. Close relationships with fathers also proved helpful, even if the father was ambivalent or pessimistic about the girl's dating potential; his interest in his daughter's life was itself an affirmation. In addition, individual personality characteristics were significant, such as being spunky or willing to take risks. Women like these and their modern-day counterparts, socially active girls with disabilities of the 1990s, warrant further study to expand our understanding of resilience. Such studies will enable us to assist future generations of girls and their parents.

Given the retrospective nature of most existing research, an important question is whether girls with disabilities today find the social scene any more receptive. For example, have the women's and disability rights movements been helpful in breaking down some of the barriers they face? The National Longitudinal Transition Study of Special Education Students conducted by SRI International indicated that, 3–5 years after leaving school, young women with disabilities had the same marriage rates and significantly higher parenting rates than girls without disabilities, which might suggest that barriers to social and sexual pursuits no longer exist (Wagner, 1992). However, a closer look at the data indicates that marriage and parenting rates for these girls varied widely, depending on the nature of their disability. Although young women with learning, emotional, and speech disabilities had higher parenting rates, young women with physical disabilities, such as orthopedic disabilities, had considerably lower rates than their nondisabled peers. They were also less likely to be married or living with a partner, suggesting that, for those young women whose bodies diverge from the cultural norms of beauty and attractiveness because of physical disability, the barriers to social success remain formidable. So have there been no advances for young women with physical disabilities? Not exactly.

In the fall of 1993, I interviewed 60 ethnically diverse adolescent girls with physical, sensory, and cognitive disabilities living in the New York City area (Rousso, 1994). Through a series of individual and group conversations, we explored such topics as the advantages and disadvantages of being a woman, social and sexual knowledge and experience, body image, and sexual abuse and harassment. These young women greatly impressed me with their openness and articulateness. Their key message was that they were girls first, not just the embodiments of their disabilities, and that they were more similar to than different from girls without disabilities. "Tell them we're girls," I heard repeatedly. It is a sorry state of affairs that these young women could not take for granted widespread recognition of their womanhood.

Their report on the social scene contained both good and bad news. The bad news is that the social scene is still difficult for young women with disabilities, particularly those with visible physical disabilities. Girls with disabilities continue to be excluded, rejected, and viewed as asexual because of their failure to meet standards of physical perfection. The good news is that many young women with disabilities have become tougher and more creative in their strategies of resistance to negative assumptions about their social potential. For example, one 14-year-old explained to me, "I may be handicapped, crippled, disabled. Whatever you think I am, I'm not. I could fight." Becoming a crackerjack fighter has been her strategy for dealing with people who stare, taunt, or reject her for having an imperfect body. Or another young woman explains, "I gave up trying to prove myself a long time ago. Now I say, 'If you want to accept me this way, then you can. And if you don't, then to hell with you.'" Both young women recognized that the source of their exclusion and oppression was outside themselves. For them, the problem was societal prejudices, not their bodies or abilities.

Like all adolescent women, adolescent women with disabilities struggle with issues of body image. Body image is interconnected with self-esteem, and to some degree with social success, although it is important to avoid blaming the victim. Even a significantly positive body image cannot serve as a complete antidote to negative societal attitudes. But young women with disabilities who have good feelings about their own bodies are better able to persist in the social arena despite rejections.

Perhaps surprisingly, the body image concerns of the girls I interviewed did not exclusively focus on their disabilities. Like all teenagers, these girls were as likely as not to complain about their weight or breast size. And not all of them were displeased with their bodies. Some had a positive view of how they looked, disability and all, and were able to offer a rather sophisticated feminist critique of the myth of the perfect body. We might wonder what enables some young women to judge the judgments about their bodies rather than judging their bodies. Some girls attributed their positive attitudes to their parents' affirmation of their beauty and value or to their access to impressive women with disabilities who served as role models, but many were uncertain about what enabled them to feel good; they simply did. We need to examine and understand the experiences of such girls on their own terms, using the lens of resilience rather than deviance from able-bodied norms. The results of such research will help us promote the positive social and sexual development of all girls, disabled or not.

One disturbing finding from the interviews was the pervasiveness of sexual abuse and harassment at home and in school, confirming findings from other studies that abuse rates for women and girls with disabilities are higher than their nondisabled counterparts (Stimpson & Best, 1991; Doucette, 1986). Almost every girl had a story to tell about abuse by a parent, attendant, van driver, or school aide. And the barriers to reporting abuse were extensive, from police stations with architectural and communication barriers to officials and counselors who doubt the credibility of the survivor with a disability. "Who would want to rape *you*?" was a painfully familiar refrain. Such abuse, as well as the trauma surrounding reporting, is likely to have a significant impact on girls' social and sexual development and their sense of self. We need to study the sexual abuse issues of girls with disabilities far more rigorously and develop effective preventive strategies so that girls with disabilities do not grow up viewing abuse and harassment as the inevitable consequences of being female and disabled.

At the conclusion of my interviews, I often asked the participants if they had any questions for me. In one particular session, a group of girls responded with the questions, "How did we do? Did we tell you enough?" My response was, "It depends on who is listening." Let us make sure we are listening. The survival and success of girls with disabilities depend on it.

REFERENCES

Bardwick, J.M. (1971). *Psychology of women: A study of biocultural conflicts.* New York: Harper & Row.

Blos, P. (1962). *On adolescence.* New York: Free Press.

Darling, R. (1979). *Families against society: A study of reactions to children with birth defects.* Beverly Hills, CA: Sage Publications.

Doucette, J. (1986). *Violent acts against disabled women.* Toronto: DisAbled Women's Network.

Duffy, Y. (1981). *All things are possible.* Ann Arbor: Garvin & Associates.

Fox, G.L. (1980). The mother-adolescent daughter relationship as a sexual socialization structure. A research review. *Family Relations, 29,* 21–28.

Katz, P.A. (1979). The development of female identity. In C.B. Kopp (Ed.), *Becoming female: Perspectives on development* (pp. 3–28). New York: Plenum.

Kris Study Group, Beres/Caldor Section. (1971, September). *The influence of early childhood illness and defect on analyzability.* Paper presented at the New York Psychoanalytic Institute, New York.

Landis, C., & Bolles, M.M. (1942). *Personality and sexuality of the physically handicapped woman.* New York: Hoeber.

Lussier, A. (1980). The physical handicap and the body ego. *International Journal of Psychoanalysis, 39,* 264–272.

Malmquist, C. (1985). *Handbook of adolescence.* New York: Jason Aronson.

Rousso, H. (1981, December). Disabled people are sexual, too! *Exceptional Parent, 11*(6), 21–25.

Rousso, H. (1984). Disabled yet intact: Guidelines for working with congenitally physically disabled youngsters and their parents. *Child and Adolescent Social Work, 1*(4), 254–269.

Rousso, H. (1988). Daughters with disabilities: Defective women or minority women? In M. Fine & A. Asch, (Eds.), *Women with disabilities: Essays in psychology, culture and politics* (pp. 139–171). Philadelphia: Temple University Press.

Rousso, H. (1994). *Girls with disabilities: Strong, proud voices.* Unpublished manuscript.

Stimpson, L., & Best, M.C. (1991). *Courage above all: Sexual assault against women with disabilities.* Toronto: DisAbled Women's Network.

Wagner, M. (1992). *Being female—A secondary disability: Gender differences in the transition experiences of young people with disabilities.* Menlo Park, CA: SRI International.

Welbourne, A.S., Lifschitz, H., Selvin, H., & Green, R. (1983). A comparison of the sexual learning experiences of visually impaired and sighted women. *Journal of Visual Impairment and Blindness, 77,* 256–259.

chapter 10

Dating and Relationship Issues

Carol J. Gill

Establishing intimate relationships is a goal that is often highlighted in the stories that women with disabilities tell about our lives (Duffy, 1981; Matthews, 1983). In this respect we differ little from men with disabilities or women without disabilities. The quest for the "right" partner, after all, is unmistakably embedded in the American dream that touches us all.

Although we learn the same romantic fairy tales and absorb the same sexualized media images as everyone else, persons with disabilities come up against strong social messages that we are not suitable romantic partners. When compared with the rest of the population, persons with disabilities wait longer in life to begin dating and to experience our first voluntary sexual contact. Fewer of us marry (Fine & Asch, 1988).

Furthermore, there is evidence to suggest that heterosexual women with disabilities encounter more devaluation in the dating arena than heterosexual men with disabilities. Although not all women with disabilities want husbands, it seems significant that fewer disabled women than disabled men get married (Bowe, 1984). This discrepancy may be partially illuminated by attitude research indicating that women in general are more accepting of disability in others—including, perhaps, prospective mates—than are men (Stovall & Sedlacek, 1983). Yet women's greater comfort with disability does not necessarily ensure romance. The limited information we have about lesbians with disabilities suggests that they, too, are less likely to establish intimate partnerships than their counterparts without disabilities.

This chapter discusses some of the difficulties encountered by women with disabilities in the establishment of intimate relationships, including societal devaluation, physical and verbal abuse, family disapproval to unions, and the practical and financial burdens placed on couples by nonaccommodation and misguided public policy.

THEORIES ON ROMANTIC
DISADVANTAGES FOR WOMEN WITH DISABILITIES

Two explanations have been proffered to explain the romantic disadvantages of women with disabilities that correlate with anecdotal data. The first is an explanation based on *aesthetics*. It argues that much of a woman's value in our society rests on her conformity with narrow prescriptions of physical attractiveness. Women with visible disabilities may be judged flawed or defective as sexual partners if they cannot fit into such traditional aesthetic gender stereotypes as the perfect doll, sophisticated model, or alluring centerfold subject. The fact that women with cognitive and learning disabilities have higher rates of marriage than other disability groups lends some support to the aesthetic argument (Safilios-Rothschild, 1977; Wagner, D'Amico, Marder, Newman, & Blackorby, 1992).

The second explanation focuses on *function*. It suggests that women who depart from the traditional role and duties delineated for them by society will be viewed as incapable partners. Women with disabilities are frequently perceived as unable to care for partners and children or as unable to coordinate households, social groups, and domestic events. Consequently, they may be viewed as useless for such relationship functions as bolstering a partner's strength or ensuring comfortable refuge. Even nontraditional women may judge a woman with a disability as unsuitable for partnership by imputing to her such unliberated characteristics as fragility, immaturity, and both emotional and physical dependency (Hanna & Rogovsky, 1986; Klein, 1992).

In my contacts with other women with disabilities, I have been impressed by my peer community's flexibility and indefatigability in approaching intimacy, despite all the obstacles. I believe many of us start out with traditional ideals regarding prospective partners, having been exposed to *Cinderella* as much as our sisters without disabilities. Somewhere along the way, however, thwarted infatuations, unsatisfying unions, and impatience with solitude prod many of us to modify and enlarge our criteria for partnership. Another impetus to refining our requirements is the improved self-knowledge we acquire over time. Like other women, we find ourselves less dazzled by a partner's physique, financial status, and ability to sweep us off our feet as our values deepen and as we develop the strength to nurture ourselves. Additionally, as we mature, some of us cultivate a positive disability cultural identity and come to prefer a partner who can respect or even share this alternative worldview.

Accordingly, it is quite common for women who have experienced unsuccessful long-term relationships with traditionally ideal partners (without disabilities) to seek a partner with a disability or from a minority culture for their "second time around." I am acquainted with a substantial number of such unions in which the woman with a disability describes her relationship as strengthened and deepened in intimacy by the shared understanding and habits of disability. Countering outsiders' judgments that she has "settled" for one of her own kind by default, she describes her partner's qualities as enhanced by the disability experience.

Even those women with disabilities who have not had prior major relationships are often quite open to the idea of having a partner with a disability. Many are, therefore, devastated and angry to discover that a good number of men with disabilities are determined to find a partner without a disability (Fine & Asch, 1988). Particularly frustrating for women with disabilities is the experience of being sought out by men with disabilities for warm friendship only to be spurned romantically in favor of a woman without a disability or a woman with a minimal disability.

Some women with disabilities have compared their devaluation by men with disabilities to the intraracial romantic rejection reported by some dark-skinned African American women. They view such disabled men as seeking a majority culture partner to offset rather than mirror their own socially devalued status, much like some African American men who prefer white women. While working as a clinical psychologist in a rehabilitation hospital, I noted another dynamic: Many recently disabled single men stated an intention to find women without disabilities who could "care for" them and assist them with daily activities. For expressed practical reasons, then, they virtually eliminated women with disabilities from romantic consideration. Again, both aesthetic and functional sources of devaluation may be operative in the rejection women with disabilities say they experience from some men with disabilities.

LIKELIHOOD FOR PHYSICAL AND EMOTIONAL ABUSE

It has been widely substantiated that women with disabilities are at high risk for emotional, sexual, and physical assault (Pelka, 1993; Sobsey, 1994). We also know that women with disabilities write and speak extensively about feeling "degenderized" or treated as asexual (Hannaford, 1985). Tragically, these two sad realities can interact to decrease women's power in relationships. The need to demonstrate and prove our essential womanhood can be a dangerous pressure to enter into relationships and stay in them, regardless of abusive treatment. Because she has fewer options for meeting potential partners due to both her social devaluation and environmental access problems, a woman with a disability in a violent relationship may view it as her only opportunity to experience sexuality, marriage, childrearing, and other rites of womanhood. She may also have internalized her social devaluation to the point that she feels too inferior as a woman to merit a better relationship. Even if she decides she wants to leave a destructive relationship, however, she may not know where to find support and may literally have no place to go. The fact that she may be relying on an assaultive partner for essential personal assistance services complicates her breaking away. Not many shelters accommodate women with physical, cognitive, or sensory disabilities.

Men, too, sometimes enter and maintain relationships with women with disabilities for all the wrong reasons. Although some men are repelled by disability, some may be, instead, drawn to a partner with a disability because they feel that her perceived vulnerability will reinforce their dominance. Such men are often controlling and paternalistic, making decisions for their partner and discouraging her independence. In rare instances men may be sexually attracted to a woman's actual disability. Women with amputations and spinal cord injury quadriplegia in particular report being pursued by men who are sexually fixated on their distinctive body parts or immobility.

MARRIAGE AND DIVORCE

Although many women with disabilities find love in the hearts of men with disabilities, this scenario is not always harmonious either. In my clinical work I encountered a number of cases in which a woman with a disability became the target of the anger of a man with a disability over his social oppression and limited choices, including his perceived inability to attract a "better" partner. This form of battering can escape outside detection for years because the man is not perceived as capable of violence. Women may find themselves enmeshed for a long time in such a relationship because they empathize with the man's rage; they fear breaking a bond of loyalty or abandoning a peer with a disability whose needs are ignored by others.

Women who acquire disabilities after marriage experience high rates of separation and divorce (Hannaford, 1985). Anecdotal evidence suggests that women who acquire progressive disabilities, such as multiple sclerosis, may have a particularly difficult time finding another relationship after disability becomes apparent.

All of that said, many women with disabilities have been quite successful in finding and keeping intimate relationships. Yet those who find love often report that some of the most troubling obstacles to a lasting relationship come from outside observers, including both family and strangers. Family members may try to talk a nondisabled loved one out of dating or marrying a partner with a disability, offering gloomy predictions of future boredom or confinement. They may "reframe" love or attraction for a disabled partner as "sympathy" and issue warnings to the nondisabled individual about "throwing your life away." When all warnings go unheeded, they may shun the couple or refuse to accommodate the partner's needs in family gatherings. Two women with physical disabilities have told me, for example, that their in-laws refused to attend the wedding because they considered it a "mistake."

One problem commonly discussed by couples in which one partner has a disability is the presumption by outsiders that the partner without a disability is the "giver" in the relationship. As one woman put it, "People imagine my husband must be a saint to stay with me; actually I deserve a medal for all I do for him!" Although such perceptions may elevate the role of the partner without a disability, they serve to denigrate the legitimacy of the love relationship itself. The union is viewed as holding together because of one party's needs and the other's sense of duty rather than from a true and equal commitment. In a crisis, the family of a woman with a disability may rush to her aid and resume decision-making responsibility, disregarding her partner as an affected party. This is particularly a hazard for heterosexual couples who are unmarried and for lesbian couples.

FAMILY, SOCIAL, AND PHYSICAL BARRIERS

Couples in which both partners have disabilities, however, are hardly immune to outside disparagement. Recently a feminist disability rights activist told an audience at a rehabilitation center how weary she felt when friends and family members enthused over her marriage to a man with a disability, implying that she had finally accepted someone with limitations similar to hers. Far from "settling" for him, she said she had found him to be the strongest and most sensitive man she had ever dated. When both partners have disabilities, it can also provoke opposition to a relationship. "How will the two of you survive? How can you take care of each other?" asked a father when his daughter announced her engagement to another wheelchair user.

The negative opinions of others take a toll on some relationships. It takes an unusually grounded union to remain undaunted by a barrage of messages insisting that the relationship lacks equity or reciprocity or even love because one partner has a disability. Similarly, it is hard to weather repeated implications that the union of two people with disabilities is either doomed or entered into by default because neither could do better.

Added to these social pressures are frequently more pragmatic problems. Although laws such as the Americans with Disabilities Act (PL 101-336) are gradually ameliorating access barriers, many still persist to try the tolerance of citizens with disabilities and the persons who fall in love with us. Access questions are annoyingly unrelentless aspects of many relationships involving a disability. Does the hotel have braille signage? Will the movie theater allow sweethearts using wheelchairs to sit together? If Dad cannot walk up the stairs to Junior's school, will Mom get the day off from work to go to first-grade Open House?

Another practical problem derives from society's continuing failure to remove policy barriers to marriage and family formation for people with disabilities. Current public policies penalize persons with extensive disabilities for marrying or even living with the man or woman they love by cutting off government funding for health coverage, adaptive equipment, and personal assistance services and shifting the inflated costs of these life necessities onto the working partner. This practice effectively crushes a new relationship under the weight of instant financial hardship. As one ventilator user lamented, "The government gave me a great choice: I could live with the man I love, or I could breathe!"

Despite the financial penalties, many couples have chosen to share households under these circumstances. In describing their relationships, they often speak of relentless money worries and material sacrifice eclipsing their happiness. Without adequate funds for hiring outside help, the nondisabled or less disabled partner is often forced to perform personal assistance duties for a significantly disabled mate. This adds the strain of fatigue and role blurring to the relationship.

In effect, by withdrawing support, government marriage penalties ensure the burdened life many people incorrectly assume is inevitable when loving a person with a disability. According to personal accounts of people with disabilities, it is often their lover's fear of financial drain, constricted lifestyle, and physical dependency that prevents her or him from making the final commitment to the relationship. Consequently, women with disabilities may find themselves in long dating relationships that either never are formalized or break up as soon as they turn serious.

Another factor that appears to contribute to the tentativeness and ambivalence of persons who are attracted to partners with disabilities is the fear of stigma contagion. Partners without disabilities commonly report that strangers treat them differently because of their association with someone who has a disability. They feel others devalue them, question their motives, or conclude that they are themselves too flawed to attract someone "normal." It is difficult for many persons without a disability to cope with disability bigotry, and some find that exposing themselves to it voluntarily is too high a price to pay for love.

Social stereotypes and cultural values are powerful variables when women with disabilities try to establish intimate relationships. Sometimes a relationship progresses smoothly, with neither partner paying much attention to society's invalidation of women with disabilities as lovers, mates, and mothers. Other times, the partners struggle with conflict and uncertainties until they work out a satisfying commitment. There are many instances, however, where socially conditioned fear and doubt mix with real disability complexities to defeat relationships. Often the final breach is precipitated by a critical decision point, such as the question of marriage or bringing children into the union. An intimate relationship can proceed for a long time when it involves only two persons in undefined affiliation, only to founder when the issue of marriage or starting a family forces the partner of a woman with a disability to reassess his or her standards for a life mate. The pressure to make a decision can expose concealed ambivalence toward a disabled partner of long standing. Many women with disabilities confront the painful reality that their partners are genuinely attracted to them yet judge them as falling short of their (or society's) standards for a spouse or parent.

CONCLUSIONS

The subject of dating and relationships for women with disabilities is one of those areas for which we have many more questions than answers, more suggested tendencies than demonstrated patterns of variables. If research pursuits reflect social values, it makes sense that a society that has long ignored or disdained the gender role of women with disabilities has invested little effort in understanding their potential for love, partnership, and motherhood.

Faced with an intolerable information void, women with disabilities have been increasingly forthright in reporting our relationship experiences, our goals, our joy, and our solitariness. The generosity of those who tell their stories has helped all of us women with disabilities to become more visible as women. There remain, however, too many unknowns. Women with disabilities want facts to guide our efforts—efforts cautiously and thriftily expended by necessity. More than ever, we feel entitled to better research studies that address our dreams.

Some of our most urgently asked questions concern relationships. What makes a woman with a disability attractive to a partner? How do you navigate the obstacles from attraction to commitment? How have some women with disabilities managed to be more successful than others in relationships? What are the relationship experiences of lesbians with disabilities? What factors determine the viability of "mixed" partnerships involving individuals with and without disabilities, and how do such persons surmount the obstacles of prejudice and frustration? What factors lead to and enhance intimacy between partners with disabilities? These are the questions of women with a growing sense of entitlement to being heard and to being adequately understood. Women with disabilities are becoming as determined to find answers as we have always been determined to find love.

REFERENCES

Americans with Disabilities Act of 1990 (ADA), PL 101-336. (July 26, 1990). Title 42, U.S.C. 12101 et seq.: *U.S. Statutes at Large, 104,* 327–378.

Bowe, F. (1984). *Disabled women in America.* Washington, DC: President's Committee on Employment of the Handicapped.

Duffy, Y. (1981). . . . *All things are possible.* Ann Arbor, MI: A.J. Garvin Associates.

Fine, M., & Asch, A. (Eds.). (1988). Introduction: Beyond pedestals. *Women with disabilities: Essays in psychology, culture, and politics* (pp. 1–37). Philadelphia: Temple University Press.

Hanna, W.J., & Rogovsky, B. (1986). *Women and disability: Stigma and "the third factor."* Unpublished paper, Department of Family and Community Development, University of Maryland, College Park.

Hannaford, S. (1985). *Living outside inside.* Berkeley, CA: Canterbury Press.

Klein, B.S. (1992). We are who you are: Feminism and disability. *Ms., 3,* 70–74.

Matthews, G.F. (1983). *Voices from the shadows: Women with disabilities speak out.* Toronto: Women's Educational Press.

Pelka, F. (1993). Rape. *Mainstream, 18,* 24–33.

Safilios-Rothschild, C. (1977, February 4). Discrimination against disabled women. *International Rehabilitation Review.*

Sobsey, D. (1994). *Violence and abuse in the lives of people with disabilities: The end of silent acceptance?* Baltimore: Paul H. Brookes Publishing Co.

Stovall, C., & Sedlacek, W.E. (1983). Attitudes of male and female university students toward students with different physical disabilities. *Journal of College Student Personnel, 24,* 325–330.

Wagner, M., D'Amico, R., Marder, C., Newman, L., & Blackorby, J. (1992). *What happens next? Trends in postschool outcomes of youth with disabilities:* The second comprehensive report from the national longitudinal transition study of special education students. Washington, DC: Office of Special Education Programs, U.S. Department of Education.

chapter 11

Mothers with Physical Disabilities

Megan Kirshbaum

Since the mid-1970s, many women with disabilities have experienced a wider range of lifestyle options as a result of the move toward deinstitutionalization, community integration, and, more recently, consumer empowerment and civil rights of people with disabilities. It is expected that the passage and implementation of the Americans with Disabilities Act (PL 101-336) will result in even more rapid social change. One particularly important change has been the dramatic increase in the number of women with disabilities who are becoming parents. In *Disability and the Family*, LaPlante (1991) used data from the National Health Interview to estimate that there are at least 8.1 million families with children in which one or both parents has a disability or work limitation, representing 10.9% of all American families. In a study analyzing the 1989 Survey of Income and Program Participation, Berkeley Planning Associates (Griss & Hanson, 1990) found that 1.25 million married couples with children under 6 included at least 1 parent with a work disability, and, in over half a million cases, a disability that was considered severe.

Yet despite the sizable numbers of families that include a parent with a disability, necessary changes in social institutions that affect such families are lacking. Integrated services may be attitudinally and physically inaccessible and may present additional problems for families with disability issues. Child protective services and family courts, for instance, often lack disability-appropriate assessment, intervention guidelines, or experience. Individuals providing specialized services for adults with disabilities often lack the expertise to assist infants/children and families of parents with

This chapter was made possible by a $400,000 per year RRTC Grant #H133B30076 from the National Institute on Disability and Rehabilitation Research, U.S. Department of Education. Its contents do not necessarily represent the policy of that agency, and the reader should not assume endorsement by the federal government.

disabilities. Practical resources, such as adaptive parenting equipment, are extremely scarce. Additional research, resources, and models are desperately needed to assist the growing numbers of parents with disabilities.

This chapter outlines deficiencies in the research to date on mothers with disabilities and then describes projects addressing a number of these issues in Through the Looking Glass's Rehabilitation Research and Training Center on Families of Adults with Disabilities.

LITERATURE REVIEW

The literature on parenting by women with physical disabilities continues to be largely anecdotal or personal in nature. Research efforts are still extremely scarce. Historically, much of the research has focused on sources of potential pathology and investigated hypotheses that are negative, such as damaged body image (Olgas, 1974). Other studies may have reflected attitudinal bias in language or content, such as that represented in the following article title: "The Mutative Impact of Serious Mental and Physical Illness in a Parent on Family Life," implying psychological damage to children of parents with disabilities that is extreme enough to be analogous to mutation (Anthony, 1970). Several books have critiqued the existing literature and suggested future research directions (Haseltine, Cole, & Gray, 1993; Thurman, 1985). These studies have shown that overgeneralization and blurring of distinctions are common. Research tends not to be gender specific and not to investigate differences between parenthood for women with disabilities versus men with disabilities. Distinctions between cultural or ethnic groups have not been examined. There is also a need for research that addresses the various stages of parenthood at different stages of the child's development (e.g., infancy, preschool-age, school-age, adolescent, and adult children). Developmental and relationship issues likewise need to be explored. Longitudinal research and the use of comparison group parents without disabilities and their children would be especially helpful.

Disability situations require differentiation. Cognitive or psychiatric components of disabilities need to be identified and specified when they are present (e.g., in research populations with physical disabilities). It is also important to distinguish recent from long-term disabilities and progressive or changing disabilities from ones that are relatively stable. A mother's grieving over recent disability losses can profoundly affect the formation of her relationship with a baby. A family that deals with a parent's progression to severe disability obviously endures particular ongoing coping difficulties, losses, and family disequilibriums that affect parents and children in a way that is very different from a mother who has had a stable disability since birth. There are also particular issues that may affect women who were disabled from birth. What is the impact of disability-related trauma on the early attachment of a girl with disabilities with her own parents and consequently on her model of a mother/infant relationship? What is the impact of being socialized in such a way that suggests that sexuality and parenting were meant for others, for people without disabilities? It is important not to blur the distinctions in timing of disability onset in relation to parenting. Did the woman have the disability before having a child? If so, for how long? How secure and well established are her coping skills, and can she extrapolate from these in the new realm of parenting? At the outset of parenthood, even the most competent woman can be shaken in her self-esteem and sense of competence. Hospitalization during birth sometimes triggers memories of disability-related trauma. One should consider whether the passage of time since the trauma is a factor.

In our clinical work and research with hundreds of such families at Through the Looking Glass over the past 13 years, we have concluded that blurred distinctions can cause us to reach inappropriate conclusions about the capability of mothers with disabilities to parent or the impact of the mother's disability on the children. For instance, one needs to isolate factors associated with the disability from the psychosocial ones. It is especially important to clearly identify women who have childhood histories of trauma and abuse and/or out of home placement with essentially no positive experience of parenting or models for secure attachment. History of this nature is frequently ignored in the literature, although it may profoundly affect a woman's capacity to parent. She may be identified solely as having a physical disability, when she actually has a dual diagnosis because of a traumatic history. If this is not recognized, her difficulties may be blamed solely on her physical disability—resulting in inappropriate generalizations about the impact of physical disability on parenting.

It is also crucial to consider the family and systems context for the mother with the disability. Varied family constellations (e.g., single mothers, couples where one partner has a disability, couples where both partners have disabilities, and intergenerational households) need to be evaluated differentially. The degree of isolation, lack of support, or undermining, as well as additional sources of stress, such as financial or sexual exploitation, abuse, and violence, needs to be determined. An example of a salient family issue is the issue of complementarity in a couple (e.g., role division where the partner with a disability underfunctions and the partner without the disability overfunctions). An increase in parental functioning by a mother with a disability, as a result of the introduction of assistive parenting equipment, may result in a difficult period of adjustment within the family system (Kirshbaum, 1995a). The transition to motherhood can also bring to the surface intergenerational conflict with grandparents who frequently question the parental ability of even the most independent and high-functioning women with disabilities (Kirshbaum, 1995b). The systems context also includes the presence or absence of appropriate social services. Negative and inappropriate services can contribute to families' problems. It is also important to consider the impact of poverty and the lack of public funding to support mothering (e.g., exclusion of in-home baby care assistance from personal assistance services, lack of funding for adaptive parenting equipment). What type of outcomes will result from adequate support, appropriate services, and an accessible environment? Despite these caveats, the field is currently in a groundbreaking, hypothesis-generating stage of research regarding mothers with disabilities and their children. Researchers will need to overcome many obstacles and utilize a variety of research approaches to address these recommendations. For instance, locally based, in-depth studies may still be faced with small and diverse populations of mothers with disabilities. This challenges the goal of clearer differentiation in studies.

RESEARCH AT THROUGH THE LOOKING GLASS

To address the need for diverse research approaches regarding parenting by persons with disabilities, the Rehabilitation Research and Training Center (RRTC) on Families of Adults with Disabilities at Through the Looking Glass is undertaking research projects that balance large quantitative national surveys with more in-depth locally focused interviewing studies, observational analyses, and longitudinal follow-up approaches. Many of the projects have practical components, and the RRTC includes a national clearinghouse for parents with disabilities, a consultation service, a newsletter, and training modules. From 1993 to 1997, the Center will include the following projects, many of which will involve mothers with disabilities:

1. Needs assessment: This project will assess the incidence and prevalence of different subpopulations of families with parents who have varying kinds of disabilities. It will also assess the types of supports that are needed by these adults and their families and the degree to which these needs are currently being met by social service systems (both integrated as well as disability-oriented services).
2. Family case studies: This project will conduct an in-depth study of families in which at least one parent has a significant disability. Researchers will select samples of families of diverse ethnic and disability backgrounds who perceive themselves as having generally positive parenting experiences. As such, this study will document financial and support strategies in successful family formation.
3. State of the nation: This project will identify, analyze, and address policy barriers to successful family life for parents with disabilities

with respect to personal assistance services, child care, and other key social service programs. The study will consider both federal and state policies to develop recommendations for policy design, change, and implementation that will enhance the participation of parents with disabilities.

4. Parents with deafness: This project will adopt and apply a Through the Looking Glass model of early intervention that integrates infant mental health work, peer teaching, and social support to families in which one or more parents is deaf. Researchers will document the effectiveness of the program, describe adaptations necessary for a deaf parented family, and develop training materials.

5. Mothers with visual disabilities: This interviewing project will explore the psychological adjustment of new mothers with visual impairments and the access to social support and resources during parenthood for women in this group.

6. A longitudinal study of children of parents with physical disabilities: This project examines the interactions between parents with physical disabilities and their children at two developmental points. Children who participated in earlier videotape analysis research during infancy (birth–3 years) will be followed during the latency period (8–10 years). Researchers will identify and develop training materials about factors that promote positive child outcomes as well as factors that increase the risk of behavior problems or psychological difficulties for children in latency.

7. Pregnancy and birthing: Using ethnographic interviewing, this project will identify problems and issues described by women with physical disabilities during pregnancy, labor and delivery, and the early postpartum period. A training module will be designed to address such problems and issues.

8. Family support model: This project is an evaluated clinical model that will respond to the problems and needs of family members of adults experiencing acute-onset or exacerbation of disabling conditions.

9. Determining the cost of living for adults with disabilities: This project will determine what a living wage should be for individuals with several different types of significant disabilities in order for them to support themselves and their families.

10. Increasing access to Head Start for parents with disabilities: This project will explore the degree to which parents with disabilities have access to Head Start for their children and how the expansion of Head Start could be shaped to improve access.

11. Assistive technology and parenting: This multifaceted research and demonstration project will include parenting equipment development

and dissemination as well as a national quantitative survey and a local qualitative study regarding the impact of assistive technology on the transition to parenthood in couples where one or both partners has a physical disability.

Our own research focus has resulted from clinical and fieldwork experience with hundreds of parenting families affected by all categories of disability: physical, medical, cognitive, sensory, and psychiatric. We invite others to derive their hypotheses and directions from their disability communities. Often dismissed, the anecdotal and personal literature could be a rich source of research ideas. Another path to cultural understanding would be initial ethnographic interviewing research. The Co-Director of Training of Through the Looking Glass's RRTC, Paul Preston, an adult child of deaf parents, has just published *Mother Father Deaf: Living Between Sound and Silence*, for which he interviewed 150 adult children of deaf parents (Preston, 1994). It is a particularly resonant book, full of research issues that are relevant to several disciplines and could be pursued through a variety of methodologies.

Observational Studies

At Through the Looking Glass we have found observational studies, using videotape analyses of mother/infant interaction, to be particularly compelling. These projects have generated many research hypotheses and informed intervention, professional training, and resource development. From 1985 to 1988, Through the Looking Glass documented how mothers with different physical disabilities dealt with basic baby care and how, without any special services or equipment, they and their babies coped with disability obstacles, from birth to toddlerhood (Kirshbaum, 1988). We analyzed how the reciprocal adaptation developed over time. One particularly engaging issue that emerged from this tape was the early adaptation often exhibited by the babies (illustrated in videotapes of babies as young as 1 month of age) and how the mothers facilitated this adaptation. In the course of performing this study, we learned a great deal about how to help other mothers with disabilities who are particularly stressed, less autonomous, or less ingenious in their problem-solving skills.

The documented ingenuity of the mothers with physical disabilities provided a foundation for Through the Looking Glass's current Field-Initiated Research Project, in which we are developing adaptive equipment to assist parents with physical disabilities to care for their babies and using videotape analysis to evaluate the impact of this equipment. Other issues that emerged from the original research are being pursued in the current RRTC. These include teamwork between parents and mothers and attendants (and how this compares with role division in parents without disabilities), the roots of behavior management during early infant care, and a longitudinal follow-up of the 11 families with infants who participated in the 1985–1988 project. Looking closely at interaction between mothers with disabilities and their babies calls attention to interactional or intervention issues for all parents and babies. The video material has been very helpful to new parents and for sensitizing professionals and training clinicians and has educated the public through national media. The research has also affected outcomes of court hearings involving child protective services or custody disputes (Mathews, 1992).

RESEARCH ON SERVICE AND EQUIPMENT NEEDS

There are currently even more critical social needs that require attention. For several years, Through the Looking Glass has been receiving approximately 1,000 calls annually from all over the country from mothers with disabilities who are desperate to obtain knowledgeable local assessments and services. These mothers urgently need adaptive parenting equipment and lack accessible housing that can accommodate children. Mothers may be facing removal of the baby. The rapidly growing population of parents with disabilities and the critical lack of accessible and appropriate local resources and services in most parts of the country underscore the potentially vulnerable situation faced by mothers with disabilities.

The following example is a dramatic illustration of one of the many social problems that can confront the most vulnerable mothers with disabilities. The Department of Social Services contacted us about a teenage African American mother who lived in a particularly hazardous Oakland housing project with her alcoholic and abusive mother. She had been given drugs by family and friends who served as attendants. Her baby had been removed at birth because a test had indicated illegal drug use during late pregnancy. This teenage mother had quadriplegia from spinal cord injury and was said to be uncooperative with substance abuse treatment. Her baby was already 6 months old when we became involved. We discovered that the mother had been referred to only two different programs, both of which were inaccessible to her wheelchair and had refused to deal with her catheter in order to do urinalyses. She had been instructed to travel to these programs on the bus, even though bus access in her town was minimal. The social worker had been unaware of disability transportation systems or of the few disability-sensitive substance abuse programs that were available. The social worker described the mother as forming no relationship to her baby during the weekly visitations. The mother had been provided no assistance since the baby had been born to make it possible for her to hold or care for her baby in any way. As a result, the baby's grandmother performed the care or left the baby in a playpen during the visits. On the first visit, the Through the Looking Glass clinician saw a depressed mother who indeed appeared estranged from and disinterested in her baby. The first visit focused on viewing videotapes of parents with disabilities, as requested by the mother. At the end of the visit, the mother asked for assistance in holding and feeding her baby. On the second visit, with the use of simple pillows and frontpacks, the mother was able to hold and feed her baby for the first time since her birth. She tenderly nuzzled and murmured to her baby, caressing her, as one greets a baby immediately after birthing (Kirshbaum, 1995a).

Early intervention services and appropriate resources can reduce, alleviate, or even prevent many problems. The impact of adaptive parenting equipment can be profound. For example, a mother with a significant disability has received services from Through the Looking Glass since her premature baby was sent home from neonatal intensive care. During home visits, we developed the adaptive parenting equipment she needed to provide totally independent care of her baby. A baby care tray attached to her motorized wheelchair kept the vulnerable baby close and minimized the stress of positional changes. Adaptations to crib, highchair, bottles, diapers, and changing table, as well as harness, safety gates, and an elevated play center, maximized the capability of the mother. Technology provision and adaptive problem solving by an occupational therapist were offered, in addition to infant mental health services, both provided through home visits. Although this mother had a high-risk childhood history of out-of-home placement, the relationship between parent and child continues to flourish (Kirshbaum, 1995a). Despite the positive impact of this project, we are frustrated by the many calls from parents with disabilities who desperately want and need our actual equipment (not merely information regarding it). However, most of these families are far beyond the geographical accessibility of our services. Additional research efforts need to focus on developing more customized adaptive parenting equipment and on moving current prototypes to the market. The legal issues regarding sharing equipment specifications need to be addressed for dissemination to be effective.

Research on Abuse and Exploitation

During the course of our extensive fieldwork over the past 13 years, another critical issue has become apparent: The functioning of a disproportionate number of mothers with disabilities is being undermined by abuse, violence, and exploitation. The problem is particularly dramatic in the lives of women labeled as developmentally disabled. In a Through the Looking Glass parenting intervention project serving 64 mothers with cognitive disabilities, many experienced abuse, neglect, violence, and sexual and/or financial exploitation. A growing body of literature substantiates our clinical observations (Nosek et al., 1994; Sobsey, 1994). Although the methodological quality of studies varies and the statistical estimates differ, it is already clear that this is an urgent problem. We therefore recommend research that targets social change regarding abuse and violence in the lives of women (and mothers) with disabilities. For instance, studies are needed on integrated and disability systems attention to these issues (e.g., current access of abuse/violence programs to women with disabilities, evaluation of training to enhance access, evaluation of model prevention programs that specialize in disability issues).

Because of the urgency of the social situation at this point, research should provide practical outcomes and resources for mothers with disabilities and their children. Such research can focus on disseminating information and training or establishing and evaluating the effectiveness of assessment and service models. Even the most abstract studies could be required to incorporate practical products or services. Statistical data could be obtained by including women with disabilities in large integrated studies and surveys, calling attention to their issues in the process. Research efforts need to reflect the dynamic changes in the lives of women with disabilities and have utility for pioneering experiences of mothers with disabilities.

CONCLUSIONS

This chapter has emphasized the gap between the growing numbers of mothers with disabilities and the lack of appropriate research and practical resources for these mothers and their families. Through the Looking Glass's work has been offered to illustrate research directions based on clinical, fieldwork, and disability community experience. Because of the critical lack of resources for mothers with disabilities, current research is encouraged that clearly contributes to improvements in the quality of family life.

REFERENCES

Americans with Disabilities Act of 1990 (ADA), PL 101-336. (July 26, 1990). Title 42, U.S.C. 12101 et seq.: *U.S. Statutes at Large, 104*, 327–378.

Anthony, E. (1970). The mutative impact of serious mental and physical illness in a parent on family life. In E. Anthony & C. Koupernick (Eds.), *The child in his family* (pp. 131–163). New York: John Wiley & Sons.

Griss, R., & Hanson, S.P. (1990). *Accessibility, adequacy, and affordability of health insurance for persons with disabilities and chronic illness*. Oakland, CA: Berkeley Planning Associates.

Haseltine, F.B., Cole, S.S., & Gray, D.B. (Eds.). (1993). *Reproductive issues for persons with physical disabilities*. Baltimore: Paul H. Brookes Publishing Co.

Kirshbaum, M. (1988). Parents with physical disabilities and their babies. *Zero to Three, 8*, 8–15.

Kirshbaum, M. (1995a). Serving families with disability issues: Through the Looking Glass. *Marriage and Family Review, 21*(1/2), 9–28.

Kirshbaum, M. (1995b). Family context and disability culture reframing: Through the Looking Glass. *Family Psychologist, 10*(4), 8–12.

LaPlante, M. (1991). *Disability and the family.* San Francisco: Institute for Health and Aging.

Mathews, J. (1992). *A mother's touch: The Tiffany Callo story.* New York: Henry Holt and Company.

Nosek, M.A., Howland, C.A., Young, M.E., Georgiou, D., Rintala, D.H., Foley, C.C., Bennett, J.L., & Smith, Q. (1994). Wellness models and sexuality among women with physical disabilities. *Journal of Applied Rehabilitation Counseling, 25,* 50–58.

Olgas, M. (1974). The relationship between parents' health status and body-image of their children. *Nursing Research, 23,* 310–324.

Preston, P. (1994). *Mother father deaf: Living between sound and silence.* Cambridge, MA: Harvard University Press.

Sobsey, D. (1994). *Violence and abuse in the lives of people with disabilities: The end of silent acceptance?* Baltimore: Paul H. Brookes Publishing Co.

Thurman, S.K. (1985). *Children of handicapped parents: Research and clinical perspectives.* New York: Academic Press.

chapter 12

Disabled Lesbians
Challenging Monocultural Constructs

Corbett Joan O'Toole

Disabled women and disabled lesbians face health care barriers that are both similar and significantly different. Both groups encounter limited access to health care, health care providers who lack even basic information about their health care needs, health care providers who refuse to provide service, prejudice, and lack of economic power to negotiate for better health care (O'Toole & Bregante, 1992; Stevens, 1994). This chapter focuses on disabled lesbians, with the underlying premise that the situation for disabled lesbians is significantly different from that of heterosexual disabled women. There is almost no research on disabled lesbians as a separate and distinct population. However, within the self-reporting literature of disabled women, there is substantial discussion by disabled lesbians of their specific experiences (Browne, Connors, & Stern, 1985; Hevey, 1992; *off our backs,* 1981).

Researchers have shown that when a population deviates from a Caucasian, European-American nondisabled male norm, their vulnerability is compounded (Cochran & Mays, 1988; Denenberg, 1992; Stevens, 1994). As Stevens (1994) points out,

This chapter is based on previous research done by Jennifer Luna Bregante and Corbett Joan O'Toole. The author wishes to thank Carol Gill, Ph.D., for her insightful comments and editorial assistance—as always, she provided invaluable mentoring; the Lyon-Martin Women's Health Services in San Francisco, pioneers in lesbian health, for their commitment to the inclusion of women with disabilities and for their editing of and research assistance with the preparation of this chapter; and Jennifer Luna Bregante, M.A., who provides daily support, reviews all my work, and without whom none of it would ever be completed.

The author is in agreement with Waxman (Chapter 15), who states, "This author uses *disability-first* language rather than the rehabilitation-oriented *people-first* language. This use of language results from the author's view of disability as a social identity, much like being African American. . . . Hence, . . . the term *disabled* is used to denote a prideful identity." For me it reflects my membership in a defined social and cultural community that has its own norms, humor, history, and culture.

[lesbians'] sense of unprotectedness seemed to be added to in geometric proportion with each identity that did not match the male, heterosexual, Euro-American, middle-class, able-bodied norm. From their perspective, exposure to adversity in health care was doubled and redoubled not only because they were lesbian, but because they were women, persons of color, low-income earners, and/or persons who suffered from chronic health conditions. (p. 224)

Even though 80% of the women in one study were generally disclosed as lesbian (i.e., "out" with friends, family, and co-workers), in health care contexts they described being more careful about information sharing. This excerpt (Stevens, 1994) describes a commonly reported consequence of disclosing information:

Some providers can't deal with finding out you are a lesbian. Like, the last physician I went to, when he asked me did I use birth control. I said I was a lesbian and his head almost spun around. He had to take a few minutes to regain his composure so that he could continue to talk to me. And in his list of questions, he had to keep hesitating because they were no longer applicable. But he didn't have a new set of questions to ask that made sense for a lesbian's health. So he did a lot of uhms and ahs. I don't really know if I got what I needed as far as the physical exam goes because he couldn't get back on track. (p. 221)

This chapter explores the issues that disabled lesbians pose within the disabled women's community. The focus is on women who are clear about their lesbian identity, live openly as lesbians, and have a permanent disability. (It is outside the scope of this chapter to discuss why women become lesbians, women who have sexual experiences with women but are not identified as lesbians, and the moral legitimacy of being a lesbian.) The need for discussion of health issues is pressing; after all, lesbians and gay men represent 10% of any population (Stevens, 1994). My favorite interpretation of this statistic is as follows:

According to Kirk and Madsen, "Many, if not most, straights would undoubtedly find it hard to believe . . . that there are nearly as many gays as blacks in America today, half again as many as Hispanics, and more than three times as many as Jews. The practice of homosexuality may be a more commonplace activity in America than, say, bowling (6 percent), jogging (7 percent), golfing (5 percent), hunting (6 percent), reading drug store romance novels (9 percent) or ballroom dancing (2 percent). (Simon, 1991, p. 11)

CULTURAL INVISIBILITY

Homophobia creates many obstacles that may not be visible to people who are sensitive only to issues of disability discrimination. As Gates (1993) says,

Prejudices don't exist in the abstract; they come with distinctive and distinguishing historical peculiarities. In short, they have content as well as form. Underplaying the differences blinds us to the signature traits of other forms of social hatred. Indeed, in judging other prejudices by the one you know best you may fail to recognize those other prejudices as prejudices. (p. 2)

These obstacles and prejudices include, for lesbians who have "come out," loss of employment, loss of housing, loss of family, and even the possibility of losing their children.

Given these risks, heterosexuals often question whether it is necessary for lesbians to announce their sexual orientation. They often suggest, with good intentions, that telling people puts a lesbian at risk—of ostracization, abandonment, rejection, and even violence. Why, they ask, couldn't she just not tell people that she is a lesbian? But such a question is a form of discrimination—they would never think this an appropriate question to a heterosexual. It is also important to note that all women, not only lesbians, are the target of homophobia. As Minkowitz (1994) reminds us,

[M]en's fear is hardly limited to the prospect that all women will be recruited into lesbianism. It encompasses the more present danger that women will become politically independent. Whether or not women opt to have sex with other women, gay rights are a prerequisite for their freedom; otherwise, homophobia can be used against any woman who declares her autonomy—or any man who refuses to enforce male power. (p. 23)

Being culturally invisible, as disabled lesbians usually are, has serious consequences—not the least of which is an almost total lack of access to any existing health services, be they geared to the general population, to the disabled community, to women, or even to disabled women specifically.

PRESUMPTION OF ASEXUALITY

Discussing sexuality-related issues is important for disabled lesbians because it is their sexual preference that removes them from the heterosexual mainstream. Disabled lesbians are presumed to be asexual. Much of the writing by disabled women attempts to invalidate this stereotype (Browne, Connors, & Stern, 1985; Luczak, 1993).

Researchers must acknowledge that disabled women are capable of deciding their own sexual orientation. This assumption is remarkably absent from many discussions of disability and sexuality. Far too often, same-sex relationships are seen as a result of a lack of opportunity for opposite sex interaction. As Fine and Asch (1988) point out,

Exempted from the "male" productive role and the "female" nurturing one, having the glory of neither, disabled women are arguably doubly oppressed—or, perhaps, "freer" to be nontraditional. Should they pursue what has been thought nontraditional, however, the decision to work, to be a single mother, to be involved in a lesbian relationship, or to enter politics may be regarded as a default rather than a preference. (p. 13)

There is tremendous resistance to the fact that not all disabled women are heterosexual. For example, the attempts to control reproduction, sometimes to the point of sterilization, and the emphasis to teach disabled women to say no to sexuality reflect nondisabled people's discomfort with disabled women's emerging independence, but also an assumption of heterosexuality (O'Toole & Bregante, 1992).

When a disabled lesbian sees a health care worker, the worker usually knows that she is disabled but is ignorant of her sexual identity. Disabled women report that the health care provider rarely asks about her sexual needs (see opening discussion of Section II). If any questions are asked, they invariably focus on birth control. Heterosexual disabled women report that even their needs for information or help are not met, because the health care worker never knows the implications of how her disability interacts with birth control methods (O'Toole & Bregante, 1992).

Disabled lesbians have much to lose by being open with homophobic workers. Indeed, many workers hold negative attitudes about both disabled people and lesbians (Stevens, 1994). As Barbara Faye Waxman (1991) reminds us,

> By disabled people stepping out of place, by asserting their very presence and refusal to take their presence elsewhere, by proclaiming that they are equal to and deserve the same rights as those of the majority, they become targets for more overt acts of hate violence. (p. 18)

However, as long as society denies any socially viable role to disabled women, there can be no room for the sexually active disabled woman. Like other lesbians, disabled lesbians have the responsibility and pressure to break the silence about sexual preference.

FAMILY

A significant commonality between disabled people and lesbians is that both grow up with the absence of important role models within their families. It is rare for there to be either disabled adults or gay or lesbian adults in the childhood homes of disabled lesbians. This is a major difference between disabled people, lesbians, and other minority groups. In a poignant statement, Gates (1993) points out, "What makes the closet so crowded is that gays are, as a rule, still socialized—usually by their nearest and dearest—into shame" (p. 44).

Birth families are often unable to assist a disabled lesbian with her struggle against ableism and homophobia. Families know that the lesbian is giving up all the privileges of heterosexuality, often including acceptance by her family (C. Thompson, 1992). Although relationships with some family members may remain positive, token support does not equal acceptance. Pearlman (1990) sought out mothers who were publicly supportive of their lesbian daughters. Yet they continued to struggle with unresolved feelings toward homosexuality. They had feelings of loss and concern over discrimination and a self-consciousness about the reality of their being mothers of lesbian daughters, and they often wished their daughters were heterosexual.

When people cannot confide in, or depend on, their family to assist them with ongoing cultural oppression, they become isolated and at risk. To survive, many lesbians have developed extensive personal and resource networks. Within the lesbian and gay communities, these are referred to as "chosen family." For many lesbians and gay men, this chosen family becomes their primary, and sometimes sole, support (Stevens, 1994). Many members of the disabled community also report that they create similar support structures (O'Toole & Bregante, 1993a).

Chosen family members are people who have first-hand experience with oppression, who have developed successful survival strategies, and who have networks to combat systematic oppression. Choosing to make a family can be complicated for disabled lesbians. They are dealing with double stereotypes that do not portray them as possible partners or parents (O'Toole & Bregante, 1993b).

If the majority of lesbians and disabled people are creating nontraditional family structures, this suggests that a reexamination of the presumptions of a heterosexual definition of family is necessary. Richard Simon (1991) wrote about his new contact with gay and lesbian families when his publication, *The Family Therapy Networker,* devoted an issue to gay men and lesbians:

> Over the past couple of months, I've come face to face with family constellations that didn't match anything in my own experience—gay men bringing up adopted children together, lesbians living as spouses while pretending to their children they are 'just friends,' gay widows afraid to tell anyone that they're in mourning. Certainly, I was generally aware of the range of family arrangements gays and lesbians create for themselves, but as I learned more about them, I was startled by my own naivete and how alien they seemed to me. My reaction is not unusual. (p. 2)

Despite the importance of the chosen family in a lesbian's life, her choice of family is usually not honored. If she is disabled, the lesbian's right to choose her family can be made dependent on her type of disability combined with the attitudes of a heterosexist and ableist legal system, as the case of Sharon Kowalski graphically demonstrates (Thompson & Andrzejewski, 1988).

Sharon Kowalski and Karen Thompson lived together as lovers for 4 years, owned a home, and considered each other as permanent partners. At this time they were both nondisabled. They were not "out" as lesbians to their families, nor did they have any paperwork—medical or legal—identifying them as partners. Sharon was hit by a drunk driver. She was permanently and severely disabled, requiring extensive hospitalization.

Her birth family presumed themselves to be Sharon's only family. Karen was systematically denied any role in Sharon's recovery. Unfortunately, Karen Thompson's experience is familiar to disabled lesbians (Anstett, Kiernan, & Brown, 1987; Bogle & Shaul, 1981; Fine & Asch, 1988). Karen came to realize that the stigma of disability and the myth of asexuality encompass her and her partner (Thompson & Andrzejewski, 1988).

Families of disabled lesbians are at risk of discrimination. Although lesbians marry and have children, their choices are not backed up legally. This can create serious problems for these women during a medical crisis. A disabled lesbian's chosen family and her birth family may not agree on treatment or placement options (O'Toole & Bregante, 1993). One particular impact of discrimination and violence against lesbians is the intentional disruption of the family. Lesbians face powerful discrimination in the courts whenever their right to parent is challenged. Each week there is a news report of another lesbian who has lost custody of her child solely because she is a lesbian.

Because this type of severe discrimination is also used against disabled mothers, the potential for legal problems for disabled lesbian mothers is enormous. This discrimination has health care consequences: If a disabled lesbian cannot be comfortable and honest with her health care worker, if important information about medical issues is not available, if her family is ignored and marginalized, she will not receive appropriate health care.

MULTICULTURAL LIVES

All disabled lesbians live multicultural lives. They usually have a primary and secondary affiliation (e.g., African American, disabled). The ways that these associations intersect depend on the life experiences of each disabled lesbian. While they have the advantages of four sets of communities, they also face four distinct sets of discrimination: homophobia, sexism, ableism, racism. As one disabled lesbian said (Stevens, 1994),

> I cannot separate my being Asian Pacific, from my being lesbian, from my being a woman who has a chronic illness. But if I look to the health care system, I'm supposed to drop one or all of these identities, depending on whose threshold I cross. (p. 227)

Yet there is little discussion within the disabled and women's communities on the problems facing disabled lesbians. As Fine and Asch (1988) point out, "To date almost all research on disabled men and women seems to simply assume the irrelevance of gender, race, ethnicity, sexual orientation, or social class. Having a disability presumably eclipses these dimensions of social experience" (p. 3). Although the experience of disability may have universality when discussing specific physical or cognitive functions, any attempt to extend its analysis to encompass disabled women across diverse age, race, and class boundaries merely obscures the specific ways that disability combines with other societal barriers to create new constructs. As the gay and lesbian movements increase their visibility, they require other movements to reexamine their premises. As Henry Louis Gates, Jr., said, "[T]he reason the national conversation on [black vs. gay oppression] has reached an impasse isn't that there's simply no comparison; it's that there's no *simple* comparison" (Gates, 1993).

Karen Thompson met with resistance from the disabled community when she asked for help for her newly disabled lover, Sharon Kowalski: "[I had] trouble getting disability groups to be willing to put their names behind the issue because they saw it as a gay rights issue. One of the leaders in the disability rights community told me, "We think Sharon's rights are being violated, but we can't afford to get involved in a gay rights issue" (K. Thompson, 1992). The lack of awareness of disabled lesbians as multicultural prompted one disabled lesbian writer to title her article, "What's It Like to Be Blind? (And please keep all that other stuff quiet. We can only deal with one minority at a time.)" (Myers, 1989–1990).

REGARD, a Canadian self-advocacy organization for disabled lesbians and gay men, articulates the need for their organization to exist:

> REGARD (campaigning organisation of disabled Lesbians and Gays) was established as a result of two processes. Rampant heterosexism in the disability movement where the lives of disabled Lesbians and Gays were invisible. Therefore no accountability or representation. Ignorance of issues resulted in bad practices including offensive terminology and negative images. To admit sexual expression of disabled people by itself challenges myths thus to embrace the sexuality of disabled Lesbians and Gays is too threatening for many disability organisations.
>
> Simultaneously the multiple oppression of disabled Lesbians and Gays was resulting in isolation and distress. Individuals' lives were being compartmentalized. At the same time valuable experience gained in other liberation struggles was being lost to the disability movement. (Gillespie-Sells, 1992, p. 111)

Solving the health care needs of disabled women will not solve the health care needs of disabled lesbians any more than the existing health clinics for nondisabled women solve the health care challenges of disabled women. The disabled, the women's, and the lesbian communities face many similar issues, differing in degree but not nature. Yet the myth that all women are equally affected by sex discrimination prevents these communities from exploring the specific ways that disabled women and disabled lesbians are affected (Women and Disability Awareness Project, 1989). These myths combine with societal invisibility to create a serious lack of access to nondisabled (Chipouras, 1981) and disabled women's services for disabled lesbians.

PROBLEMS FOR DISABLED LESBIANS IN HEALTH CARE

Disabled lesbians face three significant problems in obtaining health care:

1. There is no effort to document the experiences or problems of disabled lesbians.
2. Disabled lesbians have negative experiences with health care.
3. There are negative repercussions when disabled lesbians "come out" with health care providers.

In many cases, these three problems combine to form a circular argument: If there is nothing in the literature about disabled lesbians, then there is no need to collect any information about them. If there were a problem, lesbians would tell us. But because confronting homophobic systems is dangerous to the health of disabled lesbians, they are unlikely to take the lead.

Information Is Not Collected

Investigating the problems of disabled lesbians is difficult because of limited information. Researchers tend to see both disability and homosexuality as monocultural constructs, with neither disabled people (Davis, 1991) nor lesbians (O'Toole & Bregante, 1992) having positive societal value. Although medicine in recent years has paid increasing attention to the medical concerns of American gay men, less attention has been focused on the health issues of bisexual and lesbian women (Cochran & Mays, 1988). Accurate information about lesbians has been difficult to obtain; much of the available information has been extrapolated from studies of homosexual men, rarely addressing critical issues of lesbians (Saunders et al., 1988). Even less is known about the lives of black lesbians (Cochran & Mays, 1988).

Huge gaps exist in the public's and the medical establishment's understanding of lesbian culture and lifestyle that make it difficult to confront lesbian invisibility (Denenberg, 1992). Lesbians live in all communities; are diverse in race, ethnicity, class, and political outlook; and are not easily distinguished in health care settings (Denenberg, 1992). When lesbian and gay communities have increased their visibility in mainstream culture, the effects are not always positive. Schwanberg (1990) found that the increased attention on homosexuals resulted in increasingly negative articles in professional journals. Fine and Asch (1988) documented that two decades of work by disabled women in the women's movement did not facilitate either increased access or acceptance.

When the acquired immunodeficiency syndrome (AIDS) epidemic first received wide attention in both professional and popular literature (1983–1987), more negative images of homosexuality were evident. Much of the attention of nursing and general medicine was directed toward examining biophysical aspects of AIDS. Writers equated AIDS with stigma, gay men, and an increase in negative attitudes toward homosexuality in general (Schwanberg, 1990). Writers who addressed homosexuality by examining the complexity of human behavior, affective preference, and gender identity were more positive or neutral about gays than were writers from general medicine and nursing who dealt with issues about the AIDS epidemic (Schwanberg, 1990).

A survey of health care literature found that in a few of the articles ($n = 59$) that mentioned gay men and lesbians, the majority of them (61%) reflected negative attitudes and images (Warren, 1993). When lesbians are not being subsumed under articles about gayness that focus on gay men, they are seen relative to heterosexual women and found lacking (Magee & Miller, 1992).

An extensive literature search consistently offered only one story of a disabled lesbian—that of Sharon Kowalski and her lover Karen Thompson. Otherwise, the lives and accomplishments of disabled lesbians are completely invisible.

The problem is widespread because, as Warren (1993) states:

> Responsibility also lies with researchers who need to ask questions concerning all female sexual activity, institutions that often refuse to sponsor such research, and journals that judge articles on the topic too controversial or insignificant to publish. (p. 15)

Health Care Experiences

Health care providers have barely begun to recognize the important health care needs of nondisabled heterosexual women. A variety of elements and experiences help to determine lesbians' health status and relationship to the health care system, including their financial standing, work life, sexuality, reproductive life, and support systems (Denenberg, 1992).

When lesbians' health care needs are the same as those of other women for screening, prevention, treatment of illness, education and crisis intervention, lesbians' needs are less well met than those of heterosexuals. Less than a handful of lesbian health clinics exist (Denenberg, 1992). And when lesbians present unique problems and concerns, the medical system generally cannot or will not meet them (Denenberg, 1992). Homophobia, in the form of heterosexual presumption, is a common experience shared by all lesbians entering the health system. It is true, however, that black lesbians may be more heterosexually active than white lesbians (Cochran & Mays, 1988). Heterosexual behaviors may conceivably predispose them to a different pattern of gynecological problems than those reported by white lesbians (Cochran & Mays, 1988).

One common negative experience is that, although reproduction is the defined social role for females, most disabled females are actively discouraged from motherhood (Fine & Asch, 1988). Disabled women, more often than nondisabled women, are advised not to have children or are threatened by, or are victims of, involuntary sterilization (Fine & Asch, 1981). Many nondisabled families and professionals still frame the issue as whether or not disabled women have the right to become mothers (O'Toole & Bregante, 1992). Disabled lesbians must deal with the belief that, both as lesbians (DiLapi, 1989) and as disabled women (Holmes, 1991), they are considered "inappropriate mothers."

Another health obstacle is that lesbians often receive no preventive health care services. A 1984 survey by the National Lesbian and Gay Health Foundation and other researchers (Denenberg, 1995; Rankow, 1995) uncovered the following findings:

1. Fifty percent of lesbians surveyed had not had a Pap smear in the previous 12 months, and many of the respondents were not receiving any care for existing gynecological problems.
2. The most common health problem was depression.
3. Most women felt unable to disclose their sexual preference to their usual health care provider, yet 80% reported experiencing discrimination based on their sexual identity.
4. The most frequently reported concern regarding access to health care services was insufficient money; this was the primary reason cited for not seeking health care.

According to Haynes's projections—the first ever done for lesbians and breast cancer—one in three lesbians is likely to get the disease in her lifetime (Brownworth, 1993). This is three times the national average for all women, which the Centers for Disease Control had termed "pandemic." Breast cancer is the leading cause of death for African American women between the ages of 45 and 65 (Brownworth, 1993).

The same risk factors that increase the vulnerability for lesbians also exist for women who are disabled during their childbearing years. Additionally, many women who were disabled as children were also exposed to radiation assessments and evaluation as part of the monitoring of their disability, another risk factor. This is a very needed area of research (Rogers, 1995).

The key to treating breast cancer effectively is regular gynecological care, breast self-exam, and mammography. But Haynes found that 45% of lesbians do not have regular obstetric-gynecological care, and another 25% have only sporadic care; thus, fewer than a third of lesbians regularly get essential gynecological care. Many women simply cannot afford treatment, but Haynes adds that the majority of lesbians are also wary of the medical establishment and therefore treat themselves (Brownworth, 1993).

Researchers find that even though their sample population is educated and articulate, lesbians face difficulties (Stevens, 1994):

> The stories of the 332 health care encounters told by this multiethnic, socio-economically diverse sample of lesbians conveyed a recurrent theme across a wide range of health care facilities, health care providers, and health conditions: obtaining health care was dangerous. (p. 220)

Seventy-two percent of lesbians described negative responses from health care providers concerning sexual orientation, including inappropriate treatment, refusal of care, and sexual harassment (Warren, 1993). The collective experience of lesbians rings a bell of terror for any lesbian entering the system. It is not surprising, then, that lesbians often avoid receiving health care in traditional settings as long as it is possible for them to do so (Denenberg, 1992).

The problems lesbians often confront in dealing with the health care system—lack of health insurance, resources for health care services, and community support, the invisibility of lesbians and hostility toward the ill person's partner—all surface with particular harshness at times of immense crisis, at diagnosis, during treatment, at death. Heartbreaking stories, such as that of Sharon Kowalski, are commonplace in the lesbian community (Denenberg, 1992). A 1991 study found that more than 50% of nursing students found lesbians "unacceptable," and 15% thought lesbian sexual behavior should be made illegal (Warren, 1993). A San Diego-based study surveying levels of homophobia among California physicians showed that a whopping 31% of obstetricians and gynecologists said they were "uncomfortable" dealing with lesbians (Brownworth, 1993).

Repercussions of Being "Out"

Faced with social isolation, prejudice, and discrimination, disabled lesbians are frequently encouraged to minimize the effects of their disability and to hide their lesbianism in order to be accepted by nondisabled heterosexual people. Any attempt to hide their needs or desires, however, can have long-term consequences (O'Toole & Bregante, 1993a). Richard Simon, the heterosexual editor of *The Family Therapy Networker* magazine asks, "[I]s there a deeper divide than the one that separates the heterosexual 'us' from the homosexual 'them' (or vice versa)?" (Simon, 1991).

Economics have always determined whether or not a woman could be open about her lesbian identity. If she could support herself, she was more able to create a life that ensured her more physical safety and social support. This in turn allowed her to be openly lesbian in more aspects of her life. Studies reveal that most lesbian and bisexual women are unwilling to disclose their sexual orientation and behaviors to providers and believe that it would adversely affect health care (Warren, 1993). For African American lesbians the problem with disclosure may be twofold. If they do not inform their physicians about their sexual orientation, they are likely, as with Caucasian lesbians, to experience health care that is alienating, if not inappropriate. If they do disclose their orientation and physicians assume a pattern of health risk consistent with Caucasian lesbians, they may also receive inadequate care because physicians fail to distinguish differences in lifestyles within the lesbian community (Cochran & Mays, 1988).

Although consumers have complained about quality care issues, nurses, physicians, and psychiatrists have rarely examined their own attitudes and behaviors toward gay men and lesbian women (Schwanberg, 1990). Little effort has been directed toward evaluating the impact that stereotypes have on patient care (Schwanberg, 1990). Disabled lesbians can often receive the negative attention of health care workers because they are often considered unpopular. They may be perceived as having low moral worth or of being incurable (Kus, 1990). As one lesbian nurse documents, lesbian hospital patients are discussed in hushed tones during shift changes (Stephany, 1988). Consequences of unpopularity with nurses can be significant: withholding pain medications, ignoring call lights, staff being cool and detached, staff turning other staff against patients (Kus, 1990).

Within the health care system, homophobia radiates and creates specific constructs and barriers for both patients and staff. "Nobody seems to want to recognize that nurses like me exist," writes one lesbian nurse (Stephany, 1988). Journals may talk about gay patients but rarely speak about gay staff. Stephany (1988) contends that lesbian nurses are plentiful yet they do not come out to their co-workers because of fear of personal rejection or of losing her job. Many providers harbor beliefs that lesbians are sick, abnormal, immoral, perverse, and dangerous (Stevens, 1994).

Researchers report the experiences of lesbians during health care encounters:

> Participants commonly felt ignored, denigrated, dismissed, intruded upon, shamed, silenced, and subordinated. They recounted circumstances in which they were badgered by heterosexual assumptions, disparaged by racist epithets, and disrespected as indigent clients. They articulated the jeopardy they felt with words like: "terrified," "afraid," "betrayed," "traumatized," "abandoned," and "unsafe" (Stevens, 1994, p. 220)
>
> These experiences include sexual assault, patronizing treatment, neglect, intimidation, ignorance, and discrimination (Denenberg, 1992, p. 15)

Stevens (1994) found that in health care encounters, maintaining vigilance was integral to participants' actions. In an exacting process of environmental scanning and behavioral observation, they were intently watchful. They were attuned to subtleties in language, manner, and emotional atmosphere, monitoring for signs of ignorance, prejudice, and compromised care.

Because they did not feel safe, self-protection was a fundamental goal of participants' actions in encounters with health care providers. A repertoire of strategies intended to secure safety and guard against danger in health care contexts characterized the actions taken by these lesbian clients. The strategies were rallying support, screening providers, seeking mirrors of one's experience, maintaining vigilance, controlling information, bringing a witness, challenging mistreatment, and escaping danger (Stevens, 1994).

CONCLUSIONS

Health Care Providers Need to Serve Disabled Lesbians

The following recommendations for health care providers who wish to increase their service to lesbian and gay patients are taken from Anstett, Kiernan, and Brown (1987):

1. Ask open, direct questions.
2. Take a good sexual and social history.
3. Assist disabled lesbians in identifying peer support systems.
4. Be open to answers.
5. Remember that sexual practices influence health.
6. Remember that consumers want good care, not interference.
7. Be aware that there are different kinds of family configurations that include significant others and a support system.
8. Remember that confidentiality is an important issue because there are important insurance and employment implications.

To begin work on lesbians' concerns in clinical settings, lesbians might be identified and rendered visible by asking relevant questions and using appropriate language on health forms. For example, terms such as sexual partner or significant other are nonthreatening. Heterosexual presumption can be eliminated from history-taking, and lesbian-positive images and literature can be placed along with other educational materials in waiting rooms. Funding is needed immediately for lesbian programming, technical assistance, relevant educational materials, and advocacy (Denenberg, 1992). Additional suggestions include the following:

1. Involvement and action of the health community would hasten the development and enactment of a lesbian health agenda.
2. Identifying key issues and appropriate approaches by talking with lesbian leaders is imperative.
3. Health planning agencies need to consult lesbian health experts to determine whether or not services are targeted to, are reaching, and are acceptable to lesbian clients.
4. Slotting a seat for a lesbian on community advisory boards, medical committees, and planning boards would be helpful (Denenberg, 1992).

Other health care concerns for lesbians include (Denenberg, 1992)

1. Cancer-related services
2. Legal protection for partners and children of lesbians who face serious illness or death
3. Childbearing and parenting services (because few sperm banks are receptive to lesbians, they will use informal insemination from donors who are not screened for HIV and other sexually transmitted diseases)
4. Drug and alcohol abuse and recovery services that are lesbian sensitive
5. Mental health services
6. Gynecology—all women report suffering the abuses of unnecessary surgeries, sterilizations, and drug experimentation
7. Lesbians, like other women, are vulnerable to HIV infection and need to be rendered visible in the AIDS epidemic

Providers Must Offer Safety

In dealing with lesbians, women of color, and low-income women, health care providers of all disciplines can enhance the comfort and efficacy of health care by understanding these women's perceptions and reinforcing their use of self-protective strategies (Stevens, 1994). Finding providers who mirrored participants' life circumstances was not confined to seeking care only from those of the same gender, sexual orientation, or ethnicity; it was clear that ideal providers were those who could take the perspective of others, even those outside their own immediate life experiences (Stevens, 1994).

Disabled Lesbians Need to be Included in All Discussions of, and Research on, Disabled Women

Disabled lesbians have been totally excluded from the limited research conducted on disabled women. This means that the research will need to be undertaken again to gather any information that will assist disabled lesbians. The perspective that disabled women are a single construct needs to be reexamined. The only women who benefit from the narrow focus are the women who represent the presumed norm. Currently, nearly all work on disabled women presumes that she is Caucasian, heterosexual, and physically disabled. There is a need to study and intervene with lesbians from a multidimensional perspective, honoring them as whole persons (Stevens, 1994). Research that does not include disabled lesbians in its design or staffing will continue to perpetuate an abnormally narrow view of disabled women.

Separate Research and Discussion Is Needed on Disabled Lesbians

Research must be conducted specifically on disabled lesbians. Deriving information from general disability research and lesbian research is ineffective and flawed. Lesbians clearly experience health and illness differently from both gay men and heterosexual women, and their differing needs constitute a lesbian health agenda that must be articulated and made visible (Denenberg, 1992). As Tusler (1992) reminds us:

> For effective self-determination to occur, the family, agency, institutional and social structures which create the context of an individual's life must also be addressed. . . . Solutions determined outside the affected community are ineffective because they lack the understanding of the complete environment.

As Hevey (1992) states,

> The pious compassion shown to disabled people cannot be demonstrated to lesbians and gays. Conversely, the violent hostility shown gays and lesbians is hidden due to our disability. In a word, we are too different.
>
> However, we are proud of our non-stereotypical multi-identities, and this power will force all of our communities to expand their own horizons of the 'acceptable'. All disabled people are viewed as asexual, but we challenge that oppression twice. Our social challenge is that our sameness and our difference are included.
>
> We are in the struggle and we are OUT about it.

REFERENCES

Anstett, R., Kiernan, M., & Brown, R. (1987). The gay-lesbian patient and the family physician. *Journal of Family Practice, 25,* 339–344.

Bogle, J., & Shaul, S. (1981). Body image and the woman with a disability. In D.G. Bullard & S.E. Knight (Eds.), *Sexuality and physical disability: Personal perspectives.* St. Louis: C.V. Mosby.

Browne, S.E., Connors, D., & Stern, N. (1985). *With the power of each breath: A disabled women's anthology.* San Francisco: Cleis Press.

Brownworth, V.A. (1993, February/March). The other epidemic: Lesbians & breast cancer. *OUT,* 60–63.

Chipouras, S. (1981). Sexuality related services for disabled people. In D.G. Bullard & S.E. Knight (Eds.), *Sexuality and physical disability: Personal perspectives.* St. Louis: C.V. Mosby.

Cochran, S.D., & Mays, V.M. (1988). Disclosure of sexual preference to physicians by black lesbian and bisexual women. *Western Journal of Medicine, 149,* 616–619.

Davis, L. (1991, May). *Feminism, disability & education—for what?* Paper presented to the Women's Studies and Education Conference, North Ryde, Australia.

Denenberg, R. (1992). Invisible women: Lesbians and health care. *Health/PAC Bulletin,* Spring, 14–21.

Denenberg, R. (1995, Summer). Report on lesbian health. *Women's Health Issues, 5*(2), 81–91.

DiLapi, E.M. (1989). Lesbian mothers and the motherhood hierarchy. *Journal of Homosexuality, 18,* 101–132.

Fine, M., & Asch, A. (1981). Sexism without the pedestal. *Journal of Sociology and Social Welfare, 8*(2).

Fine, M., & Asch, A. (1988). *Women with disabilities: Essays in psychology, culture, and politics.* Philadelphia: Temple University Press.

Gates, H.L., Jr. (1993, May 17). Backlash? *The New Yorker,* 42–44.

Gillespie-Sells, K. (1992). Equality of opportunity for disabled lesbians and gays. In *Independence 92: International Congress and Exposition on Disability—Book of Abstracts* (p. 111). Vancouver, BC, Canada: Independence '92.

Hevey, D. (1992). Liberty, equality, disability—images of a movement: Five of six. In *The creatures time forgot: photography and disability imagery.* London: Routledge.

Holmes, S.A. (1991, August 23). TV anchor's disability stirs debate. *New York Times,* pp. A16, B18.

Kus, R.J. (1990). Nurses and unpopular patients. *American Journal of Nursing,* 63–66.

Luczak, R. (1993). *Eyes of desire: A deaf gay and lesbian reader.* Boston: Alyson Publications.

Magee, M., & Miller, D.C. (1992). "She foreswore her womanhood": Psychoanalytic views of female homosexuality. *Clinical Social Work Journal, 20,* 67–88.

Minkowitz, D. (1994, February 8). Mississippi is burning. *The Village Voice,* 23–28.

Myers, T. (1989–1990, Winter). What's it like to be blind? *Sinister Wisdom, 11,* 77–78.

off our backs. (1981). [Special Issue on Women and Disability.] *11*(5).

O'Toole, C.J. (1990). Violence and sexual assault plague many disabled women. *New Directions for Women, 19,* 17.

O'Toole, C.J., & Bregante, J.L. (1992). Lesbians with disabilities. *Journal of Sexuality and Disability, 10*(3).

O'Toole, C.J., & Bregante, J.L. (1993a). Disabled lesbians: Multicultural realities. In M. Nagler (Ed.), *Perspectives on disability* (2nd ed.). Palo Alto, CA: Health Markets Research.

O'Toole, C.J., & Bregante, J.L. (1993b, February). *Disabled women: The undiscovered sisterhood.* Paper presented at the Fifth International Interdisciplinary Congress on Women, San Jose, Costa Rica.

Pearlman, S.F. (1990, August). *Heterosexual mothers/lesbian daughters: Parallels and similarities.* Paper presented at the 98th Annual Convention of the American Psychological Association, Boston, MA.

Rankow, E.J. (1995, May). Lesbian health issues for the primary care provider. *Journal of Family Practice, 40*(5), 486–496.

Rogers, J. (1995). *Breast exams for physically disabled women.* Paper presented at the Conference on Breast Health for Women with Disabilities, Alta Bates Medical Center, Berkeley, CA.

Saunders, J.M., et al. (1988, October). *A lesbian profile: A survey of 1000 lesbians.* Report prepared for the National Lesbian Rights Conference, San Diego, CA.

Schwanberg, S.L. (1990). Attitudes towards homosexuality in American health care literature 1983–1987. *Journal of Homosexuality, 19,* 117–136.

Simon, R. (1991, January/February). From the Editor. *The Family Therapy Networker,* 2.

Stephany, T.M. (1988, November/December). Lesbian nurse. *Nursing Outlook,* 295.

Stevens, P.E. (1994). Protective strategies of lesbian clients in health care environments. *Research in Nursing & Health, 17,* 217–229.

Thompson, C.A. (1992). Lesbian grief and loss issues in the coming out process. *Women & Therapy, 12*(1-2), 175–186.

Thompson, K. (1992, March/April). Karen Thompson talks about the case that never should have had to happen. *Disability Rag.*

Thompson, K., & Andrzejewski, J. (1988). *Why can't Sharon Kowalski come home?* San Francisco: Spinsters/Aunt Lute.

Tusler, A. (1992, Spring). Self-determination by people with disabilities to solve the alcohol and other drug problems in their community. *The Seed,* 1–4.

Warren, N. (1993, October/November). Out of the question: Obstacles to research on HIV and women who engage in sexual behaviors with women. *SIECUS Report,* 13–16.

Waxman, B.F. (1991). Anti-disability hate crimes. *CAPH New World,* 12–18.

Women and Disability Awareness Project. (1989). *Building community: A manual exploring issues of women and disability.* New York: Educational Equity Concepts.

chapter 13

Sexual Abuse of Women with Physical Disabilities

Margaret A. Nosek

Inquiry into the sexual abuse of women with disabilities is one of the most complex, controversial, and disturbing challenges facing rehabilitation researchers. It raises a combination of many unresolved issues in the studies of abuse, disability, and the status of women. As a dimension of the general study of abuse, disability has barely been acknowledged. As a dimension of the general study of disability, abuse has only recently surfaced as a problem and has yet to be the subject of rigorous scientific inquiry. To unveil the importance of this problem and to set forth some parameters for further investigation into its magnitude and impact, this chapter reviews the literature on the sexual abuse of women with disabilities and presents the findings of a qualitative study of sexuality issues among women with physical disabilities. In this study, the experience of abuse emerged as an unexpectedly strong and ominous theme. Special attention is given to the effect of having a disability on increasing a woman's vulnerability to sexual abuse.

METHODOLOGIC ISSUES IN ABUSE RESEARCH

Before reviewing the literature on sexual abuse of women with disabilities, it is necessary to establish the framework by which abuse can be examined. The first and most fundamental of these issues is definitions. Although

The author would like to acknowledge the contribution of the research team at the Baylor College of Medicine Center for Research on Women with Disabilities in the preparation of this report: Diana H. Rintala, Ph.D., Mary Ellen Young, Ph.D., Carol Howland, B.A., Jama L. Bennett, M.Ed., and Catherine Clubb Foley, Ph.D. This research is supported by the National Institutes of Health (Grant No. 1 R01 HD30166-01). This chapter is a revised version of an earlier publication, Nosek, M.A. (1995). Sexual abuse of women with physical disabilities. In T.N. Monga (Ed.), *Sexuality and disability, physical medicine and rehabilitation: State of the art reviews, 9*(2), 487–502. Reprinted with permission.

some authors claim that there is currently no universally accepted definition of abuse (Garbarino, 1987; Laws, 1993), there have been many attempts to define it. Dorothea Glass is quoted as defining sexual assault as "any unwanted sexual activity; visual, verbal, physical, or where the victim is less than the age of consent." She further calls it

> an act of aggression and hostility against a whole person; not just a sexual act or a bodily violation, but an indignity, an invasion, and violation of a person that affects the victim physically, psychologically, and socially; an assault which does not necessarily end when the assailant leaves or is caught. (Aiello, Capkin, & Catania, 1983)

Cole (1984–1986) defines sexual abuse as "when a person is manipulated, tricked, or forced into touch or sexual contact" (p. 71).

In the literature on the sexual abuse of pregnant women, McFarlane, Parker, Soeken, and Bullock (1992) define it simply as being forced to have sexual activities. The American Medical Association, in its *Guidelines on Domestic Violence* (1992), defines sexual abuse as any form of forced sex or sexual degradation. This includes trying to make a woman perform sexual acts against her will; pursuing sexual activity when she is not fully conscious or is not asked or is afraid to say no; hurting her physically during sex or assaulting her genitals; coercing her to have sex without protection against pregnancy or sexually transmissible diseases; and criticizing her and calling her sexually degrading names.

The most thoroughly considered and practical definitions of abuse have been formulated by Finkelhor and Korbin (1988) in the context of child abuse—the portion of harm to children that results from human action that is proscribed, proximate, and preventable. By "proscribed," the authors mean action that is negatively valued at the same time it causes harm (thus eliminating harmful effects of well-intended medical procedures), but including actions that are deviant, of harmful intent, or in violation of legal or social expectations. By "proximate," they mean that action must have a direct effect and not be removed by time or space. This definition distinguishes child abuse clearly from the social, economic, and health problems of international concern. It is flexible enough to apply to a range of situations in a variety of social and cultural contexts. Finkelhor and Korbin specifically define sexual abuse of children as any sexual contact between an adult and a sexually immature (socially as well as psychologically) child for the purposes of the adult's sexual gratification; or any sexual contact to a child made by the use of force, threat, or deceit to secure the child's participation; or sexual contact to which a child is incapable of consenting by virtue of age or power differentials or the nature of the relationship with the adult. The issue of power differentials and relationships with other individuals will become salient later in the discussion of the disempowerment of people with disabilities.

Once a label of abuse has been attached to an incident, it is necessary to determine other parameters for purposes of description and comparison. Trickett and Putnam (1993) recommend that the degree of trauma related to the severity of abuse can be indexed by 1) type of abuse; 2) age at onset; 3) frequency; 4) closeness of the relationship to the abuser; and 5) presence of physical violence, pain, and threats.

The study of sexual abuse is severely compromised by issues of documentation. Estimates vary on the percent of actual cases that are reported to authorities, depending on the age of the victim. A study of 245 women with disabilities conducted by the DisAbled Women's Network of Canada (DAWN) (Ridington, 1989) found that, of the cases of abuse identified by their participants, 43% had been reported to police, social service agencies, parents, teachers, or spouses. This figure was acknowledged as high by the investigators because more than half of the participants were members of consumer advocacy groups. McFarlane, Christoffel, Bateman, Miller, and Bullock (1991) cited the Department of Justice's finding that, of actual cases of spousal abuse, 43% were not reported to the police. Their study of abused pregnant women found that 7.3% reported abuse by a partner in a paper and pencil questionnaire, but 29.3% reported abuse when interviewed by a nurse. Cases of child abuse are even more complicated to document, given a child's general lack of understanding and vocabulary related to sexual activities. For children with disabilities, particularly cognitive and communication disabilities, there are additional complicating factors related to documenting personal experiences (Light, Collier, & Parnes, 1985). In a survey of human services agencies' Child and Adult Protective Services in all 50 states, Camblin (1982) reported that 7 states had no standardized reporting form and only 26 states gathered information on preexisting disability status.

Many methodological flaws are evident in reviewing the literature on sexual abuse. Most studies violate Laws's (1993) guideline for rigorous cross-sectional studies: 1) choose subjects and controls from homogeneous populations; 2) assess sexual abuse history with an instrument that consists of multiple questions describing specific events; 3) use an explicit definition of abuse; 4) measure potential confounds such as socioeconomic status, family dynamics, psychological symptoms, history of sexual and physical abuse in childhood, and adult sexual and physical assault; 5) use valid and reliable instruments to measure comorbid medical and psychological problems; and 6) have adequate statistical power to test associations and control for confounds. Ammerman, Cassisi, Hersen, and Van Hasselt (1986) cite three shortcomings of child abuse research: 1) heterogeneous samples, 2) failure to match participant on relevant variables, and 3) use of psychometrically weak assessment instruments. In an attempt to avoid some of these shortcomings, the study reported in this chapter focuses on women with physical disabilities and attempts to describe their specific accounts of sexual abuse according to the parameters just listed. Before presenting these findings, however, it is necessary to examine previous research related to sexual abuse of girls and women with disabilities to provide a context for interpretation.

SEXUAL ABUSE OF CHILDREN WITH DISABILITIES

The most valid and respected statistic on the prevalence on childhood sexual abuse was stated by Finkelhor (1979): 25% of female children and 9% of male children. Several studies report substantially higher rates among children with disabilities, although rates vary considerably, and no attempt is made to distinguish between the experience of children with physical versus cognitive disabilities. Doucette (1986), for example, reported on a study of women with a variety of disabilities that they were about 1.5 times as likely to have been sexually abused as children compared to women without disabilities. A survey of 62 women conducted by the Ontario Ministry of Community and Social Services (1987) found that 50% of women with disabilities reported being sexually assaulted as a child compared to 34% of women without disabilities. Sobsey and Doe (1991), citing a variety of studies, report that the incidence of all types of abuse among children with disabilities appears to be 4.43 times the expected value. A Congressionally mandated study conducted by the National Center on Child Abuse and Neglect (1993) documented physical and sexual abuse twice as often in children with disabilities compared to other children. Muccigrosso (1991) claims that 90%–99% of persons with development disabilities have been sexually exploited by age 18, four times the rate in the nondisabled population. Mullins (1986) claims that 50%–90% of people with developmental disabilities are sexually abused. Despite these widely divergent estimates, the body of evidence strongly points toward a prevalence of sexual abuse of children with disabilities that far exceeds public awareness.

Much of the attention in the literature has been devoted to explaining the increased prevalence of abuse among children with disabilities. These studies, however, focus almost exclusively on children with developmental disabilities who have severe cognitive impairments. Some studies attribute causation of the abuse to stress imposed on the family by the child's disability (Bristol & Schloper, 1984). In nearly half the cases examined in the study by the National Center on Child Abuse and Neglect (1993), the disability was identified as the root of the abuse or neglect. There is a considerable body of literature, however, that fails to confirm disability itself as a risk factor in abuse, and even documents an inverse relationship between level of severity of disability and incidence of abuse (Benedict,

White, Wulff, & Hall, 1990; Benedict, Wulff, & White, 1992; Garbarino, 1987; Glaser & Bentovim, 1979; Starr, Dietrich, Fischhoff, Ceresnie, & Zweier, 1984; Zirpoli, Snell, & Lloyd, 1987). There is general agreement with Garbarino (1987) that related factors of greater importance include psychological, social, and cultural aspects of the family and characteristics of the parents, such as coping skills, parenting skills, their own history of maltreatment, interpersonal violence, and low level of social exchange. According to Sobsey and Varnhagen (1989), society's expectations and treatment of people with disabilities may contribute more to the increased risk of abuse than the disability itself. It must also be acknowledged that children with disabilities have a much greater risk of residing in institutions, where significantly higher rates of abuse are well documented (Crossmaker, 1991; Garbarino, 1987).

For all the analysis of disability as an increased risk factor in sexual abuse, little attention has been paid to the effect of child abuse on victims who have disabilities. To interpret the findings presented later in this chapter, it is helpful to understand some of the findings in the general literature on child abuse. Early writings claimed that the sexual abuse of children rarely involved coercion or violence, that the victim situation is of short duration and of minimal effect in terms of gross measure of functioning later in life (e.g., marriage and childbearing), and that even in offenses that involve a great deal of violence there is rarely a profound long-term effect (Gagnon & Simon, 1970). These statements have been soundly refuted by more recent research among psychological, sociological, and developmental investigators. Trickett and Putnam (1993) found that sexual abuse peaked in children ages 7–8 years and had a mean duration of 2 years. They documented sequelae of childhood sexual abuse to be multiple personality disorders, borderline personality disorders, somatoform disorders (especially chronic pelvic pain), eating disorders, substance abuse, and some forms of chronic psychosis. Other negative effects included low self-esteem, impaired sense of control and competence, and increased negative affect. They stated that cognitive capabilities can mediate these negative outcomes. Of women with premenstrual syndrome, 40% report histories of sexual abuse (Paddison, Gise, Lebovits, Strain, Girasole, & Levine, 1990). Researchers at Washington University found that physical abuse dramatically increases the likelihood of abnormal aggression later in life and that a significant percentage of girls developed withdrawal behavior patterns (Schwartzbeck, 1993). Garbarino (1987) was one of the few to examine the long-term effect of abuse in a disability context. He claimed that the abuse of special children (children with disabilities) results in acute and chronic medical problems that impair development and substantially increase the risk of delinquency, psychiatric disorders, and sexual dysfunction.

SEXUAL ABUSE OF WOMEN WITH DISABILITIES

The incidence of sexual abuse among women in general has been fairly well documented (American Medical Association, 1992; McFarlane et al., 1991); however, only a few studies have examined the incidence among women with disabilities. The DisAbled Women's Network of Canada (Doucette, 1986) surveyed 245 women with disabilities and found that 40% had experienced abuse, 12% of whom had been raped. Perpetrators of the abuse were primarily spouses (including ex-spouses) (37%) and strangers (28%), followed by parents (15%), service providers (10%), and dates (7%). As mentioned earlier, fewer than half were reported, mostly because of fear and dependency. Of the women, 10% had used shelters or other services, 15% reported that no services were available or they were unsuccessful in their attempt to obtain services, and 55% had not tried to get services.

The Center for Research on Women with Disabilities at Baylor College of Medicine conducted an informal survey of battered women's shelters in Houston and found 64% to be inaccessible to women in wheelchairs. Sobsey and Doe (1991) conducted a study of 166 cases handled by the University of Alberta's Sexual Abuse and Disability Project. The sample was 81.7% women—70% people with intellectual impairments—and had a very wide age range (18 months to 57 years). In 95.6% of the cases, the perpetrator was known to the victim; 44% of the perpetrators were service providers. In the National Center on Child Abuse and Neglect (1993) study and in Muccigrosso's (1991) study, 86% and 99% of the perpetrators were known to the victims, respectively. Of the individuals, 79% were victimized more than once. Treatment services were either inadequate or not offered in 73% of the cases.

The Ontario Ministry of Community and Social Services (1987) surveyed 62 women and found that more of the women with disabilities had been battered as adults compared to the women without disabilities (33% vs. 22%), but fewer had been sexually assaulted as adults (23% vs. 31%).

Although reliable statistics on the experience of sexual abuse among women with disabilities are sorely lacking, there has been some analysis of why they might experience a greater vulnerability. The combined cultural devaluation of women and persons with disabilities is a major factor (Belsky, 1980), often further confounded by devaluation based on age (Kreigsman & Bregman, 1985). Overprotection and internalized societal expectations are other significant contributors. For persons with developmental disabilities, Muccigrosso (1991) lists the by-products of living in extremely overprotected environments as 1) lack of knowledge, 2) overcompliance and socialized vulnerability, 3) the unrealistic view that everyone is a friend, 4) limited social opportunities, 5) low self-esteem, and 6) limited or no assertiveness or refusal skills. Womendez and Schneiderman (1991) characterize the experience of women with disabilities as having fewer opportunities to learn sexual likes and dislikes and to set pleasing boundaries. They may not date, go to parties, or engage in age-appropriate sexual activity, experiencing frequent rejection. Their first sexual experience may come much later in life. These limited opportunities prevent them from learning how to start a relationship; much of their information on sexuality is second-hand. Women with disabilities often perceive celibacy or violent sexual encounters as their only choices, believing no loving person would be attracted to them. Some believe that fate proclaims they deserve what they get and that bad feelings (such as pain) are better than none. There is often disassociation of the self from the parts of the body being assaulted, rooted in frequent pain inflicted by doctors and "helpers," where privacy is denied, nakedness is the norm, and women are treated as if they are not human. Few human services workers validate the abuse experienced by these women. Several studies have documented low rates of receiving sexuality counseling or information among women with arthritis (Yoshino & Uchida, 1981) and spinal cord injury (Beckmann, Gittler, Barzansky, & Beckmann, 1989; White, Rintala, Hart, & Fuhrer, 1993; Zwerner, 1982).

The vulnerability to sexual exploitation of persons with a variety of disabilities, as perceived by health care providers, was studied by Mullan and Cole (1991). Persons with a combination of mental retardation and physical disability were rated as the most vulnerable, followed by persons with mental illness, physical disability only, mental retardation only, intellectual impairment, and learning disability. The authors listed 12 ways health care providers create victims out of persons with disabilities: institutionalize, reward compliance, isolate, extend dependency, withhold information, discount signals, support or create double binds between individuals and their families, do not believe, do not regard as sexual, deny basic rights, deny privacy, and overmedicate or restrain chemically.

Many factors contribute to the vulnerability of women with disabilities to sexual abuse. Many questions remain, however, about the actual abuse experiences of these women, the role their disability plays in the abuse, and the effect the abuse has on their lives.

A QUALITATIVE STUDY

The findings from a qualitative study that details sexual abuse experiences reported in interviews with 11 women who have physical disabilities are presented in the following discussion. Although no conclusions can be drawn from this study about the relative incidence of abuse among women with disabilities compared to women without disabilities, the findings are enlightening. They illustrate the complex interweaving of personal, social, cultural, and environmental factors that allows sexual abuse of women with disabilities to take place, often with a severe negative impact.

Description of the Study

The study used the qualitative method of open-ended interviewing to identify primary themes and issues about the sexuality of women with disabilities. The research team developed a generalized interview guide (Patton, 1990) based on a literature review and their own experience. Three researchers, all with disabilities themselves and trained in interviewing techniques, used the interview guide primarily as a reference to ensure that they covered key areas.

A total of 31 adult women with disabilities that resulted in functional impairments participated in the interviews. The participants were recruited through personal contact and by fliers distributed locally and nationally. Use of theoretical sampling (Glaser & Strauss, 1967) assured that the selection of individuals represented key variables hypothesized to affect sexual functioning, such as type of disability, age at onset of disability, ethnicity, and marital status. All interviews were audiotaped and transcribed, then checked by the interviewer for accuracy. Field notes providing context to the interviews, nonverbal reactions of participants, and reactions of the interviewers were written and included within the transcripts for analysis.

The racial groups represented in the sample included Caucasian (Glaser & Strauss, 1967), Asian (Beckmann et al., 1989), Hispanic (Ammerman et al., 1986), and African American (Benedict et al., 1990). Ages ranged from 22 to 69, with ages at onset of disability ranging from birth to 52. Disabilities included cerebral palsy, postpolio, spina bifida, amputation (bilateral upper limb, unilateral lower limb), rheumatic conditions (including rheumatoid arthritis and systemic lupus erythematosus), multiple sclerosis, spinal cord injury, traumatic brain injury, and stroke. Sexual orientation included 29 heterosexuals and 2 lesbians. Of the participants, 15 were never married, 7 were divorced, and 9 were married at the time of the interview. A total of 14 had children. Level of education attained was unrepresentatively high: 10 had graduate degrees, 7 had bachelors degrees, 10 had some college, and 4 had a high school education. A total of 17 worked for pay, and 13 were considered unemployed but productive (i.e., involved in homemaking, educational, or volunteer activities). Only one was considered inactive.

Analytic induction and constant comparison (Glaser & Strauss, 1967) were the qualitative data analysis techniques employed. Analysis began with the research team reading each of the transcribed interviews and discussing the major themes, issues, and hypotheses in weekly research team meetings. As key concepts emerged from these discussions, research staff listed and grouped them into major thematic areas: sense of self, family of origin, friendship, sex education, abuse, physical sexual functioning, environmental and social barriers, abuse, health issues, dating, marriage, parenting, and personal assistance issues. After identifying these major themes, at least two researchers coded all interviews by bracketing the thematic passages on the transcripts and recording the appropriate code or codes for that passage. They resolved disagreements about coding in team meetings and refined the coding scheme itself when needed. An indication of the validity of the major themes was the lack of required modifications as the analysis of interviews neared completion. To provide the basis for a rich descriptive presentation of the major themes, staff extracted coded passages from the transcripts as "chunks" and grouped them by themes. Members of the research team then reviewed each set of thematic chunks and described of findings along with hypotheses or explanations of the phenomena under study. A review team evaluated the process and findings monthly. A panel of national experts from the fields of rehabilitation, independent living, medicine, and sexuality critiqued the preliminary report.

Procedure for Analyzing Abuse

After further analyzing themes extracted from the data, the research team identified five major thematic categories: sense of self, sexuality information, relationships, barriers, and health and physical functioning. The category of barriers consisted of factors that inhibited or prevented the development of positive sense of self, access to sexuality information, satisfactory relationships, and optimal health and physical functioning. There were three subcategories: environmental barriers, social barriers, and abuse.

The principal investigator returned to transcripts of the original interviews to identify specific reports of abuse experiences. For each abuse experience reported by each participant, the investigator determined the type of abuse as sexual, physical, or emotional, with the understanding that physical abuse includes emotional abuse, and sexual abuse includes both physical and emotional abuse. The type of abuse was charted along with the perpetrator, the age at which it occurred or began, frequency/duration (e.g., once, many times, years, lifelong), and a description of the abuse, including whether or not alcohol or drug abuse was involved. The research team examined and discussed this information until they reached consensus on designations within each parameter.

Using inductive techniques, the team processed this information with basic demographic and disability data on the participants and with a profile of each interview in order to interpret the disability-relatedness and impact of the abuse experiences. The team interpreted disability-relatedness by considering whether or not the experience occurred after the onset of disability and by asking such questions as, "Had this individual not had a disability, would the abuse have occurred?" and "Did factors related to the disability create psychological, behavioral, social, physical, or environmental conditions that made the abuse more likely to occur?" They interpreted impact as very low, low, moderate, severe, or very severe, according to predetermined guidelines based on the participants' own words. The first consideration was the length of the presentation of the experience by the participant and the number of times it was referred to throughout the interview; second was the emotional intensity expressed during the presentation of the experience; third was the degree to which the participant said the experience affected her life, physically, emotionally, or socially. The team interpreted the impact to be low for those who mentioned an event once in passing, without elaboration, with little emotional intensity, and with no statements that attributed to the experience a significant interference with developmental processes. The interpretation of severe impact was reserved for experiences that participants discussed at length or mentioned more than once in the interview, using strong, emotion-filled language and with statements indicating a serious, long-lasting interference with their physical, emotional, or social functioning.

The research team identified an abuse experience as sexual if it involved unwanted physical contact to the participant's genitals or breasts, contact of any part of her body with the genitals of the perpetrator, or if the participant used such words as "raped," "molested," or "incested" in reporting the experience. The question of exhibitionism as abuse did not arise because no such experiences were reported in this study. For young children, the question of whether or not the contact was wanted was considered moot if the participant used the language of abuse to describe it. Willfulness on the part of the perpetrator was not considered, only the participant's perception of the experience as sexual abuse.

Data Related to Sexual Abuse

Of the 31 women in the study, 11 (more than one third) reported experiencing sexual abuse. All totalled, 25 of the participants reported 55 separate experiences of abuse; 15 experiences were sexual, 17 were physical, and 23 were emotional. Brief profiles of those reporting sexual abuse follow.

Case 1: Emily, a 37-year-old, Caucasian married woman with no children, had polio at age 4 that severely affected all four limbs and her ability to breathe independently during sleep. She has a bachelor's degree and is working full time. During her college years, she met a man from out of town on an airplane and, along with her female roommate, accepted an invitation to go out to dinner with him. After they had all consumed considerable amounts of alcohol, he told her he wanted her to become his mistress because he had a good sexual experience previously with a woman who also had polio. When the roommate left to use the restroom, the man began fondling the participant's foot and placed it on his penis under the table. Because she was using her manual wheelchair instead of her power wheelchair in order to travel in his car, she was unable to pull away from his grasp. When her roommate returned, Emily talked him into taking them back to the dorm. This was the only abuse experience she reported. It was interpreted as disability related, based on the perpetrator's reasons for approaching the participant and her inability to physically escape the situation. Although it frightened her considerably at the time, and she had told only a few people about it over the years, the fact that she did not express lasting negative feelings about herself as a result of this experience indicates that it had a low impact on her development and later relationships.

Case 2: Elena, a 26-year-old Hispanic woman, had polio at age 1 that affected her ability to walk. She is married and was pregnant at the time of the interview. She had attended college and is working. Her mother raised her and two sisters in an upper-class family in South America. According to Elena, there were strong feelings of shame in the family toward her disability. As a child, her mother frequently took her to faith healers and physicians who performed numerous surgeries. She said, "I always felt that my body didn't belong to me." Her sister arranged for a boy to visit Elena in their home when Elena was 14 years old and had had no sexual experience. She hid her crutches and tried to look normal. On a later visit, he forced her to perform oral sex. When asked whether it was unusual in that culture for a young man to be that aggressive, she replied, "Oh yeah, because all the men that I knew . . . they respect the woman until they get married." Her statement about not feeling ownership of her body, combined with her statement that his behavior was uncharacteristically aggressive in their culture and social class, led the researchers to interpret this experience as disability related. The team interpreted it to have had a moderate impact, because she labeled it as an "unfortunate incident," yet used strong language such as "violent" and "totally disgusting" in describing it.

Case 3: Beatrice, a 33-year-old, never-married Caucasian woman, has had cerebral palsy since birth. She has a graduate degree, but was not working at the time of the interview. Her parents raised her in a strong Catholic environment. Her father encouraged her to overcome her shyness and invite boys she was interested in over to her house. She initially denied having any abuse experiences, but on reflection said that when she was a teenager at summer camp a boy fondled her breasts in a manner she did not like. The researchers concluded that this was not disability related in that it is often part of the developmental processes of sexual experimentation and setting boundaries. Because Beatrice thought to mention this incident only after reflection and described it in neutral terms with little detail it was considered a low-impact experience.

Case 4: Ginny, a 46-year-old Caucasian woman, is married and has two children. At her birth, her arms were broken and amputated above the elbow by an alcoholic doctor. At the time of the interview, she was attending college but not working. She was raised in a low-income, poorly educated, rural family. She said that her mother rejected her and shamed her about her disability. There were nine experiences of abuse, predominantly emotional, related in her interview. Two of the experiences were sexual: first, being molested as a child by an uncle, and second, being raped at age 12 by a stranger. The research team considered both experiences to be not disability related. Vulnerabilities related to her disability were outweighed by other risk factors in her life, such as her family demographics and persistent psychological violence. Her cursory description of the first experience indicates a low impact. The second experience, on the other hand, was interpreted as having a severe impact, because in her words, it made her feel "ashamed and dirty"; she shut off her feelings after that and was convinced that sex was the only thing men would ever want from her.

Case 5: Patsy, a 36-year-old, never-married Asian American woman, had polio at age 16 months and subsequently developed severe scoliosis. She has a master's degree and is unemployed, but volunteers at a local advocacy office. Her family was very caring and supportive during her childhood; she lived with them at the time of the interview. She has never had a romantic or sexual relationship. She came to the United States just before college and believes the doctor at the immigration physical exam may have molested her by fondling her breasts. Her description of the experience suggests a routine breast exam, but her perception was of being molested. The experience itself was interpreted by the researchers to be an ordinary occurrence that was not disability related, although her perception of it as a molestation was related to the social isolation and lack of sexuality information that resulted from her disability. She did not give many details of the experience nor describe any persistent negative feelings subsequent to it, indicating that it had a low impact.

Case 6: Josephine, a 36-year-old Caucasian lesbian, has had severe juvenile rheumatoid arthritis since age 3. She considers herself married to her lover and has been very active in a support group for lesbians with disabilities. She has a doctorate and is working. She is the eldest of three siblings in a fairly happy family, but was frequently sick and in special schools or had a home tutor until ninth grade. In addition to reporting experiences of physical and emotional abuse by personal attendants, she reported being sexually abused while in a hospital for surgery at age 7. In that her disability required her to be hospitalized frequently, thereby increasing the likelihood of experiencing sexual abuse, the researchers interpreted this experience to be disability related. She said that all the lesbians she knows were victims of incest or sexual abuse in hospitals. Her implication that lesbianism is related to sexual abuse and the impassioned language used in that discussion indicates that this experience had a severe impact.

Case 7: Heather, a 37-year-old African American woman, has had juvenile rheumatoid arthritis since age 12. She has never married, has a bachelor's degree, and is working. She was raped more than once by her stepfather before the onset of arthritis. After being raped, she reported becoming more introverted. When she told her mother about these experiences, her mother did not believe her. Neither parent ever acknowledged that the rape had occurred. She never received counseling until the 1980s, when the memories started resurfacing. Although she has had numerous dating relationships, she has never engaged in sexual activity because of religious beliefs. This abuse experience was interpreted as not disability related because it occurred before the onset of her disability. Her repression of the memories, the strong language she used in describing the experiences, and the process of dealing with it later in life indicate a severe impact.

Case 8: Geraldine, a 26-year-old Caucasian woman, incurred a spinal cord injury (resulting in paraplegia) and a traumatic brain injury in an accident at age 15. She was married twice, divorced once, and has a young daughter. She has a high school education and was not working at the time of the interview. She described herself as a juvenile delinquent and wild in her youth. In her interview four experiences of sexual abuse were described, all involving drugs or alcohol. The first three were in her teen years after acquiring a disability. In the first, she went to a bar at age 17 and met two men who were brothers with whom she drank. Afterwards, they went to the brothers' apartment to smoke marijuana. The apartment was upstairs and the brothers carried her. Once inside, they threw her on the bed, stripped her, and tried to rape her. When she stopped fighting them, they stopped and took her home. In the second and third experiences, she met men in bars on various occasions; one she referred to as the "Hatchet man" and another as the "convict." She felt coerced into sexual activity with them. The fourth experience occurred as an adult. In her words, she was "sexually harassed" into doing cocaine and having sex with a high-level official in the contracting company where she worked. In an attempt to end the sexual harassment, she married her first husband, who turned out to be physically and emotionally abusive. The first three of these experiences may be disability related because they reflect the excessive risk-taking behavior and impaired judgment that sometimes accompanies traumatic brain injury. Additionally, in the first experience her spinal cord injury limited her escape options. The fourth experience is more difficult to interpret because, although it reflects some of the same risk-taking behavior, there was nothing in her description indicating any relationship between the sexual harassment and her disability. The research team interpreted it to be not disability related. The length of her descriptions and her use of strong language in the first and fourth experiences indicate a moderate impact. She mentioned the second and third experiences almost in passing, indicating a low impact.

Case 9: Della, a 26-year-old, never-married Caucasian woman, incurred a traumatic brain injury at age 16 that requires her to use crutches for walking. She had attended college and is working. She reported one experience of abuse, a date rape in college. In describing her response to it, she said, "Nothing happened because I didn't get pregnant," and she did not let it affect her. This indicates a low impact. The experience was interpreted by the research team to be not disability related; it was viewed as a typical case of date rape.

Case 10: Sally, a 43-year-old, divorced Caucasian woman with no children, has had epilepsy and a back injury since age 24. She attended college and is working. She reported being sexually "tortured" repeatedly with a hair brush at age 5 by her 7-year-old brother and his friend. After the incidents were discovered, the whole family became overprotective of her. In her words, "it tore the family up" when she identified the brother as the perpetrator. She repressed the memory for 33 years, but for all that time she carried the hair brush around with her. Both of her parents had been sexually abused as children, and she suspected her brother had been abused by his friend's sister. Her experience was not disability related because it occurred before her back injury and the onset of epilepsy. The strong language of abuse she used to describe the experience and her efforts to deal with it later in life indicate a severe impact.

Case 11: Lin, an Asian American, 43-year-old divorced woman with two children, has had rheumatoid arthritis since age 28. She reported being sexually abused by a relative beginning at age 8 when she entered puberty. The abuse stopped only when he moved away. She said that she was caught between Eastern and Western cultures—that the Eastern way teaches children to do everything an adult says, that any adult in the house is the parent. For most of her life she would not let male friends touch her. She did not remember the abuse experiences until after her divorce. The researchers interpreted this to be non–disability related because it occurred before the onset of her disability. Her detailed discussion of this experience and her analysis of it in relation to culture, using strong language with words of frustration, indicate that it had a severe impact.

Discussion

The experiences reported by these 11 women with disabilities verify many of the observations stated in the literature. The fact that more than one third of the women interviewed in this study had experienced sexual abuse of one form or another points to a problem of significant proportions. Examining these experiences according to Trickett and Putnam's (1993) parameters—type of abuse; age at onset; frequency; closeness of the relationship to the abuser; and presence of physical violence, pain, and threats—gives greater insight into nature of the abuse.

Among the 15 experiences reported, there was considerable variety in the type of sexual abuse, including fondling (3), coerced sexual activity (3), forced oral sex (1), sexual assault (5), and rape (3). Six of these experiences occurred in childhood, six in teen years, and 3 in adulthood. The large majority were single incidents. Of the four experiences that extended over months or years, three involved abuse by a relative and one was sexual harassment in the workplace. Perpetrators were predominantly dates (7), followed by relatives (4), with single reports of abuse in a hospital and a workplace, by a stranger, and by a physician. Two experiences reported by the same individual involved alcohol and drug abuse. Twelve experiences involved violence, pain, or threats. The three that did not appeared to have a very low impact, with two occurring in a dating situation and one in a medical setting that the researchers interpreted as ordinary, but the participant interpreted as frightening.

The question of disability relatedness was clear-cut in only three experiences, where the abuse occurred before the onset of disability. In six other experiences, the researchers interpreted the situation as one common to women in general. It is important to note, however, that in the situation of Ginny, the effect of disability seemed to be far outweighed by the pervasive psychological violence in her family in creating her vulnerability to the two sexual abuse experiences she reported. Six experiences were interpreted by the research team as disability related. Important factors in these reports were the inability to escape a situation because of architectural inaccessibility (Geraldine, being carried up to a second-floor apartment) and a lack of adaptive equipment (Emily, being in a manual wheelchair she could not propel). Emily's experience also shows the effect of social stereotypes on creating vulnerable situations. Her date was attracted to her specifically because she had polio. Josephine's experience illustrates the increased risk for sexual abuse in disability-related institutional settings. Geraldine's experiences were difficult to interpret because although some may claim that high risk-taking behaviors might characterize women without disabilities, her particular behaviors may reflect impaired judgment that sometimes accompanies brain injury.

Based on the participants' own words, the researchers interpreted seven of the experiences to have had a low impact, three moderate, and five severe. All but two of the severe-impact experiences involved sexual assault or rape and tended to extend over a period of time. The manifestation of the impact was in feelings of worthlessness, dirtiness, and hopelessness regarding prospects of having future satisfying relationships.

Some interesting findings on the role of culture emerged from this study. Two of the participants specifically mention cultural factors in recounting their experience. Elena indicated that in her social class and culture (Hispanic), the man's behavior toward her was quite different from behavior she observed toward her sisters and peers. Lin stated that in Asian cultures children are taught to obey every adult very strictly, thus creating a vulnerable situation for her when she was repeatedly confronted by a malicious adult relative.

Many of the observations made by Womendez and Schneiderman (1991) about the lack of opportunity for women with disabilities to understand their sexuality and have opportunities to develop social interaction skills and a positive self-concept have been illustrated in these case examples. Several of the participants expressed feelings of helplessness to prevent the abuse and had an attitude of submission to the experience. This reflects perceptions of disempowerment, not only in situations where a power differential is evident, as in a hospital or adult authority situation, but also in dating relationships.

In the process of interviewing the 31 women participating in this study, many experiences emerged that had all the hallmarks of abuse, but could not technically be labeled abuse. A majority of the participants had experienced very frightening, frustrating, and psychologically damaging interactions with medical professionals. They reported repeated episodes of painful, insensitive handling and failure of physicians to address their questions and concerns. In addition to recounting the direct interaction as a negative event, they expressed intense feelings of abandonment and hopelessness; they were unable to perceive control of their health status and care. Technically, however, this cannot be considered abuse according to Finkelhor and Korbin's (1988) requirement that the action be proscribed. In a medical context, any action by a professional is deemed by society to be well intended. If actions by a professional have a negative impact, they could be considered malpractice, but not abuse. There is a need for clarification regarding this ethical dilemma. The severe, long-term, negative effect of inappropriate treatment in a medical context by women with physical disabilities deserves attention as an abuse issue and should not be devalued to the status of malpractice.

Previous work by the research team examined the findings of this qualitative study from the perspective of wellness (Nosek et al., 1994). Concepts of resilience and lines of resistance and defense found in the wellness models of Cowen (1991) and Neuman (1982), respectively, are particularly relevant to the investigation of abuse among women with physical disabilities. For this population, the numerous environmental and attitudinal barriers and various abuses they regularly face can be viewed as stressors, forces that can sharpen resilience or cause defeat. Constant exposure to negative feedback (women with disabilities are ugly, worthless, a burden to society, and unable to ever fulfill their proper role as women); the absence and, in some cases, withholding of information about one's body; and environmental barriers compounded by a lack of appropriate assistive technology are not factors most people have to deal with in their daily lives. Personal elements, such as strong feelings of competence and high self-esteem, and sociocultural elements, such as encouraging, supportive family and friends, have an inestimable value in counteracting these negative forces.

The setting of boundaries, or in Neuman's terms, lines of resistance and defense, emerged as an important part of the resilience displayed by some of the participants in this study. Their boundaries were constantly threatened by insensitive behaviors of medical professionals and overwhelming overprotectiveness by family. The abuse they experienced caused a hardening of defense mechanisms. Because the source of the abuse or barriers cannot be removed, the issue becomes one of management and minimizing the negative impact as much as possible.

Still, the women interviewed who experienced abuse were able to develop a positive sense of sexual self. They tended to be able to recognize their experiences as abusive and took action to reduce or eliminate them or to neutralize their impact. Some of the women interviewed had been so poorly informed about sexuality and life in general that they did not recognize the abuse until much later. The women who took action to end the abuse did so through divorce, counseling, avoidance, and escape. It is a major life challenge for women who have had these experiences to come to terms with them and develop positive sexuality in spite of them. For those with very limited life options, denial becomes the least damaging means of coping available to them.

Women in this study who exhibited characteristics of wellness had learned to reduce their vulnerability. They recognized what type of situation to avoid, be it with a date or a relative, in order to protect their emotional and physical health. Some of the participants who experienced long-term childhood abuse reported learning survival skills, such as talking their way out of it, seeking emotional support outside the family, and learning how to have back-up support available if a situation ever became life threatening.

Prevention

Discussions about strategies for preventing sexual abuse of women with physical disabilities have just begun. Researchers, clinicians, and consumers all decry the lack of attention paid to this need in families, school systems, and social service systems. The following is a list of suggestions, drawn primarily from the work of Sandra Cole (1984–86), describing actions that could be taken by social service workers and clinicians to prevent sexual abuse:

1. Learn to recognize the signs of abuse.
   a. Certain types of injuries (reported or observed)
   b. Behavioral extremes, hyperactivity, mood swings
   c. Sleep disturbances, nightmares
   d. Eating disturbances, loss of weight
   e. Somatic disorders
   f. Fear of intervention
2. Listen to, believe, and act on accounts of abuse.
3. Do everything within your power to prevent institutionalization.
4. Do everything within your power to create opportunities for quality personal assistance.
5. Acknowledge the sexuality of women with disabilities.
6. Acknowledge the basic human rights of women with disabilities.
7. Teach a healthy questioning of authority figures.
8. Teach independent behaviors.
9. Teach healthy sexuality.
10. Reinforce a positive sense of self.

CONCLUSIONS

There is an asexual, dependent, passive stereotype of women with physical disabilities that, in many ways, may lie more at the root of the vulnerability to sexual abuse faced by this population than the disability itself. There is ample evidence in the literature, as confirmed by this qualitative study, that these vulnerabilities do exist. What is seriously lacking, however, are data on the incidence and prevalence of sexual abuse in the population of women with physical disabilities. Research that analyzes the experience of abuse according to recommended definitions and parameters, in correlation with other personal, social, cultural, and environmental variables, will make a major contribution to understanding the many risk factors that disability imposes on women's lives.

REFERENCES

Aiello, D., Capkin, L., & Catania, H. (1983). Strategies and techniques for serving the disabled assault victim: A pilot training program for providers and consumers. *Sexuality and Disability*, 6, 135–144.

American Medical Association. (1992). *Diagnostic and treatment guidelines on domestic violence*. Chicago: Author.

Ammerman, R.T., Cassisi, J.E., Hersen, M., & Van Hasselt, V.B. (1986). Consequences of physical abuse and neglect in children. *Clinical Psychology Review*, *6*, 291–310.

Beckmann, C.R., Gittler, M., Barzansky, B.M., & Beckmann, C.A. (1989). Gynecologic health care of women with disabilities. *Obstetrics & Gynecology*, *74*, 75–79.

Belsky, J. (1980). Child maltreatment: An ecological integration. *American Psychologist*, *35*, 320–335.

Benedict, M.I., White, R.B., Wulff, L.M., & Hall, B.J. (1990). Reported maltreatment in children with multiple disabilities. *Child Abuse & Neglect*, *14*, 207–217.

Benedict, M.I., Wulff, L.M., & White, R.B. (1992). Current parental stress in maltreating and nonmaltreating families of children with multiple disabilities. *Child Abuse & Neglect*, *16*, 155–163.

Bristol, M.M., & Schloper, E. (1984). A developmental perspective on stress and coping in families of autistic children. In J. Blacker (Ed.), *Severely handicapped young children and their families* (pp. 91–142). Orlando, FL: Academic Press.

Camblin, L.D., Jr. (1982). A survey of state efforts in gathering information on child abuse and neglect in handicapped populations. *Child Abuse & Neglect*, *6*, 465–472.

Cole, S.S. (1984–86). Facing the challenges of sexual abuse in persons with disabilities. *Sexuality and Disability*, *7*, 71–88.

Cowen, E.L. (1991). In pursuit of wellness. *American Psychologist*, *46*, 404–408.

Crossmaker, M. (1991). Behind locked doors: Institutional sexual abuse. *Sexuality and Disability*, *9*, 201–220.

Doucette, J. (1986). *Violent acts against disabled women*. Toronto: DisAbled Women's Network.

Finkelhor, D. (1979). *Sexually victimized children*. New York: Free Press.

Finkelhor, D., & Korbin, J. (1988). Child abuse as an international issue. *Child Abuse & Neglect*, *12*, 3–23.

Gagnon, J., & Simon, W. (1970). *Sexual encounters between adults and children*. New York: Sex Information and Education Council of the United States.

Garbarino, J. (1987). The abuse and neglect of special children: An introduction to the issues. In J. Garbarino, P.E. Brookhouser, & K.J. Authier (Eds.), *Special children—special risks: The maltreatment of children with disabilities* (pp. 3–14). New York: Aldine.

Glaser, B.G., & Strauss, A.L. (1967). *Discovery of grounded theory: Strategies for qualitative research*. New York: Aldine.

Glaser, D., & Bentovim, A. (1979). Abuse and risk to handicapped and chronically ill children. *Child Abuse & Neglect*, *3*, 565–575.

Kreigsman, K.H., & Bregman, S. (1985). Women with disabilities at midlife [Special issue: Transition and disability over the life span]. *Rehabilitation Counseling Bulletin*, *29*, 112–122.

Laws, A. (1993). Does a history of sexual abuse in childhood play a role in women's medical problems?: A review. *Journal of Women's Health*, *2*, 165–172.

Light, J., Collier, B., & Parnes, P. (1985). Communicative interaction between young nonspeaking physically disabled children and their primary caregivers. *Augmentative and Alternative Communication*, *1*, 74–83.

McFarlane, J., Christoffel, K., Bateman, L., Miller, V., & Bullock, L. (1991). Assessing for abuse: Self-report versus nurse interview. *Public Health Nursing*, *8*, 245–250.

McFarlane, J., Parker, B., Soeken, K., & Bullock, L. (1992). Assessing for abuse during pregnancy: Severity and frequency of injuries and associated entry into prenatal care. *Journal of the American Medical Association, 267*, 3176–3178.

Muccigrosso, L. (1991). Sexual abuse prevention strategies and programs for persons with developmental disabilities. *Sexuality and Disability, 9*, 261–272.

Mullan, P.B., & Cole, S.S. (1991). Health care providers' perceptions of the vulnerability of persons with disabilities: Sociological frameworks and empirical analyses. *Sexuality and Disability, 9*, 221–242.

Mullins, J.B. (1986). The relationship between child abuse and handicapping conditions. *Journal of School Health, 56*, 134–136.

National Center on Child Abuse and Neglect. (1993). National Center on Child Abuse and Neglect: Study mandated by Congress: New York Times Report. *The New York Times*, October 7.

Neuman, B. (1982). *The Neuman Systems Model: Application to nursing education and practice*. Norwalk, CT: Appleton-Century-Crofts.

Nosek, M.A. (1995). Sexual abuse of women with physical disabilities. In T.N. Monga (Ed.), *Sexuality and disability, physical medicine and rehabilitation: State of the art reviews, 9*(2), 487–502.

Nosek, M.A., Howland, C.A., Young, M.E., Georgiou, D., Rintala, D.H., Foley, C.C., Bennett, J.L., & Smith, Q. (1994). Wellness models and sexuality among women with physical disabilities. *Journal of Applied Rehabilitation Counseling, 25*, 50–58.

Ontario Ministry of Community and Social Services. (1987, April 1). Disabled women more likely to be battered, survey suggests. *The Toronto Star*, F9.

Paddison, P.L., Gise, L.H., Lebovits, A., Strain, J.J., Girasole, D.M, & Levine, J.P. (1990). Sexual abuse and premenstrual syndrome: Comparison between a lower and higher socioeconomic group. *Psychosomatics, 31*, 265.

Patton, M.Q. (1990). *Qualitative evaluation and research methods*. (2nd ed.). Newbury Park, CA: Sage Publications.

Ridington, J. (1989). *Beating the "odds": Violence and women with disabilities* (Position Paper 2). Vancouver, BC, Canada: DisAbled Women's Network: Canada.

Schwartzbeck, C. (1993, May 22). Abuse makes kids aggressive. *The Houston Chronicle*.

Sobsey, D., & Doe, T. (1991). Patterns of sexual abuse and assault. *Sexuality and Disability, 9*, 243–260.

Sobsey, D., & Varnhagen, C. (1989). Sexual abuse and exploitation of people with disabilities: Toward prevention and treatment. In M. Csapo, & L. Gougen (Eds.), *Special education across Canada: Challenges for the '90's*. Vancouver, BC, Canada: Center for Human Development and Research.

Starr, R., Dietrich, K.N., Fischhoff, J., Ceresnie, S., & Zweier, D. (1984). The contribution of handicapping conditions to child abuse. *Topics in Early Childhood Special Education, 4*, 55–69.

Trickett, P.K., & Putnam, F.W. (1993). Impact of child sexual abuse on females: Toward a developmental psychobiological integration. *Psychological Science, 4*, 81–87.

White, M.J., Rintala, D.H., Hart, K.A., & Fuhrer, M.J. (1993). Sexual activities, concerns, and interests of women with spinal cord injury living in the community. *American Journal of Physical Medicine and Rehabilitation, 72*, 372–378.

Womendez, C., & Schneiderman, K. (1991). Escaping from abuse: Unique issues for women with disabilities. *Sexuality and Disability, 9*, 273–280.

Yoshino, S., & Uchida, S. (1981). Sexual problems of women with rheumatoid arthritis. *Archives of Physical Medicine and Rehabilitation, 62*, 122–123.

Zirpoli, T.J., Snell, M.E., & Lloyd, B.H. (1987). Characteristics of persons with mental retardation who have been abused by caregivers. *Journal of Special Education, 21*, 31–41.

Zwerner, J. (1982). A study of issues in sexuality counseling for women with spinal cord injuries [Special issue: Current feminist issues in psychotherapy]. *Women and Therapy, 1*, 91–100.

chapter 14

Teaching Providers to Become Our Allies

Marsha Saxton

Women with physical disabilities and chronic illness are among the most frequent consumers of medical services. Women are more likely to seek medical services than men, and people with disabilities are more likely to require medical assistance. Yet women with disabilities have often had serious difficulties finding appropriate care from health care workers because few such workers have been trained to be sensitive to our particular needs. For women with disabilities, particularly those with a developmental disability or with very severe medical difficulties from an early age, frequent exposure to patronizing attitudes and lack of awareness about the experience of disability can be overwhelming and damaging to one's sense of self-esteem and independence.

The way we as women with disabilities are treated as patients in medical care has a tremendous impact on our self-esteem and our ability to communicate our needs. Likewise, the quality of medical care is greatly affected by the quality of the patient-provider relationship. This chapter examines ways in which the relationship between health providers and women with disabilities can be improved.

HOW HEALTH PROVIDERS REGARD WOMEN WITH DISABILITIES

In the early 1990s, the Project on Women and Disability in Boston decided to address the issues of how the medical system treats women with disabilities. The first program we created offered training and support groups for women with disabilities on assertiveness in our relationships with providers. These seminars have been very successful in setting new models of empowerment for women with disabilities and in improving our health care.

However, another component needed to be addressed—namely, how to improve communication with doctors and other health care providers. First, we need to assess the level of understanding among health care providers. Accordingly, we invited a group of medical practitioners to come to our "Women and Disability Think Tank" to tell us about medical training and also about how disability issues are addressed in medical training and in continuing education for medical professionals.

Through these discussions, we realized that, by virtue of working in hospitals, doctors only see people who are ill and tend to have exposure to people with disabilities who are having medical difficulties. Many health care providers may have limited exposure to persons with disabilities outside the context of a medical setting and thus have little challenge to the stereotyped role of people with disabilities as "patients." Few medical schools have training in the social and political aspects of disability. Disability tends to be regarded solely on the basis of physical, mental, or emotional dysfunction.

RAISING AWARENESS AMONG
MEDICAL STUDENTS AND DOCTORS

The medical system in the United States has evolved to strongly emphasize cure, elimination, or at least suppression of symptoms. People with disabilities or chronic illness who cannot be "cured" of their conditions represent a kind of failure of the medical system in fulfilling its mission. The confusion of medical providers regarding disability issues reveals a fundamental denial that disability is a natural part of human life.

Armed with new knowledge and confidence and some new contacts, we approached some of the medical schools located in the Boston area to offer ourselves as speakers and trainers and to meet with students and faculty. We taught a workshop for Harvard Medical School faculty on disability awareness and basic legal and community resource issues. We started on a very small scale. To date, we have addressed two classes, one for first-year medical students and the other for residents. These orientations were well received by the students who were pleased to meet "real, live women with disabilities" and for the opportunity to interact with people with disabilities outside of the medical setting. We were interacting as peers, simply talking to each other and exchanging important information. Our research continues with regard to ways to improve medical training and how to help train medical professionals to become our allies.

DEALING WITH ANGER

An issue that has resulted from our explorations of relationships between providers and consumers, and between activists and policy makers, is the issue of anger. For many of us, some of the worst aspects of our oppression have been perpetrated by well-intentioned professionals who were truly trying to help us in their own way. Women with disabilities are typically conditioned in our culture to be passive, polite, and grateful. When we experience the abuses from the medical system discussed by other contributors in this volume, naturally we become angry. We experience our anger particularly in the context of the growing support from other women with disabilities. We are especially angry because we recognize that our feelings are legitimate. When we seek a place to vent that anger, and when we righteously rather than politely seek to make changes, it can be enormously confusing to our providers.

Medical practitioners have been trained and conditioned in the medical system to believe that as providers they know what is best for the patient. They view themselves as the experts, and because they have our best interests at heart, we women with disabilities should listen to them and comply with their approaches. Providers may become very hurt, confused, or resentful when confronted with the anger of the people whom they are eager to assist.

The conflicting perception of medical care needs is a particularly difficult issue for both health care providers and consumers. By validating our experience as a civil rights constituency, the Americans with Disabilities Act (1990) has brought to the fore previously repressed feelings of anger that may on occasion become focused on medical and human services providers. Galvanizing this anger and directing it toward new solutions to health care needs is the logical next step. The women's rights movement—with its current successes in focusing on women's health—could serve as a model for resolving this potential conflict and for creating a new model for partnership between physicians and women with disabilities. As reflected by Gill (Chapter 1), Waxman (Chapter 15), and Nosek (Chapter 2), the emergence of civil rights issues for women with disabilities has provided opportunities for empowerment and visibility.

PARTNERS IN HEALTH CARE DELIVERY

Our approach to working with medical students and other health providers sends an important message: that we are partners in the health delivery system. That is, the patient has a lot to teach the provider. Second, those of us with disabilities can also be "providers." We are represented in traditional medical areas as physicians, nurses, or physical or occupational therapists, as well as in the independent living and advocacy centers and in the self-help groups. As the number of women with disabilities becoming "providers" increases, we will be able to effect change both from within and outside the traditional health care system.

But for the present, how can providers respond to this anger? I would like to offer a point of view about dealing with the anger of individuals from a newly empowered, newly arising, civil rights constituency: When people become angry with us, it is confusing and scary, but we can also view it as an opportunity for dialogue. Indeed, these angry individuals may feel safe enough with you to try to communicate with you. What you can do is listen. Listen as undefensively as possible. Try to appreciate what they are saying in the largest context. Remember that thus far you have done the best you could to think about and respond to their needs. Get support for yourself from colleagues for your own feelings in reaction to this anger. But be open to learning more and responding even better. It is not always going to be an easy task, but ultimately the approach will open the lines of communication.

CONCLUSIONS

This chapter discusses four ways to improve the relationships between health care providers and women with disabilities. These include assertiveness training for women with disabilities, greater exposure of providers to people with disabilities outside of the medical context, increased understanding on the part of providers of the anger of people with disabilities, and ultimately greater opportunities for women with disabilities to themselves become health care providers.

FURTHER READINGS

Americans with Disabilities Act of 1990 (ADA), PL 101-336. (July 26, 1990). Title 42, U.S.C. 12101 et seq.: *U.S. Statues at Large, 104,* 327–328.

Boston Women's Health Book Collective. (1991). *Our bodies, ourselves.* New York: Simon & Schuster.

Saxton, M., & Howe, F. (Eds.). (1987). *With wings: An anthology of literature by and about women with disabilities.* New York: The Feminist Press.

Saxton, M. (1983). Peer counseling. In I.K. Zola & Nancy Crewe (Eds.), *Independent living for physically disabled people.* San Francisco: Jossey-Bass.

Saxton, M.A. (1985). Peer counseling training program for disabled women: A tool for social and individual change. In M. Deegan & N.A. Brooks (Eds.), *Women and disability: The double handicap.* New Brunswick, NJ: Transaction Books.

Saxton, M. (1991, September/October). Disability and the medical system. *Ms.,* 32–33.

Saxton, M. (1994). Confronting my foot doctor. In *Misdiagnosis: Woman as a disease* (pp. 223–227). New York: The People's Medical Society.

chapter **15**

Commentary on Sexuality and Reproductive Health

Barbara Faye Waxman

First, a note about terminology: In this discussion about formulating research priorities regarding disabled women's sexual and reproductive health, this author uses *disability-first* language rather than the rehabilitation-oriented *people-first* language. This use of language results from the author's view of disability as a social identity, much like being African American or Latina. Hence, rather than attempting to downplay this state of being, the term *disabled* is used to denote a prideful identity.

CONSIDERING THE WHOLE PERSON

In a 1994 conference, Whipple (1994) laid the foundation for a discussion of sexuality and disabled women by stating:

> Today, sexuality is seen as an important aspect of health and of personality function. It enhances the quality of life, it fosters personal growth, and contributes to personal fulfillment. When the term sexuality is viewed holistically, it refers to the totality of being; it includes all the qualities—biological, psychological, emotional, social, cultural, and spiritual—that make people who they are.

This sex-positive statement is a significant departure from past references to disabled women as sources of sexual desire, as life partners, and as childbearers. In disabled women's history, the professional literature for the most part focused on the medical management of fertility and was virtually silent on female sexual function and reproductive health. When these latter issues are still discussed within a clinical framework, the professional is often guided by sexist and heterosexist thought and by eugenic beliefs.

Indeed, as pointed out by Rousso (1994), "Whether or not we agree, the traditional measure of success of women in our culture is her capacity to attract and keep a partner, particularly a man, and to bear children." Attitudes have not changed much between 1978 and 1994. Becker (1978) pinpointed the predicament of spinal cord–injured women, when asking about their sexual function. They were told by physicians that "a female paraplegic can have intercourse more easily than a male paraplegic, since she does not have to participate actively. Although some such women have no subjective feeling of orgasm, they are perfectly capable of satisfying their husbands."

The few progressive publications that began counteracting the past ideologies have been authored by disabled women themselves. These books and articles have a unified voice that generally speaks to two points: 1) the history of medical abuse and discrimination toward disabled women's sexual and reproductive lives, and 2) an affirmative action declaration of the rights to bear and rear children and be free of sexual and reproductive violence. From these new agendas, research projects and health service models that are directed by disabled women themselves are thriving, using public and private funds.

The other sources of reformative writings, research, and reproductive health service delivery are rehabilitation professionals who have listened closely to disabled women's concerns about their feelings of invisibility as women. Jackson (1994) reported that "one female paraplegic approached me and expressed her inability to receive total health care, which included gynecological, obstetrical, and urological, as well as rehabilitative care. There were clinics for males—fertility, urology." Rehabilitation professionals like Dr. Jackson have taken action to establish women's clinics in a rehabilitation setting, meeting at least some of the voiced needs of the disabled women's community.

We hope that this book will influence the future direction of research and practice regarding disabled women's health. It plays an important role for future research in not only defining the problems, but expanding the notion of function—in sexual practices, in childbearing, in parenthood, in sexual identity, and in notions of sexual health, which will offer disabled women greater access to life choices.

However, we will not gain that knowledge and will not have access to a broader range of choices until tomorrow. Today, disabled women are still caught in a horrible dilemma of health risk. Up until now, society has not invested resources for finding answers to the following questions: How many disabled women are of childbearing age? Is sexual violence an inevitable hazard of being disabled and female? What helps or hinders disabled women's social success? What are the rates of cervical and breast cancer, sexually transmitted diseases, and infertility in the disabled women population? How do disabled mothers learn adaptive child care skills? Why do disabled lesbians have less access to health services than disabled heterosexual women? What are the interactions between hormones and disabling conditions? Which factors lead to the high rate of caeserean sections performed on disabled women in labor? How are gynecological services provided to disabled women? Why do disabled wives have a higher divorce rate than disabled husbands? Which neurological structures account for sexual responses in disabled women who have impaired sensation?

To understand the significance of the research agenda on disabled women's sexual and reproductive health presented in this section, the reader must know something about the historical basis of scientific indifference to disabled women's reproductive health. We can consider four major facts.

First, disability research has not been gender-specific. Indeed, Fine and Asch (1988, p. 3) contend, "To date, almost all research on disabled men and women seems to assume the irrelevance of gender, race, ethnicity, sexual orientation, or social class. Having a disability presumably eclipses these dimensions of social experience." However, when looking closely at disabled women's health status, these factors seem to move into prominence.

For instance, studies conclude that a woman's health status increases when her economic status improves (Taylor, 1992). Verduyn (1994) alluded to a paper out of New York that describes a pregnant spinal cord-injured woman with a decubitis ulcer. He argues that the ulcer occurred because of socioeconomic factors (i.e., not having adequate personal assistance services or enough information and access to health services). Kirshbaum (1994) came to a similar conclusion when she observed, "The literature implies that the abuse in families with heads of households who have cognitive disabilities is due to cognitive limits, and does not separate out those women with a high degree of past and current violence." The lesson to be learned from these examples is clear: the need to develop a new conceptual framework for appraising the health status of disabled women that recognizes that the fundamental restrictions disabled people face are located in the surroundings they encounter, rather than within the disabled individual.

The second fact of scientific indifference appears, with the almost exclusive focus of sexuality and disability research, on spinal cord-injured men. There are a couple of reasons for this. As Whipple (Chapter 5) points out, there are more spinal cord-injured males than females, and it is much easier to study sexual response in males, who have external genitalia. However, the social factors outweigh the physiological ones. Fine and Asch (1988) observe that, "The thrust of rehabilitation study and policy was the war-wounded or work-injured person who was invariably a male. . . . Concerns with emasculation may promote efforts directed at the locus of the masculinity/dependence contradiction, not toward those at the redundant intersection of femininity and dependence. Certainly, the social imperative seems to have been to study the wounded male" (p. 3).

The consequences of studying primarily men (especially those with traumatic or late-onset disabilities) have been that either research results have been extrapolated to the lives of disabled women, or disabled women have been missing in the literature; that is, until now. The scientific controversy of deriving conclusions about women's health from research on men, moved the National Institutes of Health to establish its Office on Women's Health Research. Finally, the controversy has come into focus within disability research with this new research agenda.

Evidence of the third fact of scientific indifference can be found in an indictment made by Kirshbaum (1994): "Historically, the research has been very pathologically focused; like whether the children of disabled mothers have poor body images." This focus exposes a societal view that disabled women are not whole women; rather, they are seen as defective women. In fact, three fourths of people surveyed believe that maternal disability is cause enough to restrict childbearing (Waxman, 1993). Many physicians conform their clinical practice to this societal view. Welner (1994) stated that "women with cognitive impairments cannot be relied upon to contracept, and that the only options are physician-controlled, long acting contraceptives such as Depo-Provera and Norplant." These findings support Verduyn's (1994) contention that medicine is, "still stuck with a social belief which can be found in major medical centers that the only option to a disabled woman's pregnancy is an abortion, then tubal ligation."

The last reason for the invisibility of disabled women in sexual and reproductive health research underpins each of the other three reasons: eugenics. Eugenics has as its objective 1) to deny people deemed biologically defective by society the rights to bear, birth, and rear children; and 2) to pressure people with desired traits to reproduce. To those ends, many disabled women have been violated with the instruments of eugenics: physical, communication, and clinical barriers to obstetrical and gynecological services; involuntary sterilization, forced abortion, sex segregation, and injections of harmful contraceptives; and the loss of child custody.

The French philosopher Michel Foucault (1980) described in his treatise *The History of Sexuality* the lives of people who are considered by society to exist outside the boundaries of reproduction—in other words, people who are not expected to reproduce or whose reproductive capacity poses a societal threat: gay men, lesbians, transsexuals, transvestites, and disabled people. O'Toole (1994) pointed out that contemporary American society segregates and stratifies its sexual minority communities, creating, in effect, a sexual caste system. For disabled women, who are at the bottom of this hierarchy, this has meant restricting voluntary sexuality and reproduction through social policies and practices.

Theoretically and pragmatically, the research agenda on disabled women's sexual and reproductive health is a force against eugenics. Within the context of this section are the principles that disabled women's reproductive health is valuable, childbearing and rearing are voluntary and personal choices, and their opportunities for and experience of sexual satisfaction are equally important. Indeed, sexuality and parenting are no longer (and in fact never were) just for other people.

SCOPE OF PRESENTATIONS

During the planning stages of the 1994 conference on sexual and reproductive health for women with disabilities, a controversy arose as to whether the physiology of sexuality and reproduction and the psychosocial-political aspects of disabled women's sexual and reproductive lives should be discussed in the same or separate groups. One voice expressed concern that physiological concerns would be overshadowed by the breadth and depth of those three other dimensions. A second voice underscored the significance of preventing the construction of artificial barriers between dynamic human functions. Fortunately, information exchanges among the participants during the priority-setting session on research encompassed the various aspects of sexual and reproductive health. Physiological health issues cannot be separated from the life situation of disabled women or anyone else, without distorting research findings. The danger of Cartesian mind-body dualism on research would lead Verduyn to instead conclude, as noted earlier, that decubitus ulcers are concomitants to the pregnancies of spinal cord-injured women or would have Kirshbaum agree that abuse of children by cognitively disabled mothers is a function of their neurological condition. As stated before, those studying disabled women's health status must consider a paradigm that recognizes that health status is affected by a person's economic, political, and social status.

Nevertheless, the scope of the presentations were categorized according to whether they were physiological in orientation or psychosocial. The approach of the panel on physiology defines disability as primarily an individual problem. These problems stem from functional limitations, which can be ameliorated by professional intervention. The intervention would correct through treatment or cure most disabilities or their functional concomitants. Corrections are attempted to be made to the point that disabled individuals could comply with the expectations and physical and behavioral attributes in order to participate in community life. Within this framework, men with diabetes, multiple sclerosis, and spinal cord injuries seek penile implants to restore their erections, and women with hip contractures who cannot have conventional intercourse have hip surgery to have intercourse in socially prescribed positions. In addition, sexual and reproductive research on disabled women has focused on those who are presumed to represent the norm: the spinal cord injured. It is also the framework of studies of disabled women's functional limitations as a means to learn more about nondisabled women's sexual function, rather than an end in itself.

The panel on psychosocial-political concerns views the major problems of disabled individuals in a disabling social and physical environment rather than as a result of any defects or deficiencies of disabled people themselves. So according to this understanding of disability, the boundaries of sexual health expand to include the unconventional, and the solutions are found in public policies and a deconstruction of the sexual and reproductive hierarchy.

What became clear as the exchange progressed is that, in order for significant changes to occur, partnerships must be forged between those who frame their research from within a medical paradigm and those who frame their research from within a psychosocial-political perspective. In fact, when describing future research priorities, most of the authors in this section incorporate psychosocial and biomedical components. For instance, with regard to how hormonal contraceptives interact with various disabilities, there are now efforts to study how the provision of contraceptive information differs between disabled and nondisabled women; and, to go deeper, among disability groups. The clinical concern of improving methods for managing labor and delivery for disabled mothers generates the sociopolitical question of how accessible obstetricians are to disabled mothers. Still another physiological question focuses on the impact of neurological disabilities on sexual response, which leads to an inquiry about how sexual beliefs about disabled women affect their opportunities to form intimate relationships. These examples demonstrate that there is a basis for collaboration between the paradigms and that such a collaboration can only enhance the work of both groups. However, many barriers still exist to that collaboration.

Among the authors of this section, there is some tension as well as disagreement over future research approaches. Most likely, the tension relates to differing theoretical models, as well as whether one worked within the established research infrastructure. Some individuals had formerly been denied access to decision making and funding for disabled women's health research. The latter group was predominantly composed of disabled women scholars and researchers.

Another source of conflict concerns traditional relationships between providers and consumers and between activists and policy makers. When the consumer is a professional at the same time, a demand to share the power and define the problems of the subject population challenges those in the research establishment to rethink their own assumptions about where disabled women's problems are rooted. This is inevitable until disabled women are finally playing a prominent role in defining and conducting the research.

Agencies such as the National Institute on Disability and Rehabilitation Research are implementing a policy on Constituency-Oriented Research and Dissemination (CORD). CORD is defined as "an approach to research, training and dissemination in which appropriate members of relevant constituencies will participate in a meaningful way at key stages of the research process." The key stages include identifying research needs; setting priorities; requesting proposal development; the application preparation process; peer review; making awards; conducting projects; dissemination; and utilization and evaluations (Zola, 1994).

CORD ushers in "a new era of a prominent role for disabled people in the formulation of disability-related research" (Zola, 1994). This new research policy grows out of an acknowledgment that disabled people have a different level of experience with disability than do researchers who are not disabled. Researchers who are part of the research establishment have not always had an accurate perspective on disability. The evidence has been in the concentration of the research on reducing functional limitations in the individual, instead of focusing on policy.

Aggravating the situation further, those in power believe disabled individuals do not have the credentials to conduct research. During the closing plenary session of one conference, a woman stood and angrily stated that disabled women must pay their dues before they can think of being awarded research grants. Many disabled women want to be or are already highly trained, but those in power have not typically opened the doors to disabled researchers. Not having access is at the foundation of oppression. If people in power wish to enhance the lives of disabled women, they will promote disabled women as leaders to influence research, policy, and service delivery.

CONCLUSIONS

The ultimate aim of sexual and reproductive research of disabled women is moving from the medical management of fertility prevention to attention to sexual pleasure and response, safe reproductive choices, safe pregnancy, labor, and delivery, and the ability to form healthy and loving relationships, healthy sexual identities, and a rich sexual culture within the disability community. The success of the research will depend on the influences of two factors. First, disabled women must define their own life problems.

Here is where initial interviewing studies can be a rich source of research ideas. Understanding the realities of disabled women's lives depends on the investigator's viewing disabled women as the experts, viewing disabled women as a unique group, and not positioning nondisabled women as the standard of measurement.

The second influence is to ensure that disabled women have access to knowledge and play a role in designing interventions that will enable them to protect their own health and safety. In the deepest sense, research will be successful when the life of a disabled woman is no longer expendable; when harmful contraceptives are replaced by those that are in harmony with her body; when obstetricians learn safe vaginal delivery techniques; when sexual violence is not an inevitable hazard of being both disabled and female; when disabled lesbians no longer live a furtive life, having fallen into a crack between the lesbian and disability communities; and when disabled girls grow up with the confidence that they have a positive sexual future.

REFERENCES

Becker, E. (1978). *Female sexuality following spinal cord injury*. Bloomington, IN: Accent Special.

Fine, M., & Asch, A. (1988). Beyond pedestals. In A. Asch & M. Fine (Eds.), *Women with disabilities: Essays in psychology, culture, and politics* (pp. 1–37). Philadelphia: Temple University Press.

Foucault, M. (1980). *The history of sexuality* (Vol. 1). New York: Vintage Books.

Jackson, A. (1994, May). *Development of research to improve management of pregnancy and delivery*. Paper presented at the conference on The Health of Women with Physical Disabilities: Setting a Research Agenda for the 90s, Bethesda, MD.

Kirshbaum, M. (1994, May). *Parenting*. Paper presented at the conference on The Health of Women with Physical Disabilities: Setting a Research Agenda for the 90s, Bethesda, MD.

O'Toole, C. (1994, May). *Lesbian issues*. Paper presented at the conference on The Health of Women with Physical Disabilities: Setting a Research Agenda for the 90s, Bethesda, MD.

Rousso, H. (1994, May). *Sense of self*. Paper presented at the conference on The Health of Women with Physical Disabilities: Setting a Research Agenda for the 90s, Bethesda, MD.

Taylor, M.L. (1992). Women's health and public policy. In R.D. Apple (Ed.), *Women, health, and medicine in America: A historical handbook* (pp. 383–402). New Brunswick, NJ: Rutgers University Press.

Verduyn, W. (1994, May). *Obstetrical issues for women with disabilities*. Paper presented at the conference on The Health of Women with Physical Disabilities: Setting a Research Agenda for the 90s, Bethesda, MD.

Waxman, B.F. (1994). Up against eugenics: Disabled women's challenge to receive reproductive health services. *Sexuality and Disability, 12*(2), 155–171.

Welner, S. (1994, May). *Gynecological issues for women*. Paper presented at the conference on The Health of Women with Physical Disabilities: Setting a Research Agenda for the 90s, Bethesda, MD.

Whipple, B. (1994, May). *Sexual response in women with physical disabilities.* Paper presented at the conference on The Health of Women with Physical Disabilities: Setting a Research Agenda for the 90s, Bethesda, MD.

Zola, I.K. (1994). Towards inclusion: The role of people with disabilities in policy and research issues in the United States—A historical and political analysis. In M. Rioux & M. Bach (Eds.), *Disability is not measles* (Chapter 3). North York, ON, Canada: Roher Institute.

STRESS AND WELL-BEING

Danuta M. Krotoski and Roberta B. Trieschmann

Studies have established that prolonged exposure to stress has a major impact on health and well-being. Women with disabilities encounter the same stressors as other women in society, yet as a consequence of their disability, they may be exposed to even greater sources of stress. They face the stress of having to function in an environment that may be attitudinally or architecturally inaccessible, of being socially disadvantaged (because, as a group, women with disabilities have some of the lowest incomes), and of facing additional prejudice as women of color or because of sexual orientation.

This section on stress and well-being was designed to explore the relationships between the physiological basis of the stress response and physical and emotional health. The section also has as its goal the identification of traditional interventions and the development of new approaches to stress amelioration and reducing the negative impact of stressors.

The experience of stress in the lives of women with disabilities has been eloquently captured by Crewe and Clarke (Chapter 16), who relate how women describe their own feelings about themselves and those around them. How can the experiences of these women be translated into more effective approaches to a more healthy lifestyle? How can these experiences be described on a biological level?

Tsigos and Chrousos (Chapter 17) provide an excellent background on the biology of the stress response by reminding us that this mechanism has evolved to allow us to cope with intermittent adversity. The stress response physiologically prepares the individual organism for heightened awareness and arousal, the proverbial "fight or flight" response, while conversely suppressing vegetative functions such as feeding and reproduction. The problem lies with the prolongation of the physiological response. Central to the response is the protein, corticotropin-releasing hormone (CRH), that mediates the "fight or flight" response but also serves in the

189

complex regulation of the immune system and in some aspects of nervous system function. Gold, Goodwin, and Chrousos (1988) have shown that prolonged stress, particularly in young women, is later followed by an increased risk of depression. Sternberger (1992) reported on studies in her laboratory that show that exposing rats to prolonged stress results in their becoming susceptible to autoimmune diseases. Information such as this may explain the anecdotal reports of increased susceptibility to urinary tract infections or depression in women with disabilities.

How the individual perceives the stressor is also important in determining its impact. Rintala, Hart, and Fuhrer (1992) (Chapter 18) described the results of the studies they have been performing to identify perceived stress in men and women with spinal cord injuries. Because the impact of an objective stressor may be mediated by the person's perception of stress, one person's long-term physiological response may be quite different from that of another individual, and gender or type of disability may play additional roles. It has been suggested (Cohen & Williamson, 1988; Rintala, Young, Hart, Clearman, & Fuhrer, 1992) that factors in the person's life, such as income, education, employment, personal relationship, and physical well-being, can have a profound effect on how the individual responds to stressful situations. Gender and hormonal status may also play an important role both in perception and in potential physiological impact of the same physiological response. Interventions that will alleviate the impact of stress must take into account the personal response.

Given that stress will always be part of each person's experience, this section explores possible approaches to reducing its impact. Baum (Chapter 19) has developed a model that can be used to reduce points of stress between an individual, the caregiver, and the physical environment. The goal of such a model is to identify interaction points and the degree of stress they may generate and then to develop strategies to reduce stressors for both parties. Although this model has been developed for persons with Alzheimer's disease, it can be modified for use in other situations. Baum's paradigm structures interventions that lead to enhanced independence on the part of the person with the disability and improved quality of life for him or her and the caregiver.

Patrick (Chapter 20) presents an overview of traditional methods that are currently utilized for stress reduction, and Trieschmann (Chapter 21) introduces a new approach to life management that includes reorienting the person's concepts of energy and life force by restructuring his or her environment.

Five major areas of inquiry are raised in this section. Little is known about the biological basis for stress and the related health consequences in people with disabilities. We also need to know more about the types of environmental stressors in the lives of women with physical disabilities, learn more about personal response styles to stress that are effective, develop effective interventions that reduce the harmful effects of stress yet build on those effects that are positive, and identify new ways of measuring positive outcomes.

Within the context of physiological responses, we need to know whether the stress syndrome has a differential impact according to the person's gender or type of disability, especially among those that vary according to duration and presence or absence of cognitive changes and whether the disability is progressive or static in nature. What is the interaction between stress and disability on the reproductive system? How are women with early-onset disabilities affected, particularly those subjected to sexual abuse as children or to public stripping as described by Carol Gill in her chapter. What is the influence of the duration of the disability on the hypothalamic–pituitary–adrenal axis? What is the relationship between the physiological basis of stress and the incidence of secondary disabilities that may occur after living 20, 30, or 40 years with a disability?

A second group of issues that require more study include environmental stressors faced by all people with disabilities. These include social and attitudinal issues, economic issues, physiologic function, environmental barriers, access issues, relationships, and geographic or urban issues. What is the influence of the number and type of roles in a person's life on their health and response study to stress? What are the differences in a person's coping styles and their long-term health consequences?

A third area of research should focus on the individual's response style to stress. How does the individual's awareness of stress affect their health, how does it vary by gender and lifestyle, and how does it vary over the long term?

Research is clearly needed to develop interventions that reduce either a person's response to stress or a person's perception of stress. Studies should include measurements of the effectiveness of current interventions, as well as identifying new alternative approaches that may include community-based programs as well as energy management techniques.

REFERENCES

Cohen, S., & Williamson, G.M. (1988). Perceived stress in a probability sample of the United States. In S. Oskamp & S. Spacapan (Eds.), *The social psychology of health: Claremont symposium on applied social psychology.* Newbury Park, CA: Sage.

Gold, P.W., Goodwin, F.K., & Chrousos, G.P. (1988). Clinical and biochemical manifestations of depression: Relation to the neurobiology of stress. *New England Journal of Medicine, 319,* 348–353 (Part 1), 413–420 (Part 2).

Rintala, D.H., Young, M.E., Hart, K.A., Clearman, R.R., & Fuhrer, M.J. (1992). Social support and the well-being of persons with spinal cord injury living in the community. *Rehabilitation Psychology, 37,* 155–163.

Sternberger, E.M. (1992). The stress response and the regulation of inflammatory disease. *Annals of Internal Medicine, 117,* 854–866.

chapter 16

Stress and Women with Disabilities

Nancy M. Crewe and Nancy Clarke

Women with disabilities contend with many stressors, including major life changes and frequent daily hassles. Some disabilities involve pain and illness as well as anxiety about the future course of the condition. Low rates of employment cause some to suffer from poverty, inadequate nutrition, and low levels of fitness. Increased vulnerability to physical and sexual abuse are further sources of stress. Limited opportunities for social interaction and support and reduced access to pleasurable experiences can affect resilience. This chapter discusses personal examples that demonstrate these factors and provides sources of information about stress management techniques.

MULTIPLE LEVELS OF STRESS

Women with disabilities are subject to double, triple, or even quadruple jeopardy with respect to stressors in their lives. They face the stress of being socially disadvantaged as women and as individuals with disabilities. In addition, some may face prejudice as women of color or because of sexual orientation. Surprisingly, these issues are not extensively addressed in the literature. Much has been written about how stress may cause illness, but little has been published about how illness or disability may produce stress.

Stress has been defined as "the nonspecific response of the body to any demand made upon it" (Selye, 1974), and stressors can be physical, psychological, and interpersonal. Walter Cannon (1932), an eminent physiologist at Harvard Medical School, was the first to describe the body's reaction to stress. Numerous changes, such as increased muscle tension, heart rate and output, blood pressure, and perspiration, prepare the body for dealing with a threat through either escape or direct confrontation.

Cannon identified this as the *fight or flight response*. Although this reaction is effective in dealing with immediate physical threats, it produces deleterious effects when one is in an ongoing state of arousal due to chronic stressors.

Hans Selye (1974), one of the foremost researchers in this area, identified three stages of stress reactivity. The physiological changes of the flight or fight response are characteristic of Selye's Stage 1, the alarm reaction. Stage 2, resistance, ensues if the stressor is compatible with adaptation. At that point, the signs of the alarm reaction fade or disappear, and resistance to stress rises above normal. After a long period of exposure, however, adaptation energy is depleted, and the person moves to Stage 3, exhaustion. A more detailed description of the physiological consequences of stress follows in Chapter 17.

Greenberg (1993) developed the following model of stress: A life situation is perceived as stressful, which leads to emotional arousal and psychological arousal, resulting in consequences to health and well-being. The following anonymous poem, written by a person with chronic disease, demonstrates the repercussions of disability-related stressors.

The Basket

The moon's soft glow
  brings little peace
In spite of heralding
  the end of day.
Another day of unmet goals,
  of broken promises,
  of shouts and tears.
Another day, stolen by pain
  and shaken by fear.
Work unfinished in hours
  stretched thin and fragile by pain.
Love unspoken in moments unsurped
  by anger and frustration.
No, I can't go to your game—
  I need to rest.
No, we can't afford it.
No, I didn't get the job.
No.
No.
The slippery barricades, the failed intentions,
  the chameleon dreams
Lie tangled in an ever-growing heap
  of threats,
Sneering at me in the morning,
Hissing in my ears at night,
Like a basket of asps
Beneath my bed.

STRESSORS FACED BY WOMEN WITH DISABILITIES

Carol Gill has said that the problems of women with disabilities are those of all women, carried to an extreme. Although not always unique, various stressors have special relevance to women with disabilities.

Life Events and Change

One frequently used measure of vulnerability to stress is a life-events scale, such as the one developed by Holmes and Holmes (1967). It identifies the number of changes, both positive and negative, that have occurred in a person's life during the past year. They include, for example, getting married, being fired from a job, and experiencing the death of a relative or close friend. Consider for a moment the number of changes faced by a woman with a new disability. She might experience involuntary admission to a rehabilitation hospital, interruption of ordinary activities, separation from family, forced involvement in new activities, inability to independently carry out self-care activities, and changes in appearance, among other things.

A woman with a more long-standing disability may face fewer changes, but even ordinary transitions typically entail more complex demands than other people would experience. For example, as a result of a move, she may need to find a new personal assistant, search for accessible housing, or obtain clearance to use special transportation systems. The need for a new physician also may involve a more difficult search than that undertaken by other newcomers.

Hassles

Kanner and Lazarus (1981) posited that everyday life hassles are even more detrimental to health than major life events. The reason is that they are chronic and unrelenting. Hassles are a major issue for persons with physical disabilities. Finding reliable personal assistants was identified by one person as the most difficult and time-consuming task in her life. For the woman with a mobility impairment, accessibility must be considered everywhere she intends to go. Transportation is likely to require advance planning and perhaps extra cost. Unshoveled sidewalks in winter can become insurmountable barriers. The effect of people staring may take a psychological toll. Every outing is likely to involve extra planning and waiting. Even when she arrives at her destination, the woman with a disability often runs the risk of being turned away by proprietors who are unwilling or unprepared to serve her. Fortunately, this overt rejection is becoming less common, thanks to passage of the Americans with Disabilities Act (PL 101-336). Time constraints constitute a chronic hassle—everything takes longer, and everything takes more effort.

Absence of Uplifts

Lazarus (1984) also identified the absence of "uplifts" (positive events) as stressful and problematic. Clearly, the common sources of uplifts for most people—relationships, social support, achievements, and pleasures—are often limited for women with disabilities. Beginning with relationships, Rousso (Chapter 9) has found that young women with early-onset disabilities must wait longer to date and to have any sexual experience compared with their peers without disabilities. DeLoach (1989), in a study of 501 University of Illinois alumni with disabilities, found that women with disabilities were less likely to be married (47.9% of women were married compared with 65.7% of the men with disabilities) and more likely to remain single (41.1% of women vs. 26.5% of men). (*Note*: The remaining members of the sample were separated, widowed, divorced, or of unknown status.) Divorce also seems to be more frequent, according to professionals who have extensive contact with women who have disabilities (Crewe, Athelstan, & Krumberger, 1979; Fine & Asch, 1988), although more reliable data on this matter are needed.

Relative isolation likewise contributes to the shortage of social support uplifts for many women with disabilities. Most women with disabilities are not employed, so they do not have this avenue for meeting new people. Further barriers for many include generalized social rejection as well as problems with accessibility and transportation.

Achievements are a powerful source of uplifts for many people, but opportunities for achievement by women with disabilities are limited because they are effectively stripped of the usual roles of worker, wife, and mother (see Gill, Chapter 10). Without these opportunities to contribute to family and society, a woman may be left with functions that seem trivial or invisible. The uplifts that come from pleasurable activities such as travel, entertainment, and the arts may be likewise unavailable because of cost.

Poverty

Employment issues are critical to understanding sources of stress for women with disabilities. According to a national poll (Harris, 1986), approximately two thirds of all persons with disabilities are unemployed. Various studies (Benefield & Head, 1984; Koestler, 1983; Vash, 1982) have found that unemployment is worst of all for the women in this group. In addition, DeLoach (1989) found significant relationships between the type of work that men and women do. She documented correlations between gender and choice of college major, gender and part-time versus full time employment, and gender and salary level. Women with disabilities are the lowest paid of any group of workers.

Inadequate Nutrition

Many women with disabilities may experience inadequate nutrition as a result of poverty. Without jobs or with poorly paying jobs, they lack money for sufficient fresh, nutritious food. Lack of readily available transportation and difficulty handling heavy parcels may also interfere with obtaining such items as produce and dairy products.

Lower Levels of Fitness

Insufficient exercise and lower levels of fitness may be related to mobility limitations that complicate movement. Lack of financial resources may also prohibit joining a health club or purchasing exercise equipment. Physical activity serves as an antidote to stress for many people, but that outlet frequently is unavailable to women with disabilities.

Pain and Illness

Pain is a chronic problem for many women with disabilities. As demonstrated in the poem reprinted earlier in this chapter, pain is clearly a direct source of stress as well as a contributor to changes in life experiences that exacerbate stress. The disability community has worked hard to demonstrate that having a disability does not necessarily mean that one is sick. Although this is certainly true for most people with stable conditions, others with chronic disease must also deal with the stress imposed by feeling ill and/or by regarding the progress of the condition with uncertainty. They may worry about the changes that could come tomorrow or in the future and how these changes will affect their abilities and quality of life. They may also fear that future changes will threaten intimate and social relationships.

Vulnerability

The reported incidence of sexual abuse among women with disabilities varies, but it is appallingly high (Moglia, 1986). One study (Finkelhor, 1994) reported that approximately 25% of women with disabilities have experienced abuse, compared with 9% of women in the general population. However, only about half of the cases may be reported (Chapter 13). The primary threat may come from family and relatives or from abusive or aggressive personal assistants. Women who require help with activities of daily living have to entrust their well-being and their very lives to those poorly paid and often transient workers, sometimes with tragic results. In addition, abusive intimate relationships may contribute to stress for an unknown number of women.

Sexual abuse and other manifestations of personal devaluation not only trigger stress in the moment, but they have a profound long-term psychological impact. Alice Riger (1993) is a psychologist with a disability who believes that a central issue for women with disabilities is that of shame—a deep, irrational shame born of early and continuing experiences with a devaluing society. Of all the sources of stress just listed, deep psychological pain must surely be the most pernicious and the one most in need of healing.

Three personal accounts by women with disabilities provide examples of various stressors and their impact on quality of life. Listening to their individual voices may further illuminate these issues prior to the discussion of possible interventions.

Cindy   Cindy is a 39-year-old Caucasian woman, married with 3 children, ages 8, 9, and 14. She has had arthritis in her knees and lower back for 7 years, and now she must use a walker or a wheelchair in order to be mobile. When we talked she had just been informed that she was going to need back surgery because of disc damage and deterioration.

"My two younger kids have never had a healthy mother. I've never gone swimming with them at the beach, never gone horseback riding with them. They've never seen me as a normal mother. They've had to help me with chores around the house since they were little, and they get mad sometimes when I can't go with them to play. My oldest daughter has had to take on tremendous responsibilities; she does the laundry, she washes the floors, and she fills in for me with the younger kids at outside games and stuff." Cindy's husband is very supportive and gave up a job in which he traveled extensively so he could be of more help around the house. Cindy says she feels guilty about what she has done to her family. She tries to make up for it by always being there for the kids whenever they need her, but she feels like it is not enough. She says her kids were entitled to a healthy mother, and instead they got her. She wonders if her kids and her husband will resent her at some point. She is afraid that her husband may find a woman he can have a "real" life with, and Cindy says she would not blame him if he does.

Cindy says she rarely relaxes. "I feel like I have to keep going, keep active, make up for all the things I can't do for my family. It's so unfair to them. I try to keep quiet about how much pain I'm in most of the time, because they don't deserve this. Then sometimes I want to scream and yell about how frustrated I am! That's when I think I'm just crazy. I can't seem to find a balance that will benefit everyone, and I owe it to my family to do that."

Cindy's husband insisted on speaking to me, after my conversation with her. He told me that Cindy is the world's best mother and wife and that the family feels privileged to have her. He and his children try to get Cindy to slow down or tell them when things are bad for her, but she will not do that. He says that the marriage and family life sometimes become strained because everyone is busy trying to figure out how everyone else is feeling. He wishes they could all just relax and enjoy their lives, but they never seem to quite get there. They are all so busy worrying about each other that it is rare for them to have a normal day.

Anna Anna is a 45-year-old African American woman, single with no children. Anna served as a nurse in Vietnam during the war and has since been diagnosed with war-related posttraumatic stress disorder (PTSD) and non-Hodgkin's lymphoma, which the Veterans Administration (VA) attributes to exposure to dioxin (Agent Orange). She has one arm amputated because of lymphoma and is now facing a lower leg amputation.

"I just never feel good. I'm either having nightmares about the war, about our hospital being overrun, or I'm deciding whether I want to live or die. Sometimes I think it would be peaceful if I die. I probably will anyway; how much more of my body can they cut off before it's all gone? . . . Stress is just a way of life for me. PTSD is normal for me. I don't sleep much, I always feel like I'm in a race against time. I don't get too close to people, because it's easier to be by myself. I've never had a romantic relationship since I left Vietnam, and now I know no man would want me anyway. Who would want a person with only half a body and a screwed-up mind? I work at the Vet Center (Veteran's Outreach and Counseling Center), I drink a lot of wine, and I read. When I'm around people I feel like they think I'm crazy. I am—and I know they don't like to look at me because my arm is gone.

"I don't cry anymore. I don't think I ever cried. If I cry, I'll never stop. What's there to cry about? Think of all the things we did to the kids over there; what right have I got to cry? I feel guilty that I went, I feel guilty about the war, and I know people hate me for going.

"It's not worth it to try to make people understand. I did that for a while, and it just made things worse for me. It made me feel like I have to prove that I'm a decent human being, and I don't want to have to do that."

Louise Louise is a 32-year-old Caucasian woman who has worked as a grant writer and administrative consultant to nonprofit organizations in the Washington, D.C., area for 5 years. One year ago Louise was diagnosed with carpal tunnel syndrome and ulnar nerve entrapment. She is on full-time disability, spends 3 days per week at physical and occupational therapy, and has been told that she will have to alter her lifestyle. Louise's work entailed extensive work on computers, which she is no longer able to do and which, she has been told, she will not be able to do in the future. She has been an avid softball and tennis player. This will be the first summer in 10 years that Louise will be unable to play in the local softball league.

When asked how this injury has affected her life, she said that most days she just feels like she does not want to get up and face another day. Her significant other is trying to be understanding, but she thinks his patience is growing thin. He does not understand why she is feeling no better and does not think her injury is "all that bad." She is afraid she may lose her relationship, along with her job.

Her daily routine consists of watching a lot of television. She is depressed, but she is also afraid to look into the future. She has recently sought counseling because "whenever I think about what's going to happen to me, I feel like I'm having panic attacks. I'm supposed to be taking it easy, relaxing as much as possible, and instead I feel like I'm anxiety-ridden all the time. I've lost my ability to earn a living, I might lose my boyfriend, I can't do the grocery shopping or drive a car, I'm too uncomfortable to have sex, and I can't do any of the things I like to do. I just can't deal with it." When asked what the panic attacks feel like, Louise says that her heart starts pounding, she gets sweaty, and she just cannot think. She lies down in bed for a few minutes, and when the anxiety subsides, she turns on the TV or calls a friend for some human contact.

Louise says she has "monster nightmares." Monsters are chasing her or holding her captive, and nobody rescues her. She says that in addition to the pain she lives with, her stress level is almost out of control. She hopes that counseling will help alleviate that, at least.

Stress Management

The true experiences that are summarized here portray convincingly the powerful role of stress in the lives of some women with disabilities. Louise is about to begin counseling in an effort to alleviate some of the problems she is experiencing, but it is not clear that the others have sought or found any substantial help to date. The remainder of this chapter briefly addresses some approaches to healing, or at least managing, the effects of disability-related stress. Patrick (Chapter 20) also provides valuable information regarding stress management techniques.

Because stress is a combination of stressors and stress reactivity, one approach to management focuses on the way that an individual interprets the stressors and responds to them—the reactivity side of the equation. Individual and group counseling are often helpful. Counseling enables people to put their fears and frustrations into words, to talk with an empathic listener, and to explore new ways of handling problems. Simply being heard and understood can often relieve stress. People tend to think in habitual ways, so they may not even recognize that they have choices in the way they react to pressures. Becoming aware of the power to modify one's response, even when the problems remain intractible, enhances freedom and reduces the experience of stress.

As an alternative or a supplement to counseling, books, tapes and videos may provide a means for self-help. Many excellent books are available for the general population that provide clear instructions for stress management techniques. For example, *The Relaxation & Stress Reduction Workbook* (Davis, Eshelman, & McKay, 1988) includes inventories to help readers understand their own reactions, as well as introductions to progressive relaxation, self-hypnosis, assertiveness training, time management, biofeedback, and other stress management techniques. At least one book, *Quick-Mini Stress-Management Strategies for You—A Person with a Disability (or Even if You Are Not Disabled—Right Now!)* (Danskin & Danskin, 1988), has been especially designed for persons with disabilities. The book provides an introduction to brief relaxation exercises, physical stretching and musculoskeletal exercises, and visualization exercises. It includes cautions to be observed in applying those procedures to specific disabling conditions. It also includes brief suggestions for diverse strategies, for example improving communication skills, gardening, and doing volunteer work. The authors suggest independent living centers as one of several places where more intensive stress management techniques might be taught.

The thrust of the "stress reactivity management" approaches is that they directly address the most controllable part of the stress equation—the individual's reaction. Cognitive-behavioral approaches to problem management are widely used by therapists, and the value of physical activity and relaxation (Benson, 1975) has been clearly demonstrated. On the flip side, the main limitation of these approaches is that they generally treat the stressors as an immutable part of the external reality. It is therefore exciting to recognize the extra dimension that the women's movement, the disability rights movement, and women with disabilities have to offer—the vision of a strategy that battles those stressors directly rather than concentrating exclusively on remediating the coping strategies of individuals. These movements proclaim, for example, that it is not enough to patch up the psyches of women who have suffered sexual abuse. We must find more effective ways to stop the abuse. It is not enough to teach women with disabilities how to stretch a dollar until it squeals—we need to build a vocational rehabilitation system that does a better job of counseling and placing women with disabilities. It is not enough to provide therapy that helps a woman accept herself and her disability—we must shout loudly enough for the whole world to hear that she is a person of inherent worth who must be treated with dignity and respect.

Some stress is inevitable; life would be flat, boring, and unproductive without it. However, the special circumstances of women with severe disabilities place them at risk for excessive doses of stress that may result in damage to physical and psychological health. Solutions lie in helping individuals to cope more effectively with stressors and also in reducing the number of stressors created for them by an insensitive society. With sufficient progress on both the individual and social fronts, the stresses experienced by women with disabilities may eventually resemble the basic challenges inherent in life.

REFERENCES

Americans with Disabilities Act of 1990 (ADA), PL 101-336. (July 26, 1990). Title 42, U.S.C. 12101 et seq.: *U.S. Statutes at Large, 104*, 327–378.

Benefield, L., & Head, D.W. (1984). Discrimination and disabled women. *Journal of Humanistic Education and Development, 23*, 60–68.

Benson, H. (1975). *The relaxation response.* New York: Avon Books.

Cannon, W.B. (1932). *The wisdom of the body.* New York: W.W. Norton.

Crewe, N.M., Athelstan, G.T., & Krumberger, J.H. (1979). Spinal cord injury: A comparison of preinjury and postinjury marriages. *Archives of Physical Medicine & Rehabilitation, 60*, 252–256.

Danskin, D.G., & Danskin, D.V. (1988). *Quick-mini stress-management strategies for you, a person with a disability (or even if you are not disabled—right now!).* Manhattan, KS: Guild Hall Publications.

Davis, M., Eshelman, E.R., & McKay, M. (1988). *The relaxation & stress reduction workbook.* Oakland, CA: New Harbinger Publications.

DeLoach, C.P. (1989). Gender, career choice and occupational outcomes among college alumni with disabilities. *Journal of Applied Rehabilitation Counseling, 20*, 8–12.

Fine, M., & Asch, A. (Eds.). (1988). *Women with disabilities: Essays in psychology, culture and politics.* Philadelphia: Temple University Press.

Finkelhor, D. (1994). Current information on the scope and nature of child sexual abuse. *Future Child, 4*, 31–53.

Greenberg, J.S. (1993). *Comprehensive stress management.* Dubuque, IA: Brown & Benchmark.

Harris, L. (1986). *The ICD survey of disabled Americans: Bringing disabled Americans into the mainstream.* New York: International Center for the Disabled.

Holmes, T.H., & Holmes, R.N. (1967). The social readjustment rating scale. *Journal of Psychosomatic Research, 11*, 213–218.

Kanner, A.D., & Lazarus, R.S. (1981). Comparison of two modes of stress management: Daily hassles and uplifts versus major life events. *Journal of Behavioral Medicine, 4*, 1–39.

Koestler, F.A. (1983). Visually impaired women and the world of work: Theme and variations. *Journal of Visual Impairment and Blindness, 77*, 276–277.

Lazarus, R.S. (1984). Puzzles in the study of daily hassles. *Journal of Behavioral Medicine, 7*, 375–389.

Moglia, R. (1986). Sexual abuse and disability. *SIECUS Report, 5*, 9–10.

Riger, A.L. (1993). *A decidedly unbeautiful woman reacts to The Beauty Myth.* Paper presented at the meeting of the American Psychological Association, Toronto, Ontario, Canada.

Seyle, H. (1974). *Stress without distress.* New York: J.B. Lippincott.

Vash, C.L. (1982). Employment issues for women with disabilities. *Rehabilitation Literature, 43*, 198–207.

chapter 17

The Neuroendocrinology of Stress

Constantine Tsigos and George P. Chrousos

Life exists by maintaining a complex dynamic equilibrium, or *homeostasis,* that is constantly challenged by intrinsic or extrinsic adverse forces, or *stressors* (Chrousos & Gold, 1992). Our physiological mechanisms for coping with adversity have not evolved appreciably over the past several thousand years. Thus, our physiological responses to the faster pace of life, increasing social pressures, and information overload of modern societies resemble those set into motion during physical danger and outright threats to survival, which were the major stressors in primitive societies. Although the concepts of stress and homeostasis can be traced back to ancient Greek history, the integration of these notions with related physiologic and pathophysiologic mechanisms and their association with specific illnesses are much more recent. In the present overview, we begin with a historical review and definition of the components of the stress response. We then focus on the cellular and molecular infrastructure of the physiological and behavioral adaptive responses. Finally, we define the pathophysiological effects of dysregulation of the stress response, which may result in vulnerability to several major disease entities, such as affective illnesses and chronic inflammatory processes.

DEFINITION OF STRESS AND HISTORICAL DEVELOPMENT

Stress is defined as a state of disharmony, or threatened homeostasis. Homeostasis is the steady state required for successful adaptation. Homeostasis is maintained by counteracting and reestablishing forces that consist of a complex repertoire of molecular, cellular, physiological, and behavioral responses, which improve chances for survival. These adaptive responses can be specific to the stressor or can be generalized and relatively nonspecific, depending on the magnitude of the threat to homeostasis.

These contemporary concepts regarding stress have evolved over the past two and a half millennia (Chrousos & Gold, 1992). In the beginning of the classic era, Heracleitus was the first to suggest that life is in constant mode of change. One hundred years later, Hippocrates equated health to a harmonious balance of the elements and qualities of life and disease to a systematic disharmony of these elements. In the years of the Renaissance, Thomas Sydenham extended this Hippocratic concept of disease, when he suggested that the systematic disharmony of disease can be potentiated by "adaptive" forces of the body turning into maladaptive ones. In the 19th century, Claude Bernard introduced the concept of the *milieu interieur,* or the principle of a dynamic internal physiological equilibrium. Walter Cannon later coined the term *homeostasis* and extended this concept to emotional as well as physical parameters. In the 1930s, Hans Selye suggested that a constellation of "stereotypic" physiological and psychological events occurring in seriously ill patients resulted from the protracted, severe, and uncontrollable application of the natural adaptive forces of the body. He referred to this state as the "General Adaptation or Stress Syndrome" and, in effect, refined Sydenham's concept of diseases of adaptation.

STRESS SYNDROME: MECHANISMS OF ADAPTATION

The stress system receives and integrates a great diversity of neurosensory (visual, auditory, nociceptive, somatosensory, visceral), blood borne, and limbic signals, which arrive through distinct pathways. The general adaptational response to stress, both behavioral and physical, is essential for survival and remarkably consistent in its presentation (Gold, Goodwin, & Chrousos, 1988a, 1988b). Behavioral adaptation includes increased arousal and alertness, heightened attention and cognition, enhanced analgesia, and appropriate aggression, with concurrent inhibition of vegetative functions, such as feeding and reproduction. Physical adaptation, on the other hand, promotes an adaptive redirection of energy. Thus, oxygen and vital substrates are directed to the central nervous system (CNS) and the stressed body site(s), where they are needed the most. Changes in cardiovascular function and metabolism are crucial elements of peripheral adaptation. In addition, the ability of the individual to quickly develop the restraining forces that prevent an overresponse, in terms of both magnitude and duration, are also major components of a successful general adaptational response and are present both in the CNS and the periphery. If the restraining or detoxifying forces of the body fail to exert timely control of the elements of the stress response, the adaptive responses turn maladaptive and contribute to development of pathology.

STRESS SYSTEM INTERACTIONS
WITH CNS COMPONENTS
REGULATING AFFECT AND PAIN SENSATION

The changes that occur in the organism during stress are subserved by several centers within the CNS, by the pituitary–adrenal axis and the systemic sympathetic and adrenomedullary systems, collectively called the stress system. Attainment of novel capabilities to adapt in a continuously changing world are crucial for self and species preservation. Thus, it is not surprising that the mild and controllable stress associated with these achievements is rewarding, pleasant, and even exciting, providing positive stimuli to the emotional and intellectual growth and development of the individual. It is of note that activation of the stress system during feeding and sexual activity links both these sine qua non functions for survival to pleasure. In contrast, activation of the stress response during threatening situations that are beyond the control of the individual can be associated with dysphoria of varying magnitude. The teleology of this phenomenon is sound, as this is the mechanism by which the individual avoids and learns to avoid situations that may be detrimental to one's existence.

The mechanism by which there is differential activation of mood depending on the type of stress is complex and not clearly understood. There are mutual interactions, however, of the stress system with three important brain areas that influence affect and anticipatory phenomena (mesocortical/mesolimbic systems); the initiation, propagation, and termination of stress system activity (amygdala/hippocampus complex); and the setting of the pain sensation (arcuate nucleus) (Gray, 1989; Nikolarakis, Almeida, & Herz, 1986; Roth et al., 1988).

EFFECTORS OF THE STRESS RESPONSE

The central components of the stress system are located in the hypothalamus and the brain stem and include the parvocellular corticotropin-releasing hormone (CRH) and arginine-vasopressin (AVP) neurons of the paraventricular nuclei (PVN) of the hypothalamus, the CRH neurons of the paragigantocellular nuclei of the medulla and the locus coeruleus (LC), and other catecholaminergic cell groups of the medulla and pons (central sympathetic system) (Chrousos, 1992). The hypothalamic–pituitary–adrenal (HPA) axis, together with the efferent sympathetic/adrenomedullary system, represent the peripheral limbs of this system (Figure 1).

Central Components of the Stress System
(CRH/AVP/Catecholaminergic Neurons)

CRH, a 41 amino acid peptide, was first isolated as the principal hypothalamic stimulus to the pituitary–adrenal axis (Vale et al., 1981). However,

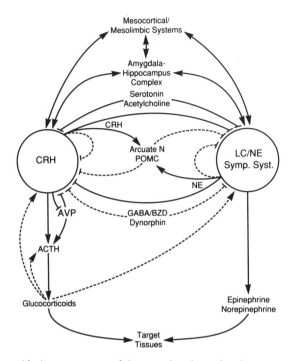

Figure 1. A simplified representation of the central and peripheral components of the stress system, whose activation leads to maintenance of basal and stress-induced homeostasis. The corticotropin-releasing hormone (CRH) and central catecholaminergic (LC/NE) neurons recipro-cally innervate and activate each other, and they exert presynaptic autoinhibition. The cholinergic and serotonergic neurotransmitter systems stimulate the central stress system, whereas gamma-aminobutyric acid/benzodiezepine (GABA/BZD) and proopiomelanocortin (POMC) systems in-hibit it. The latter is activated by the stress system and plays an important role in enhancing analgesia. Vasopressin (AVP) plays a major synergistic role in the secretion of ACTH by the pituitary and may synergize with CRH in other target tissues of the latter, including the LC/NE neurons. Solid lines, stimulation; interrupted lines, inhibition. (Adapted from Chrousos & Gold [1992].)

CRH and CRH receptors were found in many sites in the brain outside of the hypothalamus, including parts of the limbic system and the central arousal-sympathetic systems (LC-sympathetic systems) in the brain stem and spinal cord (Aguilera et al., 1987; DeSouza et al., 1985; Swanson et al., 1983). In addition, administration of CRH directly to the CNS has been shown to set into motion a coordinated series of physiological and behav-ioral responses, which included activation of the pituitary–adrenal axis and the sympathetic nervous system, as well as characteristic stress behaviors (Cole & Koob, 1991; Dunn & Berridge, 1990). Thus, CRH was shown to have a broader role in coordinating the stress response than had been sus-pected previously (Chrousos & Gold, 1992).

The central neuronal circuitry has been extensively studied, and Figure 1 provides a schematic diagram of what is currently known about the stress system. As can be seen from this heuristic representation, the control of the stress response is highly complex. Reciprocal neural connections exist between the CRH and catecholaminergic neurons (LC/noradrenergic neurons) of the central stress system, with CRH and norepinephrine stimulating each other, the latter primarily through α1-noradrenergic receptors (Calogero et al., 1988; Kiss & Aguilera, 1992; Valentino, Foote, & Aston-Jones, 1983). There is an ultra-short autoregulatory negative feedback loop on the CRH neurons exerted by CRH itself (Calogero et al., 1988a), just as there is a similar loop in the LC catecholaminergic neurons. Collateral fibers of the CRH and LC/norepinephrine neurons inhibit CRH and catecholamine secretion, respectively, via presynaptic CRH and α2-noradrenergic receptors (Aghajanian & Van der Maelen, 1982). There is also parallel regulation of both central components of the stress system by other stimulatory and inhibitory neuronal pathways. Several neurotransmitters, including serotonin and acetylcholine, excite CRH and the LC/NE neurons (Calogero et al., 1990). The negative feedback controls, however, include glucocorticoids, γ-aminobutyric acid (GABA), corticotropin, and several opioid peptides, which inhibit both CRH and LC/NE neurons (Calogero et al., 1988a, 1988b).

Each of the PVN has three main parvocellular neural divisions: a medial group, producing mostly CRH and secreting into the hypophysial portal system (HPS); an intermediate group, producing mostly AVP and also secreting into the HPS; and a lateral group, whose projections terminate in the catecholaminergic neurons of the stress system in the brain stem (Sawchenko et al., 1993). A subpopulation of parvocellular neurons synthesize and secrete both CRH and AVP. The relative proportion of this subpopulation increases significantly with stress (Whitnall, 1989). Another group of PVN CRH neurons also project to and innervate proopiomelanocortin-containing neurons in the arcuate nucleus of the hypothalamus, which in turn send reciprocal projections to the PVN CRH neurons and innervate catecholaminergic neurons of the central stress system in the brainstem, as well as neurons of pain control areas of the hind brain and spinal cord. Thus, activation of the stress system stimulates hypothalamic POMC-peptide secretion, which reciprocally inhibits the activity of the stress system and, in addition, produces analgesia (Calogero et al., 1988a; Nikolarakis et al., 1986).

Hypothalamic–Pituitary–Adrenal Axis

CRH is permissive for the secretion of ACTH by anterior pituitary corticotrophs, whereas AVP, although a potent synergistic factor of CRH, has very little ACTH secretagog activity by itself (Lamberts et al., 1984). Furthermore, it appears that there is a reciprocal positive interaction between CRH and AVP at the level of the hypothalamic-pituitary unit (Abou-Samra, Harwood, Catt, & Aguilera, 1987). Thus, AVP stimulates CRH secretion, and CRH causes AVP secretion in vitro (Antoni, 1993). In nonstressful situations both CRH and AVP are secreted in the portal system in a circadian, that is a cyclic 24-hour, pulsatile fashion, with a frequency of about two to three secretory episodes per hour (Engler et al., 1989; Redekopp et al., 1986). At baseline, resting conditions, the amplitude of the CRH and AVP pulses increase in the early morning hours, resulting finally in increases of both the amplitude and frequency of ACTH and cortisol secretory bursts in the general circulation (Horrocks et al., 1990; Iranmanesh et al., 1990).

The mechanisms within the CNS that are responsible for the circadian release of CRH, AVP, ACTH, and cortisol in their characteristic pulsatile manner are not completely understood, but appear to be controlled by one or more pacemakers, whose location is not yet known. These diurnal variations are perturbed by changes in zeitgebers (e.g., lighting, activity) and are disrupted when a stressor is imposed. During acute stress, the amplitude of the CRH and AVP pulsations increases, resulting in increases of ACTH and cortisol secretory episodes. Additional CRH, ACTH, and perhaps other factors stimulating glucocorticoid secretion are recruited during stress, potentiating the activity of the HPA axis. These include AVP of magnocellular neuron origin secreting into both the HPS via collateral neuraxons and into the systemic circulation, angiotensin II, and various cytokines and lipid mediators of inflammation (Holmes et al., 1986; Phillips, 1987).

Circulating ACTH is the key regulator of glucocorticoid secretion by the adrenal cortex. However, there is evidence that other hormones (either originating from the adrenal medulla or coming from the systemic circulation) or neuronal information from the autonomic innervation of the adrenal cortex may also participate in the regulation of cortisol secretion (Hinson, 1990; Ottenweller & Meier, 1982; Vinson et al., 1988). Glucocorticoids are the final effectors of the HPA axis and participate in the control of whole body homeostasis and the organism's response to stress. These hormones exert their effects through their ubiquitous cytoplasmic receptors (Smith & Toft, 1993). Upon binding to glucocorticoid, the glucocorticoid receptors on the cell surface translocate into the nucleus, where they interact with glucocorticoid responsive elements (GREs) of the DNA leading to the activation of appropriate hormone-responsive genes (Pratt, 1990). The activated receptors also inhibit, through protein–protein interactions, other transcription factors that lead to the production of specific gene products. Two such factors are the c-*jun*/c-*fos* heterodimer and nuclear factor κB (NF-κB), which are positive regulators of transcription of several genes involved in the activation of immune and other cells (Jonat et al.,

1990; Yang-Yen et al., 1990; Scheinman et al., 1995). In addition, gluco-corticoids change the stability of messenger RNAs and hence the rate of synthesis of several glucocorticoid-responsive proteins.

Glucocorticoids play a key regulatory role on the basal activity of the HPA axis and on the termination of the stress response by acting at extra-hypothalamic centers, the hypothalamus and the pituitary gland (de Kloet, 1991). One may speculate that attenuation of the ACTH secretory response by steroid feedback may reduce the response capacity of the HPA axis to subsequent stressors and may act to limit the duration of the total tissue exposure to glucocorticoids, thus minimizing the catabolic, antireproduc-tive, and immunosuppressive effects of these hormones. Interestingly, a dual receptor system exists for glucocorticoids in the CNS, including the glucocorticoid receptor type I, or mineralocorticoid receptor, which re-sponds to low levels of glucocorticoids and is primarily activational, and the classic glucocorticoid receptor (type II), which responds to higher lev-els of glucocorticoids and is dampening in some systems and activational in others (de Kloet, 1991).

Sympathetic/Adrenomedullary and Parasympathetic Systems

The autonomic nervous system provides a rapidly responding mechanism to control a wide range of functions. Cardiovascular, respiratory, gastro-intestinal, renal, endocrine, and other systems are regulated by either the sympathetic nervous system or the parasympathetic system or both (Gilbey & Spyer, 1993).

Sympathetic innervation of peripheral organs is derived from the ef-ferent preganglionic fibers, whose cell bodies lie in the intermediolateral column of the spinal cord. These nerves synapse in the bilateral chain of sympathetic ganglia with postganglionic sympathetic neurons, which in-nervate vascular smooth muscle cells, as well as the kidney, bladder, gut, and many other organs (Burnstock & Milner, 1992). The preganglionic neurons are cholinergic, whereas the postganglionic neurons release nor-epinephrine. The sympathetic system also has a humoral contribution. Ep-inephrine and, to a lesser extent, norepinephrine are secreted by the adrenal medulla, which can be considered as a modified sympathetic ganglion. In addition to the classic neurotransmitters acetylcholine and norepinephrine, both sympathetic and parasympathetic subdivisions of the autonomic ner-vous system contain several subpopulations of target-selective and neuro-chemically coded neurons that express a variety of neuropeptides and, in some cases, adenosine triphosphate (ATP) or nitric oxide (Benarroch, 1994). Neuropeptide Y (NPY), somatostatin, and galanin are colocalized in noradrenergic vasoconstrictive neurons, whereas vasoactive intestinal polypeptide (VIP) and, to a lesser extent, substance P and calcitonin gene-related peptide (CGRP) are colocalized in cholinergic neurons. Transmission in sympathetic ganglia is also modulated by neuropeptides released from preganglionic fibers and short interneurons (e.g., enkephalin, neurotensin), as well as from primary afferent (e.g., substance P, VIP) collaterals (Elfvin, Lindh, & Hokfelt, 1993). The particular combination of neurotransmitters, neuropeptides, and other substances in sympathetic neurons is strongly affected by the CNS and peripheral factors.

HPA AXIS-IMMUNE SYSTEM INTERACTIONS

It has been known for several decades that the stress of inflammation in the course of an infectious disease, active autoimmune inflammatory proces, and accidental or operative trauma is associated with concurrent activation of the HPA axis. In the early 1990s, it also became apparent that cytokines and other humoral mediators of inflammation are potent activators of the central stress response, constituting the afferent limb of the feedback loop through which the immune/inflammatory system and the CNS communicate (Figure 2A) (Besedovsky & del Ray, 1992; Reichlin, 1993; Sternberg et al., 1992).

The three inflammatory cytokines—tumor necrosis factor-α (TNF-α), interleukin-1, and interleukin-6—all produced at inflammatory sites and elsewhere in a cascade-like fashion can cause stimulation of the HPA axis in vivo, alone, or in synergy with each other (Akira et al., 1990; Perlstein et al., 1993). This can be blocked significantly with CRH-neutralizing an-

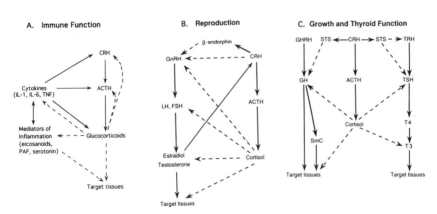

Figure 2. A simplified representation of the interactions between the hypothalamic–pituitary–adrenal axis and other neuroendocrine systems, including the immune system (A), the reproductive axis (B), and the growth and thyroid axis (C). CRH, corticotropin-releasing hormone; ACTH, corticotropin; PAF, platelet activating factor; GnRH, gonadotropin-releasing hormone; LH, luteinizing hormone; FSH, follicle-stimulating hormone; GHRH, growth hormone-releasing hormone; STS, somatostatin; TRH, thyrotropin-releasing hormone; GH, growth hormone; TSH, thyroid-stimulating hormone; T_4, thyroxine; T_3, triiodothyronine; SmC, somatomedin C. (Adapted from Chrousos & Gold [1992].)

tibodies, glucocorticoids, and prostanoid synthesis inhibitors. In addition, all three cytokines directly stimulate hypothalamic CRH secretion in vitro, in a glucocorticoid-suppressible, prostanoid-dependent manner (Busbridge & Grossman, 1991; Sapolsky et al., 1987). There is evidence to suggest that interleukin-6 (IL-6), the main endocrine cytokine, plays the major role in the immune stimulation of the axis. Interestingly, in the human, IL-6 is an extremely potent activator of the axis without the vascular leak-promoting and hypotensive side effects of the other two inflammatory cytokines (Mastorakos, Chrousos, & Weber, 1993). The elevations of ACTH and cortisol attained by IL-6 are well above those observed with maximal stimulatory doses of CRH, suggesting that AVP and other ACTH secretagogs are also stimulated by this cytokine.

Some of the activating effects of inflammation on the HPA axis may be exerted indirectly by stimulation of the central catecholaminergic pathways by the inflammatory cytokines and other humoral mediators of inflammation. Also, activation of peripheral nociceptive, somatosensory, and visceral afferent fibers would lead to stimulation of both the catecholaminergic and CRH neuronal systems via ascending spinal pathways (Figure 2A) (Matta et al., 1990).

Other inflammatory mediators may also participate in the activation of the HPA axis, in addition to the three inflammatory cytokines. Thus, several eicosanoids, platelet-activating factor (PAF), and serotonin show strong CRH-releasing properties (Bernardini et al., 1989; Fuller, 1992). It is not clear, however, which of the above effects are endocrine and which are auto/paracrine. Presence of cytokinergic neural pathways and local involvement of eicosanoids and PAF in CRH secretion are certain. Direct effects, albeit delayed, of most of the above cytokines and mediators of inflammation on pituitary ACTH secretion, on the other hand, have also been shown (Bernton, Beach, Holaday, Smallridge, & Fein, 1987), and direct effects of these substances on adrenal glucocorticoid secretion appear also to be present (Salas, Evans, Levell, & Whicher, 1990). Conversely, activation of the HPA axis has profound inhibitory effects on the inflammatory immune response because virtually all the components of the immune response are inhibited by cortisol (Figure 2A). Alterations of leukocyte traffic and function, decreases in production of cytokines and mediators of inflammation, and inhibition of the latter's effects on target tissues are among the main immunosuppressive effects of glucocorticoids (Munck, Guyre, & Holbrook, 1984).

The efferent sympathetic/adrenomedullary system apparently participates in a major fashion in the interactions of the HPA axis and the immune/inflammatory reaction by being reciprocally connected with the CRH system, by receiving and transmitting humoral and nervous immune signals from the periphery, by densely innervating both primary and secondary lymphoid organs, and by reaching all sites of inflammation via the post-ganglionic sympathetic neuron (Figure 2A) (Bellinger, Lorton, Felten, & Felten, 1992; Ottaway & Husband, 1992). When activated during stress, the autonomic system exerts its own direct effects on immune organs, which can be immunosuppressive (such as inhibition of natural killer cell activity), or both immunopotentiating and anti-inflammatory by inducing secretion of IL-6 in the systemic circulation. The latter has both proinflammatory properties and participates in the termination of the inflammatory response by stimulating the HPA axis and the acute phase reaction and by inhibiting the TNFα and IL-1 secretion (Hirano, Akira, Taga, & Kishimoto, 1990). In this context, it is interesting that 1) psychological factors, such as bereavement, depression, marital separation, and examination stress in students are associated with suppression of immune responses; 2) emotional upheaval commonly precipitates acute flare-ups of autoimmune diseases; and 3) numerous stressors alter the ability of the organism to deal with neoplasms (Kiecolt-Glaser & Glaser, 1991; Stein, Miller, & Trestman, 1991).

HPA AXIS–OTHER ENDOCRINE AXES INTERACTIONS

The systems responsible for reproduction and growth are also directly linked to the stress system and both are profoundly influenced by the HPA axis, the effector of the stress response. The reproductive axis is inhibited at all levels by various components of the HPA axis (Figure 2B) (Rabin, Gold, Margioris, & Chrousos, 1988). Thus, either directly or via secretion of arcuate POMC neuron β-endorphin, CRH suppresses the gonadotropin hormone–releasing hormone (GnRH) neurons of the arcuate nucleus of the hypothalamus. Glucocorticoids, on the other hand, exert inhibitory effects at the level of the GnRH neuron, the pituitary gonadotroph, and the gonads themselves and render target tissues of sex steroids resistant to these hromones. Cytokines also suppress reproductive function via the HPA axis and directly at various levels (Adashi, 1990; Skinner, 1991). Thus, during inflammatory stress, steroidogenesis is directly inhibited by cytokines at both ovaries and testes, with concomitant inhibition of the pulsatile secretion of the gonadotropin releasing hormone from the hypothalamus (Rivier & Rivest, 1991).

The interaction between CRH and the gonadal axis appears to be bidirectional. Vamvakopoulos and Chrousos (1993) demonstrated the presence of estrogen responsive elements in the promoter area of the CRH gene and direct stimulatory estrogen effects on CRH gene expression. This finding implicates the CRH gene and therefore the HPA axis as a potentially important target of ovarian steroids and a potential mediator of gender-related differences in the stress response/HPA axis activity. However, the activated estrogen receptor interacts with and occasionally potentiates the c-*jun*/c-*fos* heterodimer, discussed earlier in this chapter, which mediates the effects of several cytokines on their target cells (Gaub, Bellard, Scheuer, Chambon, & Sassone-Corsi, 1990). In addition, estrogen appears to stimulate adhesion molecules and their receptors in immune and immune accessory cells (Cid et al., 1994). These phenomena may explain why autoimmune diseases afflict more females than males.

The growth axis is also inhibited at many levels during stress (Figure 2C) (Dieguez, Page, & Scanlon, 1988). Prolonged activation of the HPA axis leads to suppression of growth hormone secretion and inhibition of somatomedin C and other growth factor effects on their target tissues by glucocorticoids (Burguera, Muruais, Penalva, Dieguez, & Casanueva, 1990), the latter presumably again occurring by inhibition of the c-*jun*/c-*fos* heterodimer (Jonat et al., 1990). However, acute elevations of growth hormone concentration in plasma may occur at the onset of the stress response in humans and after acute administration of glucocorticoids, presumably through stimulation of the GH gene by glucocorticoids through its GREs in its promoter region (Casanueva, Burguera, Muruais, & Dieguez, 1990). In addition to the direct effects of glucocorticoids, which are pivotal in the suppression of growth observed in prolonged stress, increases in somatostatin secretion caused by CRH, with resultant inhibition of growth hormone secretion, have also been implicated as a potential mechanism of stress-related suppression of growth hormone secretion.

A corollary phenomenon to growth axis suppression is the stress-related inhibition of thyroid axis function. Activation of the HPA axis is associated with decreased production of thyroid-stimulating hormone and inhibition of conversion of the relatively inactive thyroxine to the more biologically active triiodothyronine in peripheral tissues (the "euthyroid sick" syndrome) (Figure 2C) (Benker et al., 1990). Although the exact mechanism(s) for these phenomena is not known, both phenomena may be caused by the increased levels of glucocorticoids and may serve to conserve energy during stress (Kennedy & Jones, 1991). Inhibition of thyroid-stimulating hormone secretion by CRH-stimulated increases in somatostatin might also participate in the central component of thyroid axis suppression during stress. In the case of inflammatory stress, inhibition of TSH secretion may be in part through the action of cytokines both on the hypothalamus and the pituitary.

HPA AXIS: PATHOPHYSIOLOGY

Generally, the stress response with the resultant activation of the HPA axis is meant to be acute or at least of a limited duration. The time-limited nature of this process renders its accompanying catabolic and immunosuppressive effects temporarily beneficial and of no adverse consequences. Chronicity of stress system activation, however, would lead to the syndromal state that Selye described in 1936. Since CRH coordinates both behavioral and immunologic adaptation during stressful situations, increased and prolonged production of CRH could explain the pathogenesis of the syndrome.

The syndrome of melancholic depression also seems to represent dysregulation of the generalized stress response, leading to chronic activation of the HPA axis and the sympathetic nervous system (Gold, Goodwin, & Chrousos, 1988a, 1988b). Indeed, 24-hour urinary cortisol excretion is elevated and plasma ACTH response to exogenous CRH is decreased. These abnormalities are state-related and resolve coincident to waning psychopathology. Hypersecretion of CRH has been shown in depression and suggests that CRH may participate in the initiation or perpetuation of a vicious cycle or both.

In addition to melancholic depression, a spectrum of other conditions may be associated with increased and prolonged activation of the HPA axis (Table 1). These include anorexia nervosa (Gold, Gwirtsman et al., 1986); obsessive-compulsive disorder; panic anxiety (Gold, Pigott, Kling, Kalogeras, & Chrousos, 1988); chronic active alcoholism (Wand & Dobs, 1991); alcohol and narcotic withdrawal (Bardeleben, Heusen, & Holsboer, 1989); diabetes mellitus, especially when complicated by diabetic neuropathy (Tsigos, Young, & White, 1993); and, perhaps, hyperthyroidism. Girls who have been sexually abused have been found to have disregulation of their HPA axis (DeBellis et al., 1994). The same is true for women with the premenstrual tension syndrome (Rabin et al., 1990).

Table 1. States associated with altered hypothalamic–pituitary–adrenal axis activity and disregulation of behavioral adaptation and/or the immune/inflammatory reaction

Increased HPA axis	Decreased HPA axis
Animal models	
Fischer rat	Lewis rat
Human states	
Chronic stress	Adrenal insufficiency
Melancholic depression	Rheumatoid arthritis
Anorexia nervosa	Atypical/seasonal depression
Panic disorder	Chronic fatigue syndrome
Cushing syndrome	Fibromyalgia
Chronic active alcoholism	Hypothyroidism
Narcotic withdrawal	Nicotine withdrawal
Diabetes mellitus	Postglucocorticoid therapy
Hyperthyroidism	Post-Cushing syndrome cure
Sexual abuse	Postpartum period
Premenstrual tension	Postchronic stress
syndrome	

Decreased activation of the stress system, rather than sustained activation, in which chronically reduced secretion of CRH may result in pathological hypoarousal, also appears to exist (Table 1). Patients with seasonal depression and the chronic fatigue syndrome fall into this category (Demitrack et al., 1991; Vanderpool et al., 1991). In the depressive (winter) state of the former and in the period of fatigue in the latter, there is chronically decreased activity of the HPA axis. Similarly, patients with fibromyalgia have decreased urinary free cortisol excretion and frequently complain of fatigue (Griep, Boerdma, & de Kloet, 1993). Hypothyroid patients also have clear evidence of CRH hyposecretion (Kamilaris et al., 1987). Interestingly, one of the major manifestations of hypothyroidism is depression of the "atypical" type. Withdrawal from smoking has also been associated with decreased cortisol and catecholamine secretion (Puddey, Vandongen, Neilin, & English, 1984). Decreased CRH secretion in the early period of nicotine abstinence could explain the increased appetite and weight gain frequently observed in these patients. It is interesting that, in Cushing syndrome, the clinical picture of polyphagia and weight gain, fatigue, and anergia is consistent with the suppression of the CRH neuron by the associated hypercortisolism (Gold, Gwirtsman, et al., 1986).

Theoretically, an excessive HPA axis response to inflammatory stimuli would mimic the stress or hypercortisolemic state and would lead to increased susceptibility of the individual to a host of infectious agents or tumors, but resistance to autoimmune/inflammatory disease; a defective HPA axis response to such stimuli, however, would reproduce the glucocorticoid-deficient state and would lead to relative resistance to infections and neoplastic disease, but increased susceptibility to autoimmune/inflammatory disease. Indeed, such properties were unraveled in an interesting pair of near-histocompatible, highly inbred rat strains, named Fischer and Lewis, both selected out of Sprague-Dawley rats, respectively, for their resistance or susceptibility to inflammatory disease (Sternberg, Chrousos, Wilder, & Gold, 1989). There is an increasing body of evidence that patients with rheumatoid arthritis have a mild form of central hypocortisolism, as they have reduced 24-hour cortisol excretion, less pronounced diurnal rhythm of cortisol secretion, and blunted adrenal responses to surgical stress (Chikanza, Petrou, Chrousos, Kingsley, & Panayi, 1992). Thus, dysfunction of the HPA axis may actually play a role in the development and/ or perpetuation of autoimmune disease, rather than being an epiphenomenon.

REFERENCES

Abou-Samra, A-B., Harwood, J.P., Catt, K.J., & Aguilera, G. (1987). Mechanisms of action of CRF and other regulators of ACTH release in pituitary corticotrophs. *Annals of the New York Academy of Sciences, 512,* 67–84.

Adashi, E.Y. (1990). The potential relevance of cytokines to ovarian physiology: The emerging role of resident ovarian cells of the white blood cell series. *Endocrinological Reviews, 11,* 454–464.

Aghajanian, G.K., & Van der Maelen, C.P. (1982). α_2-Adrenoreceptor mediated hyperpolarization of locus ceruleus neurons: Intracellular studies in vivo. *Science, 215,* 1394–1400.

Aguilera, G., Millan, M.A., Hauger, R.L., & Catt, K.J. (1987). Corticotropin-releasing factor receptors: Distribution and regulation in brain, pituitary, and peripheral tissues. *Annals of the New York Academy of Sciences, 512,* 48–66.

Akira, S., Hirano, T., Taga, T., & Kishimoto, T. (1990). Biology of multifunctional cytokines: IL-6 and related molecules (IL-1 and TNF). *FASEB J, 4,* 2860–2067.

Antoni, F.A. (1993). Vasopressinergic control of pituitary adrenocorticotropin secretion comes of age. *Frontiers in Neuroendocrinology, 14,* 76–122.

Bardeleben, V., Heuser, I., & Holsboer, F. (1989). Human CRH stimulation response during acute withdrawal and after medium-term abstention from alcohol abuse. *Psychoneuroendocrinology, 14,* 441–449.

Bellinger, D.L., Lorton, D., Felten, S.Y., & Felten, D.L. (1992). Innervation of lymphoid organs and implications in development, aging, and autoimmunity. *International Journal of Immunopharmacology, 14,* 329–344.

Benarroch, E.E. (1994). Neuropeptides in the sympathetic system: Presence, plasticity, modulation, and implications. *Annals of Neurology, 36,* 6–13.

Benker, G., Raida, M., Olbricht, T., Wagner, R., Reinhardt, W., & Reinwein, D. (1990). TSH secretion in Cushing's syndrome: Relation to glucocorticoid excess, diabetes, goitre, and the "the sick euthyroid syndrome." *Clinical Endocrinology, 33,* 776–786.

Bernardini, R., Calogero, A.E., Ehlich, Y.H., Brucke, T., Chrousos, G.P., & Gold, P.W. (1989). The alkyl-ether phospholipid platelet-activating factor is a stimulator of the hypothalamic-pituitary-adrenal axis in the rat. *Endocrinology, 125,* 1067.

Bernton, E.W., Beach, L.E., Holaday, J.W., Smallridge, R.C., & Fein, H.G. (1987). Release of multiple hormones by a direct effect of interleukin-1 on pituitary cells. *Science, 238,* 519–521.

Besedovsky, H.O., & del Rey, A. (1992). Immune-neuroendocrine circuits: Integrative role of cytokines. *Frontiers in Neuroendocrinology, 13,* 61–94.

Burguera, B., Muruais, C., Penalva, A., Dieguez, C., & Casanueva, F. (1990). Dual and selective action of glucocorticoids upon basal and stimulated growth hormone release in man. *Neuroendocrinology, 51,* 51–58.

Burnstock, G., & Milner, P. (1992). Structural and chemical organization of the autonomic nervous system with special reference to nor-adrenergic, non-cholinergic transmission. In R. Bannister & C.J. Mathias (Eds.), *Autonomic failure. A textbook of clinical disorders of the autonomic nervous system* (pp. 107–125). Oxford, England: Oxford Medical Press.

Busbridge, N.J., & Grossman, A.B. (1991). Stress and the single cytokine: Interleukin modulation of the pituitary-adrenal axis. *Molecular & Cellular Endocrinology, 82,* C209–C214.

Calogero, A.E., Bagdy, G., Szemereti, K., Tartaglia, M.E., Gold, P.W., & Chrousos, G.P. (1990). Mechanisms of serotonin agonist-induced activation of the hypothalamic-pituitary-adrenal axis in the rat. *Endocrinology, 126,* 1888–1894.

Calogero, A.E., Gallucci, W.T., Chrousos, G.P., & Gold, P.W. (1988a). Catecholamine effects upon rat hypothalamic corticotropin releasing hormone secretion in vitro. *Journal of Clinical Investigation, 82,* 839–846.

Calogero, A.E., Gallucci, W.T., Chrousos, G.P., & Gold, P.W. (1988b). Interaction between gabaergic neurotransmission and rat hypothalamic corticotropin releasing hormone in vitro. *Brain Research, 463,* 28–36.

Calogero, A.E., Gallucci, W.T., Gold, P.W., & Chrousos, G.P. (1988). Multiple feedback regulatory loops upon rat hypothalamic corticotropin releasing hormone secretion. *Journal of Clinical Investigation, 82,* 767–774.

Casanueva, F.F., Burguera, B., Muruais, C., & Dieguez, C. (1990). Acute administration of corticosteroids: A new and peculiar stimulus of growth hormone secretion in man. *Journal of Clinical Endocrinology & Metabolism, 70,* 234–237.

Chikanza, I.C., Petrou, P., Chrousos, G.P., Kingsley, G., & Panayi, G. (1992). Defective hypothalamic response to immune/inflammatory stimuli in patients with rheumatoid arthritis. *Arthritis Rheumatology, 35,* 1281–1288.

Chrousos, G.P. (1992). Regulation and dysregulation of the hypothalamic-pituitary-adrenal axis: The corticotropin releasing hormone perspective. *Endocrinology & Metabolism Clinics of North America, 21,* 833–858.

Chrousos, G.P., & Gold, P.W. (1992). The concepts of stress system disorders: Overview of behavioral and physical homeostasis. *Journal of the American Medical Association, 267,* 1244–1252.

Cid, M.C., Kleinman, H.K., Grant, D.S., Schnaper, W., Fauci, A.S., & Hoffman, G.S. (1994). Estradiol enhances leukocyte binding to tumor necrosis factor (TNF)-stimulated endothelial cells via an increase in TNF-induced adhesion molecules E-selectin, intercellular adhesion molecule type 1 and vascular adhesion molecule type 1. *Journal of Clinical Investigation, 93,* 17–25.

Cole, B., & Koob, G.F. (1991) Corticotropin-releasing factor, stress, and animal behavior. In J.A. McCubbin, P.G. Kaufman, & C.B. Nemeroff (Eds.). *Stress, neuropeptides and systemic disease* (p. 119). New York: Academic Press.

de Kloet, R. (1991). Brain corticosteroid receptor balance and homeostatic control. *Frontiers in Neuroendocrinology, 12,* 95–164.

DeBellis, M., Chrousos, G.P., Dorn, L., Burke, L., Helmers, K., Kling, M.A., Trickett, P.K., & Putnam, F.W. (1994). Hypothalamic–pituitary–adrenal axis dysregulation in sexually abused girls. *Journal of Clinical Endocrinology and Metabolism, 78,* 249–255.

Demitrack, M., Dale, J., Straus, S., Laue, L., Listwak, S., Kruesi, M.J.P., Chrousos, G.P., & Gold, P.W. (1991). Evidence of impaired activation of the hypothalamic-pituitary-adrenal axis in patients with chronic fatigue syndrome. *Journal of Clinical Endocrinology and Metabolism, 73,* 1224–1234.

DeSouza, E.B., Insel, T.R., Perrin, M.H., Rivier, J., Vale, W.W., & Kuhor, M.J. (1985). Corticotropin-releasing factor receptors are widely distributed within the rat central nervous system. *Journal of Neuroscience, 5,* 3189–3203.

Dieguez, C., Page, M.D., & Scanlon, M.F. (1988). Growth hormone neuroregulation and its alterations in disease states. *Clinical Endocrinology (Oxford), 28,* 109–143.

Dunn, A.J., & Berridge, C.W. (1990). Physiological and behavioral responses to corticotropin-releasing factor administration: Is CRF a mediator of anxiety or stress response? *Brain Research Reviews, 15,* 71–100.

Elfvin, L-G, Lindh, B., & Hokfelt, T. (1993). The chemical neuroanatomy of sympathetic ganglia. *Annual Review of Neuroscience, 16,* 471–507.

Engler, D., Pham, T., Fullerton, M.J., Ooi, G., Funder, J.W., & Clarke, I.J. (1989). Studies on the secretion of corticotropin releasing factor and arginine vasopressin into hypophyseal portal circulation of the conscious sheep. *Neuroendocrinology, 49,* 367–381.

Fuller, R.W. (1992). The involvement of serotonin in regulation of pituitary-adrenocortical function. *Frontiers in Neuroendocrinology, 13,* 250–270.

Gaub, M.P., Bellard, M., Scheuer, I., Chambon, P., & Sassone-Corsi, P. (1990). Activation of the ovalbumin gene by the estrogen receptor involves the Fos-Jun complex. *Cell, 63,* 1267–1276.

Gilbey, M.P., & Spyer, K.M. (1993). Essential organization of the sympathetic nervous system. *Bailliere's Clinical Endocrinology and Metabolism, 7,* 259–278.

Gold, P.W., Goodwin, F., & Chrousos, G.P. (1988a). Clinical and biochemical manifestations of depression: Relationship to the neurobiology of stress, part 1. *New England Journal of Medicine, 319,* 348–353.

Gold, P.W., Goodwin, F., & Chrousos, G.P. (1988b). Clinical and biochemical manifestations of depression: Relationship to the neurobiology of stress, part 2. *New England Journal of Medicine, 319,* 413–420.

Gold, P.W., Gwirtsman, H., Avgerinos, P., Nieman, L.K., Galucci, W.T., Kaye, W., Jimerson, D., Ebert, M., Rittmaster, R., Loriaux, D.L., & Chrousos, G.P. (1986). Abnormal hypothalamic-pituitary-adrenal function in anorexia nervosa: Pathophysiologic mechanisms in underweight and weight-corrected patients. *New England Journal of Medicine, 314,* 1335–1342.

Gold, P.W., Loriaux, D.L., Roy, A., Kling, M.A., Calabrese, J.R., Kellner, C.H., Nieman, L.K., Post, R.M., Picker, D., Galucci, W., Avgerinos, P., Paul, S., Oldfield, E.H., Cutler, G.B., & Chrousos, G.P. (1986). Responses to the corticotropin-releasing hormone in the hypercortisolism of depression and Cushing's disease: Pathophysiologic and diagnostic implications. *New England Journal of Medicine, 314,* 1329–1335.

Gold, P.W., Pigott, T.A., Kling, M.K., Kalogeras, K., & Chrousos, G.P. (1988). Basic and clinical studies with corticotropin releasing hormone: Implications for a possible role in panic disorder. *Psychiatric Clinics of North America, 11,* 327–334.

Gray, T.S. (1989). Amygdala: Role in autonomic and neuroendocrine responses to stress. In J.A. McCubbin, P.G. Kaufman, & C.B. Nemeroff (Eds.), *Stress, neuropeptides and systemic disease* (pp. 37–53). New York: Academic Press.

Griep, E.N., Boerdma, J.W., & de Kloet, E.R. (1993). Altered reactivity of the hypothalamic-pituitary-adrenal axis in the primary fibromyalgia syndrome. *Journal of Rheumatology, 20,* 469–474.

Hinson, J.P. (1990). Paracrine control of adrenocortical function: A new role for the medulla? *Journal of Endocrinology, 124,* 7–9.

Hirano, T., Akira, S., Taga, T., & Kishimoto, T. (1990). Biological and clinical aspects of interleukin-6. *Immunology Today, 11,* 443–449.

Holmes, M.C., Antoni, F.A., Aguilera, G., & Catt, K.J. (1986). Magnocellular axons in passage through the median eminence release vasopressin. *Nature, 319,* 126–129.

Horrocks, P.M., Jones, A.F., Ratcliffe, W.A., Holder, G., White, A., Holder, R., Ratcliffe, J.G., & London, D.R. (1990). Patterns of ACTH and cortisol pulsatility over twenty-four hours in normal males and females. *Clinical Endocrinology (Oxford), 32,* 127–134.

Iranmanesh, A., Lizarralde, G., Short, D., & Veldhuis, J.D. (1990). Intensive venous sampling paradigms disclose high frequency adrenocorticotropin release episodes in normal men. *Journal of Clinical Endocrinology & Metabolism, 71,* 1276–1283.

Jonat, C., Rahmsdorf, H.J., Park, K-K, Cato, A.C.B., Gebel, S., Ponta, H., & Herrlich, P. (1990). Antitumor promotion and anti-inflammation: Down modulation of AP-1 (fos/jun) activity by glucocorticoid hormone. *Cell, 62,* 1189–1204.

Kamilaris, T.C., DeBold, R.C., Pavlou, S.N., Island, D.P., Hoursanidis, A., & Orth, D.N. (1987). Effect of altered thyroid hormone levels on hypothalamic-pituitary-adrenal function. *Journal of Clinical Endocrinology & Metabolism, 65,* 994–999.

Kennedy, R.L., & Jones, T.H. (1991). Cytokines in endocrinology: Their roles in health and in disease. *Journal of Endocrinology, 129,* 167–178.

Kiecolt-Glaser, J.K., & Glaser, R. (1991). Stress and immune function in humans. In R. Ader, D.L. Felten, & N. Cohen (Eds.), *Psychoneuroimmunology* (2nd ed., pp. 849–867). San Diego: Academic Press.

Kiss, A., & Aguilera, G. (1992). Participation of α_1-adrenergic receptors in the secretion of hypothalamic corticotropin-releasing hormone during stress. *Neuroendocrinology, 56,* 153–160.

Lamberts, S.W.J., Verleun, T., Oosterom, R., DeJong, F., & Hackeng, W.H.L. (1984). Corticotropin releasing factor and vasopressin exert a synergistic effect on adrenocorticotropin release in man. *Journal of Clinical Endocrinology and Metabolism, 58,* 298–303.

Mastorakos, G., Chrousos, G.P., & Weber, J. (1993). Recombinant interleukin-6 activates the hypothalamic-pituitary-adrenal axis in humans. *Journal of Clinical Endocrinology and Metabolism, 27,* 1690–1694.

Matta, S.G., Singh, J., Newton, R., & Sharp, B.M. (1990). The adrenocorticotropin response to interleukin-1β instilled into the rat median eminence depends on the local release of catecholamines. *Endocrinology, 127,* 2175–2182.

Munck, A., Guyre, P.M., & Holbrook, N.J. (1984). Physiological functions of glucocorticoids in stress and their relation to pharmacological actions. *Endocrinological Reviews, 5,* 25–44.

Nikolarakis, K.E., Almeida, O.F.X., & Herz, A. (1986). Stimulation of hypothalamic β-endorphin and dynorphin release by corticotropin-releasing factor. *Brain Research, 399,* 152–155.

Ottaway, C.A., & Husband, A.J. (1992). Central nervous system influences on lymphocyte migration. *Brain, Behavior, and Immunity, 6,* 97–116.

Ottenweller, J.E., & Meier, A.H. (1982). Adrenal innervation may be an extrapituitary mechanism able to regulate adrenocortical rhythmicity in rats. *Endocrinology, 111,* 1334–1338.

Perlstein, R.S., Whitnall, M.H., Abrams, J.S., Mougey, E.H., & Neta, R. (1993). Synergistic roles of interleukin-6, interleukin-1, and tumor necrosis factor in adrenocorticotropin response to bacterial lipopolysaccharide *in vitro. Endocrinology, 132,* 946–952.

Phillips, M.I. (1987). Functions of angiotensin in the central nervous system. *Annual Review of Physiology, 49,* 413–435.

Pratt, W.B. (1990). Glucocorticoid receptor structure and the initial events in signal transduction. *Progress in Clinical & Biological Research, 322,* 119–132.

Puddey, J.B., Vandongen, R., Neilin, L.J., & English, D. (1984). Haemodynamic and neuroendocrine consequences of stopping smoking: A controlled study. *Clinical & Experimental Pharmacological Physiology, 11,* 423–426.

Rabin, D., Gold, P.W., Margioris, A., & Chrousos, G.P. (1988). Stress and reproduction: Interactions between the stress and reproductive axis. In G.P. Chrousos, D.L. Loriaux, & P.W. Gold (Eds.), *Mechanisms of physical and emotional stress* (pp. 377–387). New York: Plenum Press.

Redekopp, C., Irvine, C.H.G., Donald, R.A., Livesey, J.H., Sadler, W., Nicholls, M.G., Alexander, S.L., & Evans, M.J. (1986). Spontaneous and stimulated adrenocorticotropin and vasopressin pulsatile secretion in the pituitary venous effluent of the horse. *Endocrinology, 118,* 1410–1416.

Reichlin, S. (1993). Neuroendocrine-immune interactions. *New England Journal of Medicine, 329,* 1246–1253.

Rivier, C., & Rivest, S. (1991). Effect of stress on the activity of the hypothalamic-pituitary-gonadal axis: Peripheral and central mechanisms. *Biology of Reproduction, 45,* 523–532.

Roth, R.H., Tam, S.Y., Ida, Y., Yang, J., & Deutch, A.Y. (1988). Stress and the mesocorticolimbic dopamine systems. *Annals of the New York Academy of Sciences, 537,* 138–147.

Salas, M.A., Evans, S.W., Levell, M.J., & Whicher, J.T. (1990). Interleukin-6 and ACTH act synergistically to stimulate the release of corticosterone from adrenal gland cells. *Clinical and Experimental Immunology, 79,* 470–473.

Sapolsky, R., Rivier, C., Yamamoto, G., Plotsky, P., & Vale, W. (1987). Interleukin-1 stimulates the secretion of hypothalamic corticotropin releasing factor. *Science, 238,* 522–526.

Sawchenko, P.E., Imaki, T., Potter, E., Kovacs, K., Imaki, J., & Vale, W. (1993). The functional neuroanatomy of corticotropin releasing factor. In *Corticotropin-releasing factor: Ciba Foundation Symposium 172* (pp. 5–29). Chichester, England: John Wiley and Sons.

Scheinman, R.I., Gualberto, A., Jewell, C.M., Cidlowski, J.A., Baldwin, A.S., Jr. (1995). Characterization of mechanisms involved in transrepression of NF-KB by activated glucocorticoid receptors. *Molecular Cell Biology, 15,* 943–953.

Skinner, M.K. (1991). Cell-cell interactions in the testis. *Endocrinological Reviews, 12,* 45–77.

Smith, D.F., & Toft, D.O. (1993). Steroid receptors and their associated proteins. *Molecular Endocrinology, 7,* 4–11.

Stein, M., Miller, A.H., & Trestman, R.L. (1991). Depression, the immune system, and health and illness. *Archives of General Psychiatry, 48,* 171–177.

Sternberg, E.M., Chrousos, G.P., Wilder, R.L., & Gold, P.W. (1992). The stress response and the regulation of inflammatory disease: NIH combined clinical staff conference. *Annals of Internal Medicine, 117,* 854–866.

Sternberg, E.M., Young, W.S., Jr., Bernardini, R., Calogero, A.E., Chrousos, G.P., Gold, P.W., & Wilder, R.L. (1989). A central nervous defect in the stress response is associated with susceptibility to streptococcal cell wall arthritis in Lewis rats. *Proceedings of the National Academy of Sciences USA, 86,* 4771–4775.

Swanson, L.W., Sawchenko, P.E., Rivier, J., & Vale, W.W. (1983). Organization of ovine corticotropin-releasing factor immunoreactive cells and fibers in the rat brain: An immunohistochemical study. *Neuroendocrinology, 36,* 165–186.

Tsigos, C., Young, R.J., & White, A. (1993). Diabetic neuropathy is associated with increased activity of the hypothalamic-pituitary-adrenal axis. *Journal of Clinical Endocrinology and Metabolism, 76,* 554–558.

Vale, W.W., Spiess, S., Rivier, C., & Rivier, J. (1981). Characterization of a 41-residue ovine hypothalamic peptide that stimulates secretion of corticotropin and beta-endorphin. *Science, 213,* 1394–1397.

Valentino, R.J., Foote, S.L., & Aston-Jones, G. (1983). Corticotropin-releasing hormone activates noradrenergic neurons of the locus ceruleus. *Brain Research, 270,* 363–367.

Vamvakopoulos, N.C., & Chrousos, G.P. (1993). Evidence of direct estrogen regulation of human corticotropin releasing hormone gene expression: Potential implications for the sexual dimorphism of the stress response and immune/inflammatory reaction. *Journal of Clinical Investigation, 92,* 1896–1902.

Vanderpool, J., Rosenthal, N., Chrousos, G.P., Wehr, T.A., Skwerer, R., Kasper, S., & Gold, P.W. (1991). Evidence for hypothalamic CRH deficiency in patients with seasonal affective disorder. *Journal of Clinical Endocrinology and Metabolism, 72,* 1382–1387.

Vinson, G.P., Whitehouse, B.J., Henvill, K.L., et al. (1988). The actions of α-MSH on the adrenal cortex. In M.E. Hadley (Ed.), *The melanotropic peptides: Biological roles* (Vol. II, pp. 87–133), Boca Raton, FL: CRC Press.

Wand, G.S., & Dobs, A.S. (1991). Alterations in the hypothalamic-pituitary-adrenal axis in actively drinking alcoholics. *Journal of Clinical Endocrinology and Metabolism, 72,* 1290–1295.

Whitnall, M.H. (1989). Stress selectively activates the vasopressin containing subset of corticotropin-releasing hormone neurons. *Neuroendocrinology, 50,* 702–707.

Yang-Yen, H-F, Chambard, J-C, Sun, Y-L, Smeal, T., Schmidt, T.J., Drouin, J., & Karin, M. (1990). Transcriptional interference between c-jun and the glucocorticoid receptor: Mutual inhibition of DNA binding due to direct protein-protein interaction. *Cell, 62,* 1205–1215.

chapter 18

Perceived Stress in Individuals with Spinal Cord Injury

Diana H. Rintala,
Karen A. Hart, and Marcus J. Fuhrer

Stress has long been found to be related to physical and psychological well-being (Benjaminsen, 1981; Brown & Harris, 1978; Jacobs & Charles, 1980; Tennant & Andrews, 1976). It has been hypothesized that a mediator between objective stressors, such as major life events, and well-being is a person's perception of stress (Lazarus, 1966; Lazarus & Folkman, 1984). The question is whether the occurrence of an objectively stressful event has an effect on a person's well-being if the person does not interpret the event as being stressful. Cohen and Williamson (1988) developed and evaluated the Perceived Stress Scale (PSS) to facilitate investigations of the role of perceived stress. They found that some groups of people were more likely to experience higher levels of perceived stress. These groups included persons with lower income, less education, more children, and larger households; persons who were unemployed; those in occupations with relatively low degrees of status and control; people who were divorced, separated, or never married; racial and ethnic minorities; females; and younger persons. They also found that frequency of serious illnesses and serious and nonserious symptoms of illness were greater with increased perceived stress. Higher PSS scores were also associated with several health practices—shorter periods of sleep, infrequent consumption of breakfast, smoking cigarettes, decreased frequency but increased quantity of alcohol consumption, less frequent physical exercise, and increased frequency and variety of legal drug use.

Cohen and Williamson also reported higher perceived stress in persons with disabilities. Their classification of a person having a disability was

This study was conducted under the auspices of the Rehabilitation Research and Training Center on Community-Oriented Services for Persons with Spinal Cord Injury, supported by Grant #H133B80020 from the National Institute on Disability and Rehabilitation Research.

based on responses to a single question regarding how many times in the past month illness or injury had caused them to be either absent from work, to be unable to perform routine activities, or to have difficulty performing routine activities. Chronicity of the disability was not a factor.

Perlin and Schooler (1978) hypothesized that continuing problems referred to as "life strains" may have an independent effect on physical and psychological well-being beyond the effect of discrete life events. Turner and Wood (1985) postulated that chronic physical disabilities are one type of life strain. In a study of persons with a variety of self-reported long-term or permanent disabilities, chronic strain was assessed by combining four factors: 1) extent of functional limitations imposed by the impairment, 2) a global self-assessment of these limitations, 3) self-reports of the intensity and frequency of pain and the limitations imposed by the pain associated with the impairment, and 4) the self-perceived severity of the impairment. They found that both chronic strain and discrete life events were significantly related to depression. A multiple regression analysis indicated that these two sources of stress made independent contributions to explained variance in depression after controlling for demographic factors and duration of disabling condition. Turner and Wood did not address the issue of perceived stress as a mediator between objective stressors and psychological well-being.

To our knowledge, there have been no previously published studies using the PSS with persons with a severe chronic disability such as spinal cord injury (SCI). In the remainder of this chapter we present and discuss the findings regarding perceived stress in a community-based sample of persons with SCI.

METHOD

Sample

This investigation was a component of the Baylor College of Medicine Life Status Study of persons with SCI. The purpose of this study was to assess the status and needs with regard to many life areas of persons with SCI living in the community. In preparation for that study, a population sampling frame was established of 661 persons with SCI who resided in a 13-county area that included Houston and Galveston, Texas. Candidates for the community-based frame were solicited via a variety of media and by contacting them through lists of names obtained from area hospitals and organizations for persons with disabilities. To be included, an individual had to have a traumatic SCI sustained at least 9 months prior to enrollment in the frame, have residual motor disability at least severe enough to require use of an assistive device for walking (if the person was ambulatory), and be at least 17 years old.

The Life Status Study design called for a sample of 100 men and 40 women. Women were to be oversampled to assure an acceptable number for statistical analyses. Candidates for inclusion in the sample were randomly selected from the sampling frame, contacted by telephone or letter, and invited to participate. That process continued until the desired numbers of men and women agreed to participate. Characteristics of the sample are displayed in Tables 1 and 2.

Procedure

After being introduced to the study by telephone, participants were sent a packet of questionnaires and standardized instruments covering a large number of topics regarding various areas of life. The completed packets were collected at the time of an interview conducted in the participant's residence. Participants underwent a medical examination at The Institute for Rehabilitation and Research, including a standardized set of laboratory tests. In addition to the free examination and tests, participants received $100 upon completion of all parts of the study, and all associated costs were paid (e.g., transportation, meals).

Three years following the first phase of data collection, the men were invited to participate in a second phase of the study. Of the 100 men who participated in Phase 1, 89 agreed to participate in Phase 2. A total of 3 men had died in the interim, 4 men could not be contacted, and 4 men declined the opportunity to participate in Phase 2. Women were not included in Phase 2 because of funding restrictions and time restrictions imposed by the grant period. However, a current study on community integration involves the women who participated in Phase 1 and incorporates many of the same measures.

Measures—Phases 1 and 2

The following measures were used.

Demographic and Injury-Related Measures Participants reported their age, gender, race/ethnicity, education, veteran status, personal monthly income, age at onset of SCI, time since onset of SCI, and the cause of their injury.

Perceived Stress The Perceived Stress Scale (PSS; Cohen, Kamarck, & Mermelstein, 1983) is a 10-item instrument that measures the degree to which respondents find their lives to be unpredictable, uncontrollable, and overloading. Each item is rated on a 5-point scale ranging from 0 to 4 with regard to the frequency with which the person felt or thought a certain way (e.g., nervous, things were going your way) in the past month (never, almost never, sometimes, fairly often, very often). It has been shown to have high internal reliability (alpha coefficient = .78) and acceptable evidence of validity (Cohen & Williamson, 1988).

Table 1. Characteristics of the sample

Characteristic	Mean			Standard deviation			Range		
	Total	Women	Men	Total	Women	Men	Total	Women	Men
Age (years)	37.0	37.1	36.9	11.5	11.5	11.6	19–77	21–76	19–77
Age at onset of SCI (years)	26.4	25.8	26.7	11.0	12.5	10.4	Birth–68	Birth–58	14–68
Time since SCI (years)	10.6	11.3	10.2	7.8	7.7	7.9	.75–48	2–36	.75–48
Monthly personal income*	$1,235	$771	$1,426	$2,145	$490	$2,508	$0–22,000	$0–2,448	$0–22,000

Significant gender differences *p < .05.

Table 2. Further characteristics of the sample

Characteristic	Number			Percent		
	Total	Women	Men	Total	Women	Men
Race / Ethnicity						
White	95	27	68	67.9	67.5	68.0
African-American	28	9	19	20.0	22.5	19.0
Hispanic	15	4	11	10.7	10.0	11.0
Other	2	0	2	1.4	0.0	2.0
Education**						
Less than high school	24	8	16	17.1	20.0	16.0
High school graduate	41	19	22	29.3	47.5	22.0
Some college	75	13	62	53.6	32.5	62.0
Veteran*	23	2	21	16.4	5.0	21.0
Level and completeness of injury						
Quadriplegia / functionally motor complete	58	14	44	41.4	35.0	44.0
Paraplegia / functionally motor complete	60	18	42	42.9	45.0	42.0
Quadriplegia or paraplegia / functionally motor incomplete	22	8	14	15.7	20.0	14.0
Cause of injury						
Motor vehicle crash	70	20	50	50.0	50.0	50.0
Acts of violence	27	11	16	19.3	27.5	16.0
Sports	23	4	19	16.4	10.0	19.0
Falls	10	2	8	7.1	5.0	8.0
Other	10	3	7	7.1	7.5	7.0

Note: The sum of percentages does not equal 100 for cause of injury ($N = 140$) due to rounding.
Significant gender differences: $**p < .01$, $*p < .05$.

Depressive Symptomatology The Center for Epidemiological Studies Depression Scale (CES-D) is a 20-item, self-report scale designed to measure symptoms of depression in the general population (Radloff, 1977). Each item was rated on a scale ranging from 0 to 3 according to how often the person experienced certain feelings (e.g., depression, hopefulness) during the past week (less than 1 day, 1–2 days, 3–4 days, 5–7 days). Scores for positive feelings were reversed. A high level of internal consistency was found by Radloff (1977), with alpha coefficients ranging from .84 to .90. Radloff also reported correlations with other measures of depression ranging from .50 to .70, indicating moderately good concurrent validity.

Life Satisfaction The 18-item Life Satisfaction Index A (LSIA) is designed to measure zest for life; fortitude; congruence between desired and achieved goals; physical, psychological, and social self-concept; and mood tone (Adams, 1969). The respondent indicates whether he or she agrees, disagrees, or is uncertain about each statement. In Schulz and Decker's (1985) study of persons with SCI, the scale had an alpha coefficient of .76, indicating acceptable internal consistency. Lohman (1977) found the index to have satisfactory concurrent validity with other measures of life satisfaction.

Handicap To measure various dimensions of handicap, the Craig Handicap Assessment and Reporting Technique (CHART) was administered to participants (Whiteneck, Charlifue, Gerhart, Overholser, & Richardson, 1992). The five dimensions were Physical Independence, Mobility, Occupation, Social Integration, and Economic Self-Sufficiency. Physical Independence is the individual's ability to sustain a customarily effective independent existence. Mobility is the individual's ability to move about effectively in his or her surroundings. Occupation is the individual's ability to occupy time in the manner customary to that person's sex, age, and culture. Social integration is the individual's ability to participate in and maintain customary social relationships. Economic Self-Sufficiency is the individual's ability to sustain customary socioeconomic activity and independence.

Scores on each dimension could range between 0 and 100, with the higher value indicating absence of handicap. A total CHART score was obtained by summing the scores on the five dimensions. Test-retest reliability coefficients reported by Whiteneck et al. are Physical Independence, .92; Mobility, .95; Occupation, .89; Social Integration, .81; and Economic Self-Sufficiency, .80. As a validity check, Whiteneck et al. compared CHART scores with rehabilitation professionals' ratings of the level of handicap of the members of the sample. Individuals rated as having a high level of handicap had, on average, total CHART scores that were significantly lower (reflecting more handicap) than people rated as having a low level of handicap. The validity of the separate CHART dimensions, except for Economic Self-Sufficiency, was supported in a similar manner. Only the Mobility, Occupation, and Social Integration dimensions are included in the present report.

Living Arrangement Participants were asked whether they lived alone or with others. If they lived with others, they were asked to describe their relationship (e.g., spouse, parent, child) to each person in the household.

Social Support Social support was assessed during the home interview using the procedures of Schulz and Decker (1985). Each participant was asked to name persons whom he or she deemed to be important sources of help, support, and guidance. The participant then rank-ordered this list of persons with regard to importance. The satisfaction of the participant with the relationship with each of the five top-ranked persons was assessed on a 5-point scale ranging from 1 (very dissatisfied) to 5 (very satisfied). Next, the participant indicated on 5-point, Likert-type scales the frequency with which each of the five top-ranked persons provided each of 11 kinds of support. Included were items regarding affective, cognitive, and instrumental types of support. The rating scale was: 1 (not at all), 2 (rarely), 3 (on some occasions), 4 (often), and 5 (very frequently). A total social support score was derived by summing ratings on the 11 scales across all supporters within a participant's network, resulting in scores that could range from 0 (no support) to 275 (extensive support). The internal consistency of the total score was found by Schulz and Decker (1985) to be high (coefficient alpha = .90).

Self-Assessed Health Status Self-assessed health status was measured on a four-point, Likert-type scale using the descriptors of excellent, good, fair, and poor. Schulz and Decker (1985) used this measure as a correlate of subjective well-being but not as an outcome measure.

Morbidity Index An index was derived from self-reports on whether any of a large number of health conditions had occurred in the past 12 months prior to taking part in the study. Many problems were counted as occurring only if they interfered with daily activities or occurred more than once a month. Each type (not each occurrence) of health problem that had occurred added 1 point to the index.

Urinary Tract Infection Urinalysis and urine cultures were conducted to assess possible urinary tract infections (UTIs). Presumptive evidence of a UTI for research purposes included a urine colony count above specified levels according to the type of urinary management system utilized by the participant.

Pressure Ulcers A thorough inspection of the skin over the whole body was performed during the physical examination to assess the absence or presence of pressure ulcers. The location and severity of each ulcer was also noted. A 4-point grading scheme, consistent with that used by the National Spinal Cord Injury Statistical Center database (Stover & Fine, 1986), was used to assess severity of each ulcer—I) limited to superficial and dermal layers, including redness that did not blanch to touch and redness that required no intervention; II) involving epidermal and dermal layers extending into adipose tissue; III) extending through superficial structure and adipose tissue down to and including muscle; and IV) destruction of all soft tissue structures and communication with bone or joint structures.

Impairment Degree of paralytic impairment was assessed during the physical examination by means of the ASIA Total Motor Index Score (American Spinal Injury Association, 1987). This score is the sum of ratings for 10 key muscle segments on each side of the body. Each muscle segment was rated on a 6-point scale ranging from 0 (total paralysis) to 5 (normal). Total scores could range from 0 to 100 (50 for each side).

Participants also were categorized by a combination of their level of injury and the completeness of the injury. First, those whose injuries were in the cervical area were categorized as having quadriplegia. The remainder were categorized as having paraplegia. Second, participants were divided into those who had some motor function below the level of injury (i.e., functionally motor incomplete) and those who did not (i.e., functionally motor complete). Finally, three groups were formed by combining level and completeness of injury—Quadriplegia/Functionally Motor Complete, Paraplegia/Functionally Motor Complete, and Quadriplegia or Paraplegia/Functionally Motor Incomplete.

Disability A self-report version of the Functional Independence Measure (FIM; Hamilton, Granger, Sherwin, Zielezny, & Tashman, 1987) was administered during the home interview to assess level of disability. This prototype instrument for the FONE FIM (Smith, Hamilton, & Granger, 1989) was developed by Andres, Robinson, Sand, Weyford, and Mills (1988). Each participant's degree of independence was assessed on a 7-point scale for each of 13 activities of daily living (i.e., walking or using a wheelchair; transferring to and from tub or shower; bathing; grooming; dressing upper body; dressing lower body; feeding; transfer to and from the toilet; bladder management; bowel management; and toileting). A total score was derived by summing the ratings across the 13 activities. Scores could range from 13 (totally dependent) to 91 (totally independent).

Personal Assistance Received Participants were asked whether they received any personal assistance with activities of daily living. If they did, they were asked whether they received 1 hour or less per day or more than 1 hour per day.

Measures—Phase 2 Only

Several additional measures were used in Phase 2.

Hassles Hassles are relatively minor stressors encountered in daily life as described by Crewe and Clarke earlier in this volume (Chapter 16). Scores on the Hassles Scale (Kanner, Coyne, Schaefer, & Lazarus, 1981) have been shown to be related to self-reported health status, functional status, subjective well-being, and objective health outcomes. The respondent indicated how much of a hassle, annoyance, or bother each item had been in the past month on a 4-point scale ranging from 0 to 3 (none or not applicable, somewhat, quite a bit, a great deal). The original Hassles Scale contained 53 items. We added four items that, based on previous research findings, we believed may be a source of stress for persons with disabilities—personal assistance, assistive equipment, transportation, and accessing the environment.

Life Events The Life Events Scale (Avison & Turner, 1988) is a checklist of events such as "Problems with children," "Serious illness," and "Close friend died." The original instrument devised by Avison and Turner contained a list of 30 items. We added two items that we believed may be important events for some persons with disabilities—"Loss of a caregiver" and "Loss or reduction of benefits." Each item that happened to the respondent during the past 12 months was checked. A count of the items checked provided a measure of objective stress caused by relatively discrete life events.

Personal Independence The Personal Independence Profile (PIP; Nosek, Fuhrer, & Howland, 1992) assesses four broad aspects of independence: perceived control over one's life, psychological self-reliance, physical functioning, and environmental resources. Explicitly included in its purpose is measurement of self-direction. The control portion of the PIP is a 10-item scale that assesses the degree of control over a life area (e.g., material comforts, participation in active recreation, close relationships) that a person perceives himself or herself to have. Each item was rated on a 5-point scale ranging from 1 to 5 (no control, little control, some control, a lot of control, complete control).

Satisfaction with Personal Assistance The Personal Assistance Satisfaction Index (PASI; Nosek, Quan, & Potter, 1995) assesses how satisfied a person is with various aspects of their personal assistance (i.e., cost, control, availability, quality). Each item was rated on a 5-point scale ranging from 1 to 5 (not at all satisfied, slightly satisfied, somewhat satisfied, very satisfied, extremely satisfied). The original PASI contains 16 items. We added one item assessing satisfaction with the availability of substitute personal assistants if the usual assistant cannot be available.

Social Support The Interpersonal Support Evaluation List (ISEL, Cohen, Mermelstein, Kamarck, & Hoberman, 1985) is a 40-item list of statements concerning the perceived availability of potential social resources. The respondent indicated whether each item was true or false about himself or herself. The ISEL has proven reliability (Cronbach's alpha = .77) and validity.

RESULTS—PHASE 1

Perceived Stress

Women reported significantly more perceived stress than men (women, 18; men, 14; Table 3). These findings, when compared with the results of the national sample of the general population (Cohen & Williamson, 1988), indicate that both men and women with SCI reported more perceived stress, on average, than their counterparts in the general population (Figure 1). However, the difference was much larger for women. In the general population, the mean score on the PSS for women was 14 and 13 for men.

Table 3. Phase 1 means, standard deviations, and ranges

Measure	Mean			Standard deviation			Range		
	Total	Women	Men	Total	Women	Men	Total	Women	Men
Perceived stress**	15.1	18.0	13.9	7.2	6.0	7.4	0–33	6–29	0–33
CES-D*	12.1	14.7	11.0	9.7	9.0	9.9	0–40	0–40	0–40
LSIA	8.8	8.1	9.1	4.3	4.7	4.1	0–18	0–17	1–18
Morbidity index	6.4	7.2	6.1	4.0	3.8	4.0	0–16	1–16	0–15
Mobility (CHART)*	79.5	71.9	82.6	23.7	24.4	22.8	5–100	10–100	5–100
Occupation (CHART)	60.2	63.7	58.7	37.7	38.0	37.7	0–100	6–100	0–100
Social integration (CHART)	81.2	84.2	80.0	24.7	25.2	24.5	10–100	10–100	15–100
Social support	182.3	186.1	180.8	46.3	44.7	47.1	40–271	85–271	40–266
Satisfaction with social support	4.7	4.6	4.7	0.5	0.5	0.5	2–5	3–5	2–5
ASIA total motor index score	43.7	43.0	44.1	22.5	19.5	23.6	0–95	0–85	0–95
Self-reported FIM	59.5	57.3	60.4	20.9	19.9	21.4	17–90	17–83	20–90
Number of pressure ulcers on day of examination	0.7	0.5	0.7	1.2	0.8	1.3	0–7	0–3	0–7

Note: CES-D, Center for Epidemiological Studies Depression Scale; LSAI, life satisfaction. Significant gender differences: **$p < .01$, *$p < .05$.

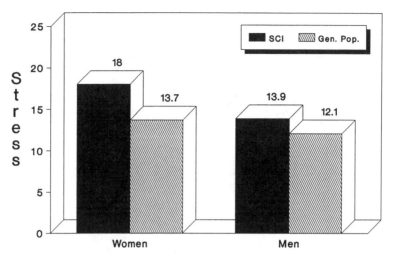

Figure 1. Perceived stress: SCI versus general population by gender.

Correlates of Perceived Stress

A number of correlates of perceived stress were identified. Variables that were not significantly related are not described in detail. However, results are presented in various tables.

Depressive Symptomatology Women had higher scores on the CES-D scale than men (women, 15; men, 11; Table 3). These compared unfavorably with the means for general population samples that range from 7 to 9. Scores on the CES-D were significantly correlated with scores on the PSS for both women and men (Figure 2). People who had more depressive symptomatology perceived more stress.

Life Satisfaction Women and men did not differ significantly on the LSIA (women, 8; men, 9; Table 3). Their scores compared poorly with the mean of 13 found in a study of the general population. Life satisfaction was significantly related to perceived stress for both women and men (Figure 2). People who were less satisfied with their lives reported more perceived stress.

Morbidity Index Women had a mean morbidity index of 7 and men had a mean of 6—not a significant difference (Table 3). In other words, women had 7 of the problems counted in the index and men had 6 of the problems, on average. No other studies have used this index. The morbidity index was significantly related to perceived stress for men but not for women (Figure 2). Men who had more health problems perceived more stress.

Social Integration On the Social Integration dimension of the CHART, women had a mean of 84 and men had a mean of 80—not a

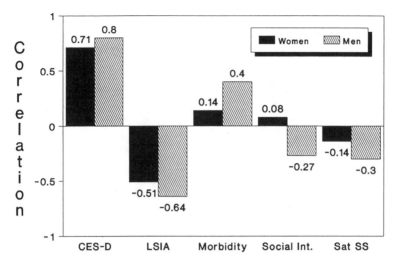

Figure 2. Phase 1 correlates of perceived stress by gender. (CES-D, Center for Epidemiological Studies Depression Scale; LSIA, Life Satisfaction Index A; Int., Integration.; Sat SS, Satisfaction with Social Support.)

significant difference (Table 3). A score of 100 indicates absence of handicap (i.e., similar to the general population). For men, perceived stress was significantly related to social integration. This was not the case for women (Figure 2). Men who were less well integrated socially perceived more stress.

Satisfaction with Social Support   Women and men had nearly equal mean ratings of their satisfaction with their social support (women, 5; men, 5; Table 3). These ratings indicated a very high level of satisfaction with support persons, in general. Perceived stress was significantly related to satisfaction with social support for men but not for women (Figure 2). Men who were less satisfied with their social support reported more perceived stress.

Self-Assessed Health   Ratings of their own health by women were excellent, 15%; good, 65%; fair, 18%. Only one woman rated her health as poor. Ratings of health for men were excellent, 17%; good, 69%; and fair, 14% (Table 4). Perceived stress was significantly related to the self-assessed health ratings for both women and men. The better the health rating, the lower the stress score, on average (Figure 3).

Severity of Worst Pressure Ulcer   Women and men did not differ on the severity of pressure ulcers (Table 5). Ten percent of the women and 15% of the men had at least one severe pressure ulcer (stage III or IV), and another 20% of the women and 19% of the men had at least one mild pressure ulcer (stage I or II). For women, perceived stress

Table 4. Frequency distributions of living situation and health data

Measure	Number			Percent		
	Total	Women	Men	Total	Women	Men
Living arrangement						
Live alone	23	5	18	16.4	12.5	18.0
Live with spouse	45	11	34	32.1	27.5	34.0
Live with parent(s)	32	5	27	22.9	12.5	27.0
Live with child(ren)**	41	21	20	29.3	52.5	20.0
Self-assessed health						
Excellent	23	6	17	16.4	15.0	17.0
Good	95	26	69	67.9	65.0	69.0
Fair	21	7	14	15.0	17.5	14.0
Poor	1	1	0	0.7	2.5	0.0
Personal assistance received						
None	70	20	50	50.0	50.0	50.0
1 hour or less per day	20	5	15	14.3	12.5	15.0
More than 1 hour per day	50	15	35	35.7	37.5	35.0

Note: Separate analyses were performed for each type of person in household because participants could indicate more than one type.
Significant gender differences: **$p < .01$.

was significantly related to the severity of their worst pressure ulcer, but this was not true for men (Figure 4). Women who had severe pressure ulcers perceived more stress than women with mild ulcers.

Variables Unrelated to Perceived Stress

Many other variables were examined for relationships with perceived stress; however, none of these were significantly related for either men or women. They included age, race or ethnicity, education, veteran status, persons with whom one lived, cause of SCI, age at onset, time since onset, ASIA Total Motor Index, self-reported FIM, amount of personal assistance received with activities of daily living, amount of social support, the Mobility and Occupation dimensions of the CHART, personal income, having a pressure ulcer or not on examination, number of pressure ulcers found on examination, and having presumptive evidence of a UTI based on laboratory results (Tables 1–5).

Summary of Phase 1

Gender Differences The Phase 1 results indicate that women with SCI have more perceived stress than men with SCI and more than women in the general population. Women also reported more depressive symptomatology than men, and they were more likely to be living with a child. Men with SCI had higher personal incomes, more education, and greater mobility than women with SCI. Men were also more likely to be veterans (Tables 1–4).

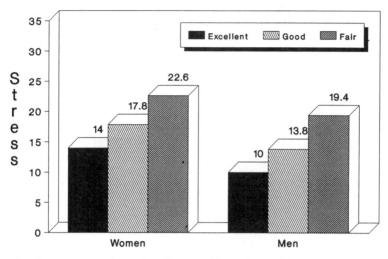

Figure 3. Phase 1 perceived stress by self-assessed health by gender.

Correlates of Perceived Stress Correlates of perceived stress for women included depressive symptomatology, life satisfaction, self-assessed health, and the severity of pressure ulcers. Correlates for men were depressive symptomatology, life satisfaction, the morbidity index, self-assessed health, the Social Integration dimension of the CHART, and satisfaction with their social support.

RESULTS—PHASE 2

Perceived Stress

The men who participated in Phase 2 had a mean perceived stress score of 14, which was almost identical to the mean stress score for these same

Table 5. Frequency distributions of urinary and pressure ulcer data

	Number			Percent		
Measure	Total	Women	Men	Total	Women	Men
Presumptive evidence of a UTI on day of examination	50	15	35	35.7	37.5	35.0
Presence of at least one pressure ulcer on day of examination	46	12	34	32.9	30.0	34.0
Severity of worst pressure ulcer						
None	94	28	66	67.1	70.0	66.0
Mild (Stage I or II only)	26	8	18	18.6	20.0	18.0
Severe (Stage III or IV)	19	4	15	13.6	10.0	15.0
Missing Severity Rating	1	0	1	0.7	0.0	1.0

Note: UTI, urinary tract infection.

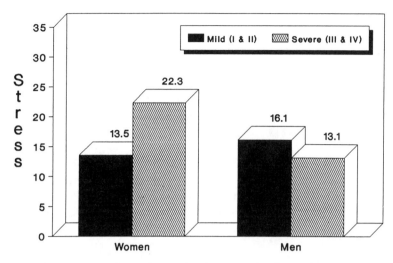

Figure 4. Phase 1 perceived stress by severity of pressure ulcer by gender.

89 men for Phase 1 (Table 6). However, scores for some individual men changed dramatically; change scores ranged from a decrease of 19 to an increase of 22.

Correlates of Perceived Stress

Correlates of perceived stress in Phase 2 were identified.

Depressive Symptomatology In Phase 2 the men had a mean score on the CES-D of 10 compared with a score of 11 for these men in Phase 1 (Table 6). Men who had more depressive symptoms also perceived more stress.

Life Satisfaction The mean LSIA score for the men in Phase 2 was 9, almost identical to their score in Phase 1 (Table 6). Life satisfaction

Table 6. Phase 2 means, standard deviations, and ranges

Measure	Mean	SD	Range
Perceived stress	14.1	7.9	1–33
CES-D	10.4	9.5	0–42
LSIA	9.2	3.8	0–18
Hassles scale	34.1	22.9	0–103
Morbidity index	5.5	4.3	0–16
Life events scale	2.4	2.2	0–10
ISEL	32.3	7.1	12–40
PIP	37.8	7.1	20–50
PASI (n = 36)	59.7	12.4	32–85

Note: SD, standard deviation; CES-D, Center for Epidemiological Studies Depression Scale; LSIA, Life Satisfaction Index A; ISEL, Interpersonal Support Evaluation List; PIP, Personal Independence Profile; PASI, Personal Assistance Satisfaction Index.

continued to be significantly related to perceived stress. Men who were more satisfied with their lives perceived less stress.

Hassles Scale The men in Phase 2 had a mean Hassles score of 34, or 20% of possible points (Table 6). This is twice as high as the 10% of possible points found in a study of the general population. Hassles were significantly correlated with perceived stress (Figure 5). Men who reported more hassles also reported more perceived stress.

Morbidity Index Men in Phase 2 had a mean morbidity index score of 6, very close to their score in Phase 1 (Table 6). The morbidity index was significantly related to perceived stress (Figure 5). Men with higher morbidity index scores reported higher levels of perceived stress.

Life Events Scale The average life events score was 2.4 (Table 6). This was higher than the score of 1.4 found in a group of persons with and without physical disabilities. The correlation with perceived stress was significant (Figure 5). Men who experienced more life events reported more perceived stress.

Interpersonal Support Evaluation List The men in Phase 2 had a mean score on the ISEL of 32 (Table 6). This is comparable to means ranging from 33 to 34 obtained in studies of the general population. There was a significant relationship between the ISEL and the PSS (Figure 5). Men with more social support perceived less stress.

Personal Independence Profile The mean score on the PIP was 37 (Table 6). No other mean scores have been reported for this measure. Men who reported being more in control of their lives had lower stress scores (Figure 5).

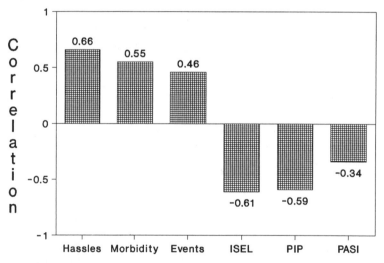

Figure 5. Phase 2 correlates of perceived stress. (ISEL, Interpersonal Support Evaluation List; PIP, Personal Independence Profile; PASI, Personal Assistance Satisfaction Index.)

Personal Assistance Satisfaction Index For the 36 men who received personal assistance, the mean score on the PASI was 60 (Table 6). This is similar to the mean score of 59 obtained for a national sample of consumers with a variety of physical disabilities selected by 10 independent living centers. Men who were more satisfied with their personal assistance reported less perceived stress (Figure 5).

Stepwise Multiple Regression Analyses

A multiple regression analysis was performed to determine which of the variables introduced in Phase 2 that had significant bivariate relationships with perceived stress accounted for the most variance (Table 7). Hassles entered first and accounted for 43% of the variance in perceived stress. Personal independence (PIP) accounted for 13% additional variance, life events accounted for 4% of the variance, and social support, as measured by the ISEL, accounted for 3% of the variance. The Morbidity Index did not enter the equation. The total amount of variance accounted for (R^2) was 63% with an adjusted R^2 of .61.

A second multiple regression analysis was done using data only from the 36 men who received personal assistance in order to determine the variance accounted for by satisfaction with personal assistance (PASI; Table 8). Social support (ISEL) accounted for 37% of the variance, the Morbidity Index accounted for 13% of the variance, and Hassles accounted for an additional 7%. The PASI, PIP, and Life Events scores did not enter the equation.

Summary of Phase 2

Average levels of perceived stress remained stable across the 3 years between Phase 1 and Phase 2. However, some individuals' scores changed dramatically. More perceived stress was associated with more depressive symptomatology, less life satisfaction, higher morbidity, more hassles, more life events, less social support, and less control over one's life. For men with personal assistance, more perceived stress was related to less satisfaction with the assistance.

Table 7. Stepwise multiple regression of phase 2 correlates of perceived stress for all male subjects

Variable	R	R^2	R^2 change
Hassles scale	.66	.43	.43
Personal independence profile (PIP)	.75	.56	.13
Life events scale	.77	.60	.04
Interpersonal support evaluation list (ISEL)	.79	.63	.03
Morbidity index	Did not enter equation		

Note: N = 89. Adjusted R^2 = .61.

Table 8. Stepwise multiple regression of phase 2 correlates of perceived stress for male subjects, using personal assistance services

Variable	R	R^2	R^2 change
Interpersonal support evaluation list (ISEL)	.61	.37	.37
Morbidity index	.71	.50	.13
Hassles scale	.76	.57	.07
Personal independence profile (PIP)	Did not enter equation		
Personal assistance satisfaction index (PASI)	Did not enter equation		
Life events scale	Did not enter equation		

Note: N = 36. Adjusted R^2 = .53.

The multiple regression analysis for all 89 men indicated that hassles accounted for the most variance in perceived stress, followed by personal independence, life events, and social support. The multiple regression analysis for the 36 men receiving personal assistance demonstrated that, for these men, social support accounted for the most variance in perceived stress, followed by the Morbidity Index and Hassles.

CONCLUSIONS

Because of the significantly higher perceived stress reported by the women in this study, it is very important to identify the causes of the stress. Once the causes are identified, interventions must be designed and evaluated to attempt to alleviate the causes of stress or to help women with disabilities manage their stress effectively.

The results of Phase 2, which for reasons of limited time and funding included only men, suggest additional variables (e.g., hassles, life events, personal independence) that need to be investigated for relationships with perceived stress for women. Sources of stress for men cannot simply be assumed to be the same as sources of stress for women. For both men and women, the predictors of change in perceived stress scores may help to identify potential areas for interventions. Such analyses of the men's data are planned. Once a second wave of data collection for women that is in progress has been completed, these analyses also will be possible for women.

REFERENCES

Adams, D.L. (1969). Analysis of a life satisfaction index. *Journal of Gerontology*, 24, 470–474.

American Spinal Cord Injury Association. (1987). *Standards for Neurological Classification of Spinal Injury Patients.* Chicago: Author.

Andres, J., Robinson, P., Sand, M., Weyford, M., & Mills, J. (1988). *The modified FIM guide: Behavioral flow chart.* Kansas City, MO: Truman Medical Center East.

Avison, W.R., & Turner, R.J. (1988). Stressful life events and depressive symptoms: Disaggregating the effects of acute stressors and chronic strains. *Journal of Health and Social Behavior, 29,* 253–264.

Benjaminsen, S. (1981). Stressful life events preceding the onset of neurotic depression. *Psychological Medicine, 11,* 369–378.

Brown, N.B., & Harris, T. (1978). *Social origins of depression: A study of psychiatric disorder in women.* London, England: Tavistock Publications.

Cohen, S., Kamarck, T., & Mermelstein, R. (1983). A global measure of perceived stress. *Journal of Health and Social Behavior, 24,* 385–396.

Cohen, S., Mermelstein, R., Kamarck, T., & Hoberman, H. (1985). Measuring the functional components of social support. In I.G. Sarason & B.R. Sarason (Eds.), *Social support: Theory, research and application.* Dordrecht, The Netherlands: Martinus Nijhoff.

Cohen, S., & Williamson, G.M. (1988). Perceived stress in a probability sample of the United States. In S. Oskamp, & S. Spacapan (Eds.), *The social psychology of health: Claremont symposium on applied social psychology.* Newbury Park, CA: Sage Publications.

Hamilton, B.B., Granger, C.V., Sherwin, F.S., Zielezny, M., & Tashman, J.S. (1987). A uniform national data system for medical rehabilitation. In M.J. Fuhrer (Ed.), *Rehabilitation outcomes: Analysis and measurement* (pp. 137–147). Baltimore: Paul H. Brookes Publishing Co.

Jacobs, T.J., & Charles, E. (1980). Life events and the occurrence of cancer in children. *Psychosomatic Medicine, 42,* 11–24.

Kanner, A.D., Coyne, J.C., Schaefer, C., & Lazarus, R.S. (1981). Comparison of two modes of stress measurement. *Journal of Behavioral Medicine, 4,* 1–39.

Lazarus, R.S. (1966). *Psychological stress and the coping process.* New York: McGraw Hill.

Lazarus, R.S., & Folkman, S. (1984). *Stress, coping, and adaptation.* New York: Springer-Verlag.

Lohman, N. (1977). Correlation of life satisfaction, morale, and adjustment measures. *Journal of Gerontology, 32,* 73–75.

Nosek, M., Fuhrer, M.J., & Howland, C.A. (1992). Independence among people with disabilities: II. Personal Independence Profile. *Rehabilitation Counseling Bulletin, 36*(1), 21–36.

Nosek, M., Quan, H., & Potter, C. (1995). The Personal Assistance Satisfaction Index: An assessment tool for individuals with severe physical disabilities. Manuscript in preparation.

Perlin, L.I., & Schooler, C. (1978). The structure of coping. *Journal of Health and Social Behavior, 19,* 2–21.

Radloff, L.S. (1977). The CES-D scale: A self-report depression scale for research in the general population. *Applied Psychological Measurement, 1,* 385–401.

Schulz, R., & Decker, S. (1985). Long-term adjustment to physical disability: The role of social support, perceived control and self-blame. *Journal of Personality and Social Psychology, 48,* 1162–1172.

Smith, P., Hamilton, B.B., & Granger, C.V. (1989). *Functional independence measure decision tree: The FONE FIM.* Buffalo: Research Foundation of the State University of New York.

Standards for Neurological Classification of Spinal Injury Patients. (1987). Chicago: American Spinal Injury Association.

Stover, S.L., & Fine, P.R. (Eds.). (1986). *Spinal cord injury: The facts and figures.* Birmingham: University of Alabama at Birmingham.

Tennant, C., & Andrews, G. (1976). A scale to measure the stress of life events. *Australian and New Zealand Journal of Psychiatry, 10,* 27–32.

Turner, R.J., & Wood, D.W. (1985). Depression and disability: The stress process in a chronically strained population. *Research in Community and Mental Health, 5,* 77–109.

Whiteneck, G.G., Charlifue, S.W., Gerhart, K.A., Overholser, J.D., & Richardson, G.N. (1992). Quantifying handicap: A new measure of long-term rehabilitation outcomes. *Archives of Physical Medicine and Rehabilitation, 73*(6), 519–526.

chapter 19

Women as Care Providers and Care Receivers

Effective Strategies

Carolyn M. Baum

As we consider the issues of women and disability, it is important to look at the issues of women who because of a disability may require the assistance of a family member to remain engaged in their daily activities. Women are usually the providers of such daily care, particularly when the person has sustained a cognitive loss. It is important to explore the caregiving process and how it is possible to manage new, and perhaps changing, responsibilities that support the function of loved ones without either person having to face undue stress or decreased function. The model that forms the basis of this chapter was developed on a sample of persons with Alzheimer's disease; future work will be carried out on persons with other cognitive deficits, particularly stroke and head injury. Although the focus of this book is on physical disabilities, often cognitive loss affects physical performance. In addition, when accidents occur, physical and mental deficits can coexist, especially with traumatic brain injuries. This issue therefore warrants discussion.

Many women who survive accidents, and particularly those who sustain an injury with a resulting cognitive loss, need help. Caring for such people requires specialized knowledge and skills. Without training, people are not prepared for this role (Acorn, 1993). Most of what is currently known about managing persons with cognitive loss within the family unit has evolved from studies of older adults, not from studies of younger women. Future studies must look at the needs of families managing persons

This work was supported in part by the National Institute on Aging, Grant #A603991 and The Norman J. Stupp Foundation. It was conducted as a part of the Memory and Aging Project at the Alzheimer's Disease Research Center at Washington University School of Medicine, St. Louis.

of all ages. Also, rather than looking only at the provision of care, another goal should be facilitating independence in those who have the potential to make continuing progress.

The current system of care relies heavily on the family. Of the care needed by a person with an impairment, 85% is given by the family system (Brody, 1990); 83% of all caregivers are female, 39% are daughters, and 34% are employed (Lawton, Brody, & Saperstein, 1989). These women's assistance comes at an enormous physical and financial cost. Clearly it deserves the attention of rehabilitation professionals, who must consider patients in the context of their families if rehabilitation is to achieve significant and permanent outcomes. The pivotal link that these women play between the person with the disability and the formal (and informal) social and health services must be understood.

The time commitment of care is significant. Montgomery, Gonyea, and Hooyman (1985) report that families provide 36.7 hours of care per week to frail older adults, and 20% have given that care for more than 5 years. They report that 75% of the daughters devote a part of the day to caregiving activities, 7 days a week. An even greater commitment of time is involved when the person has a cognitive deficit. Families provide 56 hours of assistance per week to older adults with cognitive loss (Birkel & Jones, 1989) and are constantly forced to adapt and adjust to new problems (Chenworth & Spencer, 1986). In addition to time, a caregiver's commitments include heavy physical labor, with tasks of transferring family members and in some cases lifting (Miller, McFall, & Montgomery, 1991). The process of care causes strain in work, finances, and the emotional and physical status of the caregiver (Cantor, 1983; Robinson, 1983). Thus, rehabilitation professionals must consider the needs of the family, and particularly women, as care is planned for persons with disabilities. The family plays an important role in the rehabilitation process by providing the environmental, social, and emotional support to challenge independence and continued recovery in their family member who has impairments.

The Rehabilitation Research Plan of the National Center for Medical Rehabilitation Research (National Institutes of Health, 1993) was designed to foster the development of better medical rehabilitation treatments for people with disabilities. The following priorities of the plan address issues of the family:

- Identify coping strategies and support mechanisms, including service provision and family education, that promote successful adjustment and community integration for both children and adults with disabilities. (p. 61)
- Identify the factors that contribute to the successful long-term integration of persons with functional impairment into their families and communities. (p. 61)

The goal of rehabilitation should therefore be twofold: maximizing the function of the person with the disabling condition and minimizing the stress on the caregiver and family. The following discussion summarizes a study designed to identify the factors guiding the development of intervention strategies for persons with Alzheimer's disease. The processing deficits experienced by older adults with cognitive loss of this type can offer insight to the problems that must be addressed with persons with head injuries and strokes.

The NCMRR model was used to frame this study (Figure 1). By incorporating measures across the levels of impairment, functional limitation, disability, and societal limitation, it was possible to study the problem of cognitive loss and how it affects the actions and interactions of the person with the impairment and the family.

The goal of this study was to examine the importance of activity in maximizing the function and minimizing the disturbing behaviors of the person with cognitive loss and how both activity and disturbing behaviors affect the burden experienced by the caregiver. A structural equation model is employed.

Figure 2 describes the hypothesized relationships. With the exception of the measure of engagement in instrumental, leisure, and social activities, the factors and the measurements that support them have been examined in previous research.

METHOD

Sample

This study included 34 females and 38 males with Alzheimer's disease and their spouses selected from the patient registry of the Washington University Alzheimer's Disease Research Center. These individuals were enrolled in longitudinal studies conducted by the Center; many of them have provided data for other research reports. They were selected because they were married couples living in the community and had received the functional testing and caregiver interview that provided the data necessary for this analysis. Recruitment, clinical diagnostic procedures, and criteria have been described elsewhere (Berg et al., 1983). Individuals with other medical, neurologic, or psychiatric disorders that could impair cognition were excluded.

Each person enrolled in the patient registry was assigned a clinical dementia rating (CDR) (Berg, 1988) based on an individual and a collateral source (in these subjects, the spouse) interview, as well as a neurological examination of the participant. Assessments were conducted by a trained research physician. All of the subjects were Caucasian, even though efforts were made to recruit persons of other races. The social class was distributed through the top five positions as classified by Hollingshead and Red-

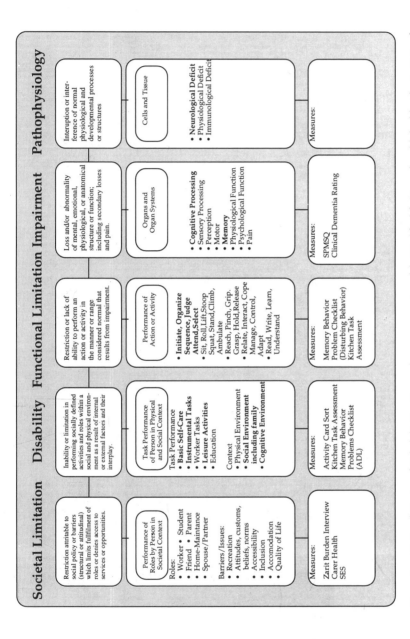

Figure 1. National Center of Rehabilitation Research measurement model. (Modified from work published by the Institute of Medicine in *Disability in America*, 1991, and in National Institutes of Health, 1993.)

lich (1958). Table 1 describes the population sample, which includes people across all stages of dementia (questionable, mild, moderate, and severe) and their caregivers.

Procedure

Informed consent was obtained from each participant and from the spouse. Data were collected from the subject and the caregiver at the same time by a trained individual who was blind to the CDR rating. The subjects completed the Kitchen Task Asessment and The Short Portable Mental Status Questionnaire. The caregivers completed the Memory Problems Behavior Checklist and the Zarit Burden Interview and The Activity Card Sort, reporting on the activities of their impaired spouse. The conditions of the statistical procedure were met, as there were no missing data. The measurement of variables was conducted with the following assessment tools.

- *The Kitchen Task Assessment* (Baum & Edwards, 1993) represents the variable for describing the executive skill deficit and serves as an objective measure of a person's cognitive performance on an instrumental task.
- *The Short Portable Mental Status Questionnaire* (Pfeiffer, 1975) represents the memory variable in the model.

Table 1. Demographic characteristics ($N = 72$)

Subject information	Sex	N	%
Impaired person	Male	34	47
	Female	38	53
Caregiver	Male	38	53
	Female	34	47
Age			
Impaired person	71.4 years (range 55–85)		
Spouse	66.4 years (range 53–84)		
Years of education			
Impaired person	13.1 years (range 5–21)		
Spouse	12.1 years (range 8–20)		
Socioeconomic status:			
Hollingshead Index of Social Position	3.20 (range 1–5)		
Subject's stage of dementia		N	%
CDR[a] 0.5	Questionable	12	16.4
CDR 1	Mild	29	39.7
CDR 2	Moderate	15	20.5
CDR 3	Severe	16	23.3

[a]CDR, clinical dementia rating.

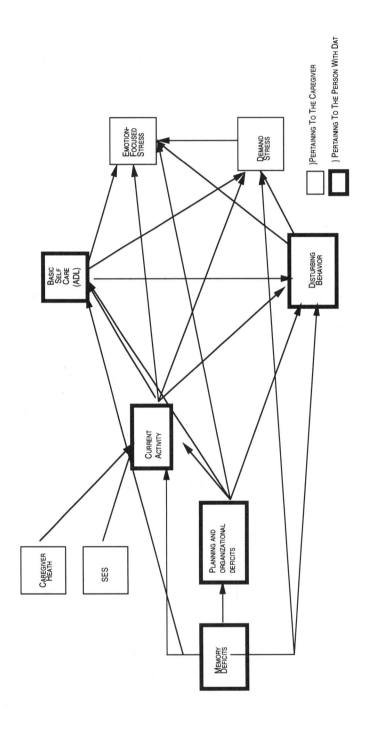

EMOTION-FOCUSED STRESS

DEMAND STRESS

BASIC SELF CARE (ADL)

DISTURBING BEHAVIOR

CURRENT ACTIVITY

CAREGIVER HEATH

SES

PLANNING AND ORGANIZATIONAL DEFICITS

MEMORY DEFICITS

) PERTAINING TO THE CAREGIVER

) PERTAINING TO THE PERSON WITH DAT

Figure 2. Hypothesized relationships. The following references support the variables in the model. *Carer Health to Current Activity:* Baumgarten et al. (1992), Birkel and Jones (1989), Horowitz (1985), Miller et al. (1991), Ory et al. (1985), Pratt et al. (1985). *SES to Current Activity:* Relationship not established, parameter being examined. *Memory to Current Activity:* Almli (1993), Baum and Edwards (1993), Duchek (1991), Edwards et al. (1991), Kielhofner (1992), Kulund (1982), Lawton (1990), McArdle et al. (1986), Pearlin et al. (1990), Sharpe et al. (1987). *Memory to Disturbing Behavior:* Miller et al. (1991), Teri and Gallagher-Thompson (1991). *Memory to Basic Self-Care:* Christiansen (1991). *Planning to Current Activity:* Almli (1992), Baum and Edwards (1993), Edwards et al. (1991), Filder and Fidler (1963), Kielhofner (1992), Lawton (1990), Mayer et al. (1986), Sharpe et al. (1987), Sullivan et al. (1989). *Planning to Disturbing Behavior:* Miller et al. (1991), Teri and Gallagher-Thompson (1991). *Planning to Basic Self-Care:* Christiansen (1991), Diller (1986), Kielhofner (1992), Mayer et al. (1986). *Planning to Emotion-Focused Stress:* Miller et al. (1991), Teri and Gallagher-Thompson (1991). *Current Activity to Emotion-Focused Stress:* Pearlin et al. (1990). *Current Activity to Basic Self-Care:* Almli (1992), Baynes et al. (1992), Bronfenbrenner (1979), Christiansen (1991), Kielhofner (1992), Sharpe et al. (1987). *Current Activity to Disturbing Behavior:* Baynes et al. (1992), Pearlin, Turner, and Semple (1990). *Basic Self-Care to Disturbing Behavior:* Relationship not established, parameter being examined. *Basic Self-Care to Emotion-Focused Stress:* Montgomery et al. (1985). *Basic Self-Care to Demand Stress:* Cantor (1983), Miller, McFall, and Montgomery (1991), Pearlin, Turner, and Semple (1990), Poulshock and Deimling (1984), Robinson (1983), Vitaliano et al. (1990). *Disturbing Behavior to Emotion-Focused Stress:* Pearlin, Turner, and Semple (1990). *Disturbing Behavior to Demand Stress:* This parameter is being tested because most studies related to stress do not differentiate between emotion-focused and demand stress and it will be important to begin the process of differentiation. *Demand Stress to Emotional Stress:* Coyne and Holroyd (1982), Csikszentmilhalyi (1988), Pearlin et al. (1981).

- *The Memory and Behavior Problem Checklist* (MBPC; Zarit, Reever, & Bach-Peterson, 1980) was used to capture the basic self-care skills and the disturbing behavior of the person with Alzheimer's disease.
- *The Activity Card Sort* (ACS; Baum, 1993) records the impaired person's level of engagement in activities compared with those performed before the onset of the disease.
- *The Zarit Burden Interview* (Zarit et al., 1980) reports the burden experienced by the caregiver in managing the person with cognitive impairment.
- *Carer Health Self-Report* is a measure of carer health, the carer responded to whether he or she had any of 23 illness or chronic diseases.
- *Hollingshead Index of Social Position* (Hollingshead & Redlich, 1958) determines a social class from the occupational scale of the head of household and the educational scale of the subject.

DATA ANALYSIS

All of the variables were examined to determine if they were consistent with the assumptions of multivariate normality and their correlations were reviewed prior to the analysis. The Covariance Analysis of Linear Structural Equations (CALIS) procedure was used for the analysis. Linear structural equations build on correlation studies and permit the construction of models that incorporate and correct for measurement error. They allow the objective evaluation of the fit of a theoretical model to the data, as indicated by the degree to which the matrix of interrelations among observed variables reproduced by the hypothesized model differs from the sample counterpart (Alwin, 1991).

The CALIS procedure allows the hypothesized model to be formulated as a system of equations relating key variables to assumptions about the variance and covariance of the variables. This results in structural coefficients, which express the degree of change in the outcome variable expected from a unit change in causal variables in the model. The resulting equations can be used to learn what to expect from interventions.

RESULTS

A series of analyses were performed to evaluate and improve the fit of the model. The best fit is determined by reviewing the χ^2, the adjusted goodness of fit (AGFI), and the Schwarz's Bayesian criterion (SBC). The χ^2 should not be significant, the AGFI should be a number close to 1.0, and the SBC should be the smallest number (Raykov, Tomer, & Nesselroade, 1991). The initial analysis tested the hypothesized model and identified a model where the parameters were restricted by the low degrees of freedom and 12 paths that did not have significant t values ($\chi^2 = 8$ [$df = 12$], $p = .7899$ AGFI $= .91$, SBC $= -43.38$). Further analysis was required. Each parameter that did not reach a level of significance was removed one by one until the model was determined to have the best fit.

The best fit model ($\chi^2 = 20.93$ [$df = 23$], $p = .5853$, AGFI $= .89$, SBC $= -77.43$) is described in Figure 3. There are several indicators to consider in assessing the fit between the specified model and the data. Low values of χ^2 relative to the degrees of freedom are interpreted as suggesting adequate fit (indicating that the data do not significantly differ from the proposed model). For this model the χ^2 is 20.93 and the $df = 23$. The ratio of χ^2 to degrees of freedom is .91. On the basis of the χ^2 measure, the model does fit the data. A second assessment of fit is obtained from the goodness of fit adjusted for sample size. The AGFI has a range of 0 to 1, with the higher number the stronger fit. The AGFI for this model is .89. The SBC is used to compare models with different numbers of parameters (the lower the number the better the fit). The SBC for the best fit model is -74.43, reduced from -43.38 in the hypothesized model.

Rather than express the degree of change, in a cross-sectional design the structural coefficient represents the expected differences in the downstream variable associated with one unit of difference in the causal variable (Loehlin, 1992). The data from the structured equation model can be interpreted as follows. If the other variables in the model remain stable, the following will occur:

- An increase in *executive skills* would result in the person giving up less activity and would result in a decrease in the help needed to perform basic self-care.
- An increase in *memory ability* would result in the person giving up less activity.
- An increase in *current activity* would be reflected by a decrease in the disturbing behavior and require less help in performing self-care.
- An increase in *disturbing behavior* would increase the demand stress and the emotion-focused stress.
- An increase in the *demand stress* would increase the emotion-focused stress.

This can be interpreted to mean that, if the caregiver helps the person with cognitive loss to perform an activity, the assistance would bypass the poor executive skills and the person could remain active. Additionally, the person would require less help with self-care and demonstrate fewer disturbing behaviors, and the caregiver would experience less stress as a result of the fewer disturbing behaviors. The data also highlight the importance that disturbing behavior plays in the stress of the person who is responsible for care.

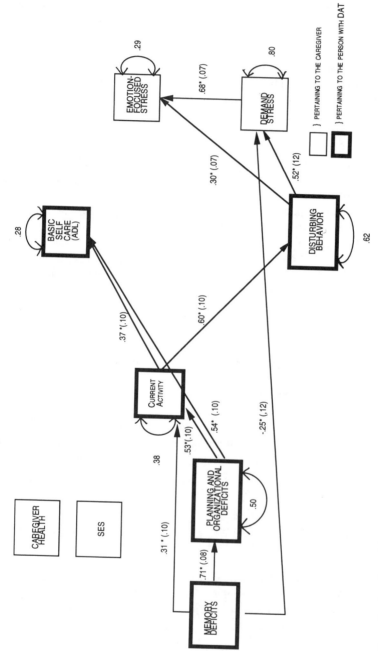

Figure 3. Best fit model. Measure of fit: $\chi^2 = 20.93$ ($df = 23$), $p = 0.5853$, AGFI = .8876, SBC = −77.43.

This model validates the importance of designing intervention programs to train family members to support the activities of their loved one with cognitive loss. These family members must learn to recognize that difficult behaviors will affect the entire family. Thus, various strategies can be used to minimize behaviors that will be disturbing to the persons providing care.

DISCUSSION

Individuals who remained engaged in activities displayed fewer disruptive behaviors and fewer occurrences of difficulty with dressing, feeding, bathing and grooming. When disturbing behaviors were minimized, there was less demand and emotion-focused stress in the caregiver. For individuals to remain engaged in activities, it is necessary for the caregiver to compensate for the executive skill deficits and memory loss experienced by the person with Alzheimer's disease. The caregiver must provide the organizational strategies and memory supports that the person with the impairment can no longer provide for him or herself. These strategies take the form of environmental modifications, verbal cues, physical assistance, building daily routine to tap the procedural memory for overlearned tasks, among others. The caregiver becomes an enabler so the person has the assistance to compensate for his or her cognitive impairment.

According to this model, the rehabilitation professional should help families acquire the skills to support the performance of their loved ones in activities that are important to them. This support will help increase the function of the person with the cognitive loss and at the same time decrease the burden they will experience in providing the support.

Families need assistance so that those who choose to care for their loved ones can successfully manage them in the community and can support their loved ones' dignity and independence. This assistance can take the form of information, skills, and/or formal support, such as day care or respite care. Families who provide care and professionals working or consulting with formal service delivery programs need information to guide their actions. This study suggests that continued engagement in activity can reduce the disturbing behaviors of the person with cognitive loss, which in turn can reduce the stress of the caregiver. How these activities are supported depends on the caregiver's skills to construct environments to overcome the neurological deficits associated with the disease. To properly train caregivers, the clinician must be skilled in identifying the specific neurological deficits and in clinical strategies to compensate for deficits that interfere with performance.

Many caregivers are not sufficiently trained to manage complex behavioral problems associated with neurological deficits. If the person with the impairment has a deficit such as apraxia, agnosia, or aphasia, it would be important to teach the caregiver how to bypass these deficits in performing tasks so the caregiver can minimize those behaviors that emerge from frustration. Diller (1986) describes the process of teaching the caregiver of a person with a head injury. He suggests that mastery of skilled acts requires the integration of many subroutines, even for people with intact nervous systems. Addressing the behavioral problems is complex because the person with the impairment may have a poor grasp of what is expected. The behavioral symptom must be seen in a context rather than as an isolated target behavior to be altered. The task must be presented in a structured way that will produce a successful response by the person with the impairment.

The person with a neurological deficit presents many problems that are not easy to grasp. It is important for people caring for individuals with cognitive deficits to acquire skills themselves. This training would best be carried out in the home by skilled rehabilitation clinicians who are knowledgeable about successful strategies to assist the caregiver. The professional should be equipped to apply cognitive strategies unique for the person with cognitive loss to help him or her accomplish activities that are meaningful. Seeing the person perform tasks may make it possible for caregivers to understand how their family member can be successfully engaged in activities and fosters optimism.

Limitations of the Study

Structural equation methods are usually employed in longitudinal research designs where the research questions involve analysis of change and its explanation. They can be used in cross-sectional designs if there is theoretical support for the parameters. The parameters in this study were supported with previous studies and strong assumptions about the importance of activity. This study was conducted on a sample of people with Alzheimer's disease, and because those with head injury and stroke experience similar cognitive deficits, the theoretical model was applied. Studies are needed to test the model on persons with head injuries and stroke. Samples should include persons of all ages to specifically guide interventions that can be useful across the life span.

CONCLUSIONS

The field of rehabilitation involves team members from many disciplines. It is virtually impossible to separate one discipline's contributions from the contribution of another if a team approach is used effectively. Studies like this one, which consider all the variables in one model, can help the team look at the complexity of a problem and determine the points at which various professionals might target their interventions to focus on the needs of the person with the disability. Structured equation models offer important opportunities for the rehabilitation team to understand the potential implication of their interventions. These models additionally provide a new method to evaluate effectiveness by employing the technique in longitudinal designs.

This study has implications for men and women, but women disproportionately provide the care to people who need such care. Thus, providing comprehensive rehabilitation services that include the family will minimize stress in the women that provide the care for their family members. By helping these women acquire the skills to help their loved ones, professionals help provide them with greater skills to support the independence of their family member.

REFERENCES

Acorn, S. (1993). Head-injured survivors: Caregivers and support groups. *Journal of Advanced Nursing, 18,* 39–45.

Alwin, D.F. (1991). Structured equation models in research on human development and aging. In K.W. Schaie, R.T. Campbell, W. Meredith, & S.C. Rawlings (Eds.), *Methodological issues in aging research* (pp. 70–71). New York: Springer-Verlag.

Baum, C.M. (1993). *The effect of occupation on behaviors of persons with senile dementia of the Alzheimer's type and their carers.* Dissertation, Washington University, St. Louis, MO.

Baum, C.M., & Edwards, D.F. (1993). Cognitive performance in senile dementia of the Alzheimer's type: The kitchen task assessment. *American Journal of Occupational Therapy, 47,* 431–436.

Berg, L. (1988). Clinical dementia rating (CDR). *Psychopharmacology Bulletin, 24,* 637–638.

Berg, L., Hughes, C.P., Cohen, L.A., Danziger, W.L., Martin, R.L., & Knesevich, J. (1982). Mild dementia of the Alzheimer type: Research diagnostic criteria, recruitment and description of a study population. *Journal of Neurology, Neurosurgery and Psychiatry, 45,* 962–968.

Birkel, R.C., & Jones, C.J. (1989). A comparison of the caregiving networks of dependent elderly individuals who are lucid and those who are demented. *Gerontologist, 29,* 114–119.

Brody, E.M. (1990). The family at risk. In E. Light & B.D. Lebowitz (Eds.), *Alzheimer's disease treatment and family stress: Directions for research* (pp. 2–49). New York: Hemisphere Publishing Co.

Bronfenbrenner, U. (1979). Purpose and perspective. In U. Bronfenbrenner (Ed.), *The ecology of human development* (pp. 1–15). Cambridge, MA: Harvard University Press.

Cantor, M.H. (1983). Strain among caregivers: A study of experience in the United States. *Gerontologist, 23,* 597–604.

Chenworth, B., & Spencer, B. (1986). Dementia: The experience of family caregiver. *Gerontologist, 26,* 267–272.

Christiansen, C. (1991). Occupational therapy: Intervention for life performance. In C. Christiansen & C. Baum (Eds.), *Occupational therapy: Overcoming human performance deficits* (pp. 41–43). Thorofare, NJ: Slack.

Coyne, J., & Holroyd, K. (1982). Stress, coping and illness: A transactional perspective. In T. Millon, C. Green, & R. Meagher (Eds.), *Handbook of clinical health psychology* (pp. 103–127). New York: Plenum Press.

Csikszentmihalyi, M. (1988). A theoretical model for enjoyment. In M. Csikszentmihalyi, *Beyond boredom and anxiety* (pp. 35–54). San Francisco: Jossey-Bass.

Diller, L. (1986). Cognitive remediation—some questions and answers. *Rehabilitation Report, 2,* 1–4.

Duchek, J. (1991). Cognitive dimensions of performance. In C. Christiansen & C. Baum (Eds.), *Occupational therapy: Overcoming human performance deficits* (pp. 284–303). Thoroughfare, NJ: Slack.

Edwards, D.F., Baum, C.M., & Deuel, R.M. (1991). Constructional apraxia in senile dementia: Contributions to functional loss. *Physical and Occupational Therapy in Geriatrics, 9,* 53–68.

Fidler, G., & Fidler J. (1963). *Occupational therapy: A communication process in psychiatry.* New York: Macmillan.

Hollingshead, A.B., & Redlich, F.C. (1958). *Social class and mental illness: A community study.* New York: John Wiley & Sons.

Horowitz, A. (1985). Sons and daughters as caregivers to older parents: Differences in role performance and consequences. *Gerontologist, 25,* 612–617.

Kielhofner, G. (1992). *Conceptual foundations of occupational therapy.* Philadelphia: F.A. Davis.

Kuland, D.N. (1982). *The injured athlete.* Philadelphia: J.B. Lippincott.

Lawton, M.P. (1990). Environmental approaches to research and treatment of Alzheimer's disease. In E. Light, & B.D. Lebowitz (Eds.), *Alzheimer's disease treatment and family stress: Directions for research* (pp. 340–362). New York: Hemisphere Publishing Co.

Lawton, M.P., Brody, E.M., & Saperstein, A.R. (1989). A controlled study of respite service for caregivers of Alzheimer's patients. *Gerontologist, 29,* 8–16.

Loehlin, J.C. (1992). *Latent variable models: An introduction to factor, path, and structural analysis* (2nd ed.). Hillsdale, NJ: Lawrence Erlbaum Associates.

Mayer, N.H., Keating, D.J., & Rapp, D. (1986). Skills, routines, and activity patterns of daily living: A functional nested approach. In B. Uzzell & J. Gross (Eds.), *Clinical neuropsychology of intervention* (pp. 205–222). Boston: Martinus Nijhoff.

McArdle, W.D., Katch, F.L., & Katch, V.V. (1986). *Exercise physiology: Energy, nutrition and human performance* (2nd ed.). Philadelphia: Lea & Febiger.

Miller, B., McFall, S., & Montgomery, A. (1991). The impact of elder health, caregiver involvement and global stress on two dimensions of caregiver burden. *Journal of Gerontology, Social Sciences, 46*(1), S9–S19.

Montgomery, R.J.V., Gonyea, J.G., & Hooyman, N.R. (1985). Caregiving and the experience of subjective and objective burden. *Family Relations, 34,* 19–26.

National Institutes of Health. (1993). *Research Plan for the National Center for Medical Rehabilitation Research* (NIH Publication No. 93-3509). Washington, DC: U.S. Government Printing Office.

Ory, M.G., Williams, T.F., Emr, M., Lebowitz, B., Rabins, P., Salloway, J., Sluss-Radbaugh, T., Wolff, E., & Zarit, S. (1985). Families, informal supports, and Alzheimer's disease, current research and future agendas. *Research on Aging, 7,* 623–644.

Pearlin, L.I., Lieberman, M., Menaghan, E.G., & Mullen, J.T. (1981). The stress process. *Journal of Health and Social Behavior, 22,* 337–356.

Pearlin, L.I., Turner, H., & Semple, S. (1990). Coping and the mediation of caregiver stress. In E. Light & B.D. Lebowitz (Eds.), *Alzheimer's disease treatment and family stress: Directions for research* (pp. 196–217). New York: Hemisphere Publishing Co.

Pfeiffer, E. (1975). SPMSQ: Short portable mental status questionnaire. *Journal of the American Geriatric Society, 23,* 433–441.

Poulshock, S.W., & Deimling, G.T. (1984). Families caring for elders in residence: Issues in the measurement of burden. *Journal of Gerontology, 39,* 230–239.

Pratt, C.C., Schmall, V.L., Wright, S., & Cleland, M. (1985). Burden and coping strategies of caregivers to Alzheimer's patients. *Family Relations, 34,* 27–33.

Raykov, T., Tomer, A., & Nesselroade, J.R. (1991). Reporting structural equation modeling results in *Psychology and Aging:* Some proposed guidelines. *Psychology and Aging, 6,* 499–503.

Robinson, B. (1983). Validation of a caregiver strain index. *Journal of Gerontology, 38,* 344–348.

Sharpe, P.E., Barnes, C.A., & McNaughton, B.L. (1987). Effects of aging on environmental modulation of hippocampal evoked responses. *Behavioral Neuroscience, 101,* 170–178.

Sullivan, E.V., Sagar, H.J., Gabrieli, J.D., Corkin, S., & Growdon, J.H. (1989). Different cognitive profiles on standard behavioral tests in Parkinson's disease and Alzheimer's disease. *Journal Clinical Experimental Neuropsychology, 11,* 799–820.

Teri, L., & Gallagher-Thompson, D. (1991). Cognitive-behavioral interventions for treatment of depression in Alzheimer's patients. *Gerontologist, 31,* 413–416.

Vitaliano, P.P., Russo, J., Breen, A.R., Vitiello, M.V., & Prinz, P.N. (1986). Functional decline in the early stages of Alzheimer's disease. *Psychology of Aging, 1*(1), 41–46.

Zarit, S.H., Reever, K.E., & Bach-Peterson, J. (1980). Relatives of the impaired elderly, correlates of feeling of burden. *Gerontologist, 20,* 649–655.

Zarit, S.H., Todd, P.A., & Zarit, J.M. (1986). Subjective burden of husbands and wives as caregivers: A longitudinal study. *Gerontologist, 26,* 260–266.

chapter 20

Traditional Approaches to Stress Reduction Through Skills Training

George D. Patrick

Part of being alive is accepting that things are changing all the time. One of life's challenges is to respond flexibly and creatively to these changes. There is a naive expectation that our physical bodies will stay the same, even after several decades. We are surprised when changes, even inevitable ones, occur. When faced with illness or chronic disability, one must deal with one of the greatest challenges to our ability to accept change. The threat of physical vulnerability dramatically raises an issue most of us must confront at some time in our lives: facing who we are when it is no longer possible to continue in our familiar roles. This challenge is intensified by another issue that surfaces with an illness—our own mortality (Cantor, 1993).

The onset of a serious illness or adventitious disability can result in the loss of a sense of security and predictability (Watson, 1983). Vulnerability has often been seen as a personal weakness rather than as an act of courage. Within families or other close relationships, people in our culture often make an unspoken agreement with each other to guard against exposing their vulnerability. An illness insists that our common vulnerability be recognized. The integrity of the relationship then requires that the original (unspoken) agreement be replaced by a new one that promises mutual acceptance of each other's susceptibilities as well as appreciation of each other's strengths (Heiss, 1988).

The psychological impact of life-threatening disease has received intensive study. Both cross-sectional and longitudinal research suggest that the psychosocial functioning of cancer patients differs little over the long run from that of individuals who are disease free (e.g., 2–5 years; Cassileth et al., 1984; Penman et al., 1986; Vinokur, Threatt, Caplan, & Zimmerman, 1989). However, clinical experience indicates that some patients demonstrate symptomatology (anxiety, stress, depression) serious enough to warrant medical attention. Similarly, the responses to traumatic disability have been studied thoroughly (Cassileth & Cassileth, 1982; Patrick, 1984; Wright, 1960). For persons suffering chronic illness or disability, stress is a frequent and unwelcome secondary result requiring intervention if optimal clinical outcome (quality of life) is to be fully achieved (Cantor, 1993; Linkowski & Dunn, 1974; Moos, 1979).

STRESS MANAGEMENT

Stress management is an active, directive, educational form of therapy. The individual often describes his or her difficulties, then works collaboratively with the therapist to understand the presenting complaints and what they signify in the context of that person's life (Lehrer & Woolfolk, 1993). Although stress management is taught in a consulting room, it is practiced primarily in the natural environment. Virtually all forms of stress management assume the model of skills training. Stress management techniques do not make stress vanish, nor do they confer permanent immunity to stressors; instead, they provide tools that aid individuals in work that is perennial.

TRADITIONAL TECHNIQUES

In the discussion that follows, several techniques for stress management are explained. The focus of the approaches is on women with disabilities, who are often faced with numerous and complex stressors.

Cognitive Training

Typical stress management includes identification of personal stress by the individual to characterize what stress means to her. Although the woman with a disability is ultimately the one who perceives stress, she may need to be led to a fuller understanding of stress in terms of the physiological concomitants of arousal. Furthermore, she may need to understand and identify real-life examples of eustress and distress (Selye, 1974). Through cognitive training she learns to identify the *physical signs and symptoms* of stress, especially those that are specific reactions she experiences. These may include increased heart rate; pounding heart; elevated blood pressure; sweaty palms; tightness of the chest, neck, jaw, and back muscles; headache; diarrhea; constipation; urinary hesitancy; trembling, twitching; stuttering and other speech difficulties; nausea and vomiting; sleep disturbances; fatigue; shallow breathing; dryness of the mouth or throat; itching; being easily startled; and chronic pain.

In addition, the individual often needs to learn the *emotional signs and symptoms* of stress, which may include irritability, angry outbursts, hostility, depression, jealousy, restlessness, withdrawal, anxiousness, diminished initiative, feelings of unreality or overalertness, reduction of personal involvement with others, lack of interest, tendency to cry, being critical of others, self-deprecation, nightmares, impatience, decreased perception of positive experiences or opportunities, narrowed focus, obsessive rumination, reduced self-esteem, insomnia, and changes in eating habits.

Similarly, she may need to identify the *cognitive/perceptual signs and symptoms* of stress, such as forgetfulness, preoccupation, blocking, blurred vision, errors in judgment, diminished or exaggerated fantasy life, reduced creativity, lack of concentration, diminished productivity, lack of attention to detail, orientation to the past, disorganization of thought, negative self-esteem, negative self-statements, lack of control/need for too much control, and negative evaluation of experiences.

Finally, the person needs to identify *behavioral signs and symptoms* of stress in her life, including increased smoking, aggressive behaviors (such as in driving), increased alcohol or drug use, carelessness, under- or overeating, withdrawal, listlessness, hostility, accident proneness, nervous laughter, compulsive behavior, and impatience.

The role of perception and attribution in interpreting stressful events is shaped by our past experiences, personality, cultural background, moral values, family background, social support network, gender, lifestyle, and personal belief system. These factors influence an individual's cognitive appraisal of a stressor (Lazarus, 1981). In addition to change, uncertainty, and overload (so-called "real" stressors), unnecessary worry can cause stress responses.

In a thorough stress management course, the individual's previous attempts to handle stress will be evaluated. Both failed and successful attempts to cope with stress are very important keys to developing a successful plan for each individual.

Skills Training Techniques

The focus of this chapter is on the stress reduction skills that can be learned by women living with a disability that, when practiced, are effective in reducing stress. This chapter specifically excludes other effective stress management techniques such as medication, hypnosis (except self-hypnosis), and massage because the skills presented and learned can be implemented by the client alone. Of course, once skills are learned, the woman will be faced with adherence to and maintenance of behavior change—no small task for those familiar with the difficulties related to other behavioral alterations such as smoking cessation and dieting. The main advantages of self-practiced stress management skills are the enhanced sense of self-efficacy and the concomitant nondependence on a therapist. The major skills that are reviewed here are progressive relaxation, relaxation response, autogenic training, yoga, meditation, aerobic exercise, weight training, and leisure activity participation.

Nonvigorous Behavioral Approaches

Progressive Relaxation First devised by Edmund Jacobson (1938), and later modernized by Bernstein and Borkovec (1963) this is a widely used method. It is perhaps more familiar to psychotherapists than any other stress management technique (Lehrer & Woolfolk, 1993). Although there are key differences and interpretations in the application of progressive relaxation, the similarities include teaching the individual the from the very beginning to 1) perceive the most subtle of muscle proprioceptions and to voluntarily eliminate even the most minute traces of skeletal muscle tone, and 2) eliminate unnecessary tension continuously during everyday activities. The more recent versions have not focused so much on awareness of tension as on the production of relaxation. Where the Jacobson technique (1938) refrained from suggestion of relaxation, Bernstein and Borkovec (1963) make full use of suggestion, including telling the trainee the sensations that might be felt, using voice modulation, and using some hypnotic-like relaxation suggestions.

Bernstein and Carlson (1993) have thoroughly described their "abbreviated progressive relaxation training" (APRT). APRT begins with a 45-minute session that alternatively tenses and relaxes 16 muscle groups. With practice, by the sixth session the skillful individual will have reduced the number of muscle groups to just four. By the tenth and final session, counting to 10, which takes less than a minute, the client will be able to induce deep relaxation. For reasons of time efficiency, the APRT is recommended for clinical application over the original progressive relaxation model.

Relaxation Response This is a widely used meditative technique synthesized by Benson (1975) and can be considered the "respiratory one method" (ROM) in that the trainee repeats the word "one" (or another word or phrase) to herself, while at the same time intentionally linking this word with each exhaled breath. As with other relaxation techniques, the ROM is best learned in a comfortable, quiet, and low-stimulation environment. Other meditative techniques include, but are not limited to, yoga, Buddhist "mindfulness," positive affirmations, clinically oriented meditation (Carrington, 1978), and repetitive prayer/chanting.

Autogenic Training Developed in 1932 by Schultz and Luthe in Germany, but promulgated on this side of the Atlantic Ocean by Linden (1990), autogenic training (AT) is one of the earliest Western systems of physiological self-regulation. AT is essentially a collection of autosuggestive exercises whose focus is somatic and cognitive. AT has been aptly described as the "legitimate daughter" of hypnosis. The images of "warm" and "heavy" are two of the suggestions prescribed in this training. It does not offer a singular technique, as Bernstein and Borkovec (1963) or Benson (1975) do, and it cannot provide a manual or tape to facilitate relaxation practice for the trainee. Autogenic techniques teach the stressed mind and body to return from an "alarm state" to a relaxed state. After tailoring the adjustment (reduction or augmentation) of specific autonomic arousal, AT teaches the person to abbreviate the process and encourages self-regulation.

AT literature describes a phenomenon of "autogenic discharges." Although AT is presumed to have an overall gentle, slow effect on autonomic self-regulation, AT practitioners report a phenomenon described as a short burst of central nervous system activity. Trainees are likely to report these as unwanted, bothersome side effects of AT. As with other adverse effects, these must be interpreted by the instructor to the trainee in sensible, comforting explanations. Other relaxation techniques describe similar phenomena as "relaxation-induced anxiety" (APRT) and "side effects of tension release."

Hatha Yoga   This relaxation technique is one branch of Indian philosophy and practice. "Yoga" means union or yoke, referring to the communion of body, mind, and soul. Hatha yoga uses the physical pathway to this communion, but yoga is categorized in the nonvigorous category because it only requires only such low energy output activities as controlled breathing and stretching. Hatha yoga participants regulate the mind and body through

1. A total of 14 different breathing exercises, of which simple abdominal breathing is only the first exercise
2. Over 200 balanced physical postures developing flexibility, suppleness, and tone
3. Mobilizing the body's stored energy

The latter is least well understood by traditional stress management, but needs greater attention by researchers (Patel, 1993). Breathing is the cornerstone of hatha yoga; more specifically, controlled, deep diaphragmatic breathing. Finally, yoga is an attitude toward life that engenders the practice of deep muscle relaxation.

Meditation   This state has been practiced in religious contexts for 5,000 years. Benson (1975) reported the relaxation benefits of a variety of meditative states. Meditation can be classified as either "concentrative" or "nonconcentrative." Like autogenic strategies, most meditation begins with a quiet environment, a passive uncritical attitude, and a rhythmic breathing cadence. In concentrative meditation, stimulus input is limited by directing attention to a single unchanging or repetitive stimulus (e.g., watching a candle or repeating the word "one"). Most Western forms of meditation are concentrative. A nonconcentrative technique (Kabat-Zinn, Lipworth, & Burney, 1985) expands the meditator's field of attention to include as much of his or her conscious mental activity as possible (e.g., Buddhist "mindfulness").

Transcendental meditation (TM), while having popular acceptance, has found little use in clinical settings. Carrington (1978) has promulgated a "clinically standardized meditation" (CSM) that is devoid of cultic features. A trainee selects a sound from a standard list of sounds and then repeats this sound mentally, without intentionally linking the sound to the breathing pattern or pacing it in any structured manner. CSM is relatively permissive and less complex when compared with the relaxation response.

Meditation has many forms, including repeated prayer, chanting, or visual focus on an object (icon, waterfall, or sunbeam). T'ai Chi and some dance forms (e.g., modern dance, line dancing, even whirling dervishes) are examples of moving meditations. Some people will prefer to meditate, others to relax muscles, and others to talk about their thoughts and feelings. Still others will want to exercise, so it should be a matter of preference as to which modality is better for a specific client. However, "on the average, meditation is one of the most motivational techniques" (Lehrer & Woolfolk, 1993, p. 533).

Vigorous Physical Activity

Over the last several decades, participation in regular physical exercise has been espoused for health benefits such as weight control and prevention of cardiovascular disease. Anecdotal claims of psychological benefits were frequently associated with regular exercise enough to encourage a variety of scientific investigations. Since the mid-1980s, many studies have supported the stress reduction efficacy of chronic exercise (Fillingim & Blumenthal, 1992; Morgan, 1985; Van Doornen & DeGeus, 1989). These studies indicate that acute and chronic exercise enhance mood in normal and clinical populations, but the definitive explanation of cause (physiological or psychological) remains elusive to researchers. DePauw (see Chapter 32) describes the importance of physical activity for women with disabilities. A growing body of evidence (Haskell, 1987) suggests that physical exercise reduces psychophysiological stress responses, although the mechanisms are not well known.

Aerobic Exercise   Aerobic exercise refers to the repetitive movement of large muscle groups in which energy is derived from aerobic metabolism. Activities such as walking, wheelchair propulsion, swimming, and jogging are considered aerobic. A training effect occurs over a period of time (8–12 weeks) when the exerciser participates 3 times a week for at least 30 minutes at an intensity equal to Maximum Heart Rate − Resting Heart Rate × .75 + Resting Heart Rate ±6. The American College of Sports Medicine published guidelines for exercise (1986) and its testing that have become the "gold standard" for prescribing exercise, including contraindications. Adapted exercises have been developed and are available through the National Handicap Sport and Recreation Association. Santiago, Coyle, and Kinney (1993) demonstrated that aerobic exercise had a positive impact on individuals with disabilities.

From a clinical perspective, aerobic exercise as a stress reduction regimen offers a number of advantages. Exercise may appeal to a number of individuals for whom cognitive relaxation techniques have not been successful. Exercise approaches usually require closer contact with physicians and exercise physiologists, an advantage it has over less regimented techniques for individuals suffering stress.

Furthermore, concomitant health benefits of cardiovascular fitness and weight loss may become self-reinforcing enough to ensure adherence. Aerobic exercise, both acute and chronic, tends to enhance mood by reducing depression and anxiety and increasing feelings of vigor (Fillingim & Blumenthal, 1993).

Progressive Resistance Training This is another term for weight training and is used by individuals claiming anecdotal stress reduction benefits. Weight lifting mirrors the tension–relaxation cycling of Jacobson's (1938) progressive relaxation training. Less systematic investigation has been conducted on stress reduction from weight training, but comparative studies show that superior effects are found with aerobic training. Personal communication (T.K. Cureton, 1965) indicated unexpected positive psychological effects from taking a shower during the middle of the workday. Both clinicians and researchers ought to look at more than specific activity for developing a stress reduction response. It appears that any break in the ongoing routine of life's stressful events has a salutary effect.

Leisure as Stress Reduction

The concepts of leisure and health are being broadened to include more subjective notions. The residual definition of health (e.g., the absence of disease) is limited, just as a residual definition of leisure (e.g., absence of obligated time) has basic limitations. Clearly, leisure and health, especially when broader subjective definitions are used, share many of the same characteristics. Health, like leisure, cannot be defined in exact measurable terms because its presence is largely a matter of subjective judgment. About as precise as one can get is that "health is a relative affair that represents the degree to which an individual can operate with effectiveness within the particular circumstances of . . . heredity and . . . physical and cultural environment" (Mansourian, 1992, p. 1). Definitions that embrace the concept of "absence of disease" in reality are misleading, for all living things are diseased in varying degrees. Furthermore, chronic diseases that now account for the majority of debilitating and life-threatening conditions are not amenable to medical solutions. Rather, they are largely attributable to lifestyle and environmental conditions.

There is strong evidence that what an individual does during leisure time significantly affects illness, disease, and even longevity (Orstein & Sobel, 1990; Wankel & Berger, 1990). To experience leisure with the characteristics of perceived freedom, competence, self-determination, satisfaction, and perceived quality of life is to experience a subjective state of health. In this sense, the development of a broad repertoire of leisure skills to facilitate rich, meaningful experiences provides the foundation for extending such holistic quality experiences to all of life (Csikszentmihalyi & LeFevre, 1989). Personal initiative, choice, meaningful involvement, and enjoyable, supportive social networks—key aspects for leisure—also have important implications for well-being (Coleman & Iso-Ahola, 1993).

On the practical side, each individual should be encouraged to cultivate leisure experiences (hobbies, events, and skills) that can relieve stress. For example, research exists to support the stress reduction qualities of pets. Even the seemingly innocuous placement of a fish tank in an apartment complex lobby reduced the blood pressure of the residents significantly (Schriver & Cutler-Riddick, 1988). Similarly, gardening has shown stress reduction benefits, as has music listening (Maranto, 1993). Choral singing combines a felicitous mixture of deep breathing, music, and social support that might prove beneficial to individuals so inclined. Daydreaming ("unguided imagery") has the advantages of portability, no equipment, and low cost. It appears that most individuals have the ability to self-select leisure experiences that have beneficial effects because the nonreinforcing experiences tend not to be repeated.

Leisure is so self-reinforcing that compliance, resistance, and maintenance issues would seem nonexistent. Such is *not* the case. Individuals do not always embrace lifestyle changes easily. Our culture has not always supported the importance of leisure (e.g., "finish your homework first"; "once you start a job, finish it"). Furthermore, many individuals do not know how to enjoy leisure time. Individuals suffering stress overload have notoriously difficult times in decision making, behavioral change, and attempts at self-regulation; therefore, it is to be expected that persons with disabilities suffering stress will need assistance in leisure education.

CONCEPTUAL ISSUES

Cognitive Appraisal

Stress is a real phenomenon that is dependent upon the perception of the individual. The way an individual appraises a situation determines its strength as a stressor. We are always active participants in a continuing process that includes successive appraisals of the external situation and the risks, costs, and gains of a particular response. When our vital interests appear to be at stake, the cognitive process provides a highly selective conceptualization. Beck (1993) presented a cognitive model of stress and its associated emotionality and psychopathology. However, any approach to stress management that fails to acknowledge the causal role of cognitive appraisal in the genesis of stress falls short. Certainly, the treatment of stress requires education on the nature of stress and training in identification of the circumstances that trigger stress (Basler, Brinkmeier, Buser, Haehn, & Molders-Kober, 1982). Cognitions can be restructured: stressors can be reframed, rational problem solving can be practiced, and salutary self-statements can be substituted for those that are stress inducing. Clearly, positive changes in cognitive appraisal have enormous potential to contribute significantly to the reduction of an individual's stress burden.

Coping Process Versus Style

An assumption too frequently found in the stress management literature is that individuals develop relatively stable coping strategies—a coping style (e.g., an individual may use an avoidance style when faced with stressful situations, choosing to disengage from an overwhelming task). According to the cognitive appraisal model (Beck, 1993; Lazarus & Folkman, 1984), coping is generated in response to the evaluation of environmental or internal demands as well as the coping options. A major issue in theory development and the measurement of coping concerns whether coping style (or disposition) is more salient than context-specific decisions. Bouffard and Crocker (1992) have presented strong data suggesting "that individuals with disabilities did not consistently use the same coping skill strategies across settings" (p. 410).

Moos (1992) emphasizes two basic coping responses: approach and avoidance. In general, approach coping is problem focused; it reflects cognitive and behavioral efforts to master or resolve life stressors. In contrast, avoidance coping tends to be emotion focused; it reflects cognitive and behavioral attempts to avoid thinking about a stressor and its implications or to manage the affect associated with it.

Moos states that avoidance coping may be an effective way to cope with a short-term stressor, such as blood donation, where there is little or no opportunity for behavioral coping. Nonetheless, persistent use of avoidance strategies may compound problems and delay stressor resolution. In a study by Cronkite and Moos (1984), women were more likely to use avoidance coping than men were. However, averages and tendencies are not important clinically or for the individual because the only relevant number is one.

Changing Behavioral Responses

Particularly with individuals who have a history of either nonproductive or counterproductive stress coping strategies, behavioral response changes come dearly. One successful model in helping people change is stress inoculation therapy (SIT), proposed by Meichenbaum (1993). He has developed a conditioning framework to reduce emotional reactions such as anxiety or anger. This cognitive–behavioral approach uses prolonged imaginal and behavioral exposure and rehearsal to provide the female client with "data" indicating that she is indeed able to cope with distressing events. Such repeated exposure provides opportunities to practice coping skills, or, in SIT terms, to "inoculate" themselves against future stressful encounters.

SIT uses training opportunities to help develop an adaptive personal narrative (positive "self-talk") about their ability to cope with stressful life events. Some women with disabilities may have internal dialogue characterized by feelings of helplessness, victimization, and demoralization, as well as a belief system that has been seriously challenged if not invalidated. SIT employs diverse experiential learning trials directed at affect-laden situations in order to nurture more adaptive and resourceful personal narratives. SIT has proven helpful in clinical and nonclinical populations (Walton, 1990). One way of overcoming some individuals' resistance to entering a stress management training program may be to repackage (reframe) it as a course in "mental toughness." Regardless of how effective changing a person's response to stressors might be, there must also be a real effort to change the environment in order to reduce the stress load. Realizing just how many persons drop out of aerobic exercise programs in spite of all the putative benefits reminds us of how difficult it is to change personal behavior.

Assessment Issues

For researchers and program evaluators, several excellent psychological measurement devices for stress are worthy of consideration:

- Profile of Mood States (McNair, Lorr, & Droppelman, 1971)
- State-Trait Anxiety Inventory (Spielberger, Gorsuch, & Luchene, 1970)
- Optimism Scale (Seligman, 1992)
- Hopelessness Scale (Beck, Weissman, Lester, & Trexler, 1974)
- Coping Response Inventory (Moos, 1992)
- Leisure Diagnostic Battery (Witt & Ellis, 1987)

Clearly, stress reduction has physiological consequences that can be measured either as feedback from the client (how well am I reducing the stress response?) or as a measure of instructional efficiency. Physiological measures (galvanic skin response, heart rate, blood pressure, blood measures such as cortisol) are also indirect indices of stress reduction. Nonetheless, further research could use a combination of psychological and physiological measurements to note their impact on long-term outcomes (quality of life, robustness of immune system, and longevity).

CONCLUSIONS

Stress is a normal part of life. However, at times the stress burden is almost more than one can bear. When chronic stress overload occurs, health suffers. Efforts are needed to change the individual's environment, but stress management techniques can also improve the capacity of the individual to tolerate health-endangering stress levels. This goal is attainable by changing one's perception of the situation and by teaching the body and mind to relax and to buffer the physical responses to stress. Women with disabilities face an additional set of stressors (see Chapter 16). Stress reduction has an important role in minimizing negative outcomes secondary to the illness or disability.

REFERENCES

American College of Sports Medicine (ACSM). (1986). *Guidelines for exercise testing and prescription* (4th ed.). Philadelphia: Lea & Febiger.

Basler, H., Brinkmeier, U., Buser, K., Haehn, K., & Molders-Kober, R. (1982). Psychological group treatment of essential hypertension in general practice. *British Journal of Clinical Psychology, 21,* 295–302.

Beck, A. (1993). Cognitive approaches to stress. In P. Lehrer & R. Woolfolk (Eds.), *Principles and practice of stress management* (2nd ed., pp. 333–372). New York: Guilford Press.

Beck, A., Weissman, A., Lester, D., & Trexler, L. (1974). The measurement of pessimism: The Hopelessness Scale. *Journal of Consulting and Clinical Psychology, 42,* 861–865.

Benson, H. (1975). *The relaxation response.* New York: Morrow.

Bernstein, D., & Borkovec, T. (1963). *Progressive relaxation training: A manual for helping professions.* Champaign, IL: Research Press.

Bernstein, D., & Carlson, C. (1993). Progressive relaxation: Abbreviated methods. In P. Lehrer & R. Woolfolk (Eds.), *Principles and practice of stress management* (2nd ed., pp. 53–88). New York: Guilford Press.

Bouffard, M., & Crocker, P. (1992). Coping by individuals with physical disabilities with perceived challenge in physical activity: Are people consistent? *Research Quarterly for Exercise and Sport, 3*(4), 410–417.

Cantor, N. (1993). *Advance directives and the pursuit of death with dignity.* Bloomington: Indiana University Press.

Carrington, P. (1978). *Clinically standardized meditation (CSM) instructor's kit.* Kendall Park, NJ: Pace Educational Systems.

Cassileth, B., & Cassileth, P. (1982). *Clinical care of the terminal cancer patient.* Ann Arbor, MI: Books on Demand.

Cassileth, B., Lusk, E., Strouse, T., Miller, D., Brown, L., Cross, P., & Tenaglia, A. (1984). Psychosocial status in chronic illness: A comparative analysis of six diagnostic groups. *New England Journal of Medicine, 311,* 506–511.

Coleman, D., & Iso-Ahola, S. (1993). Leisure and health: The role of social support and self-determination. *Journal of Leisure Research, 25,* 111–128.

Cronkite, T., & Moos, R. (1984). The role of predisposing and moderating factors in the stress-illness relationship. *Journal of Health and Social Behavior, 25*, 372–393.

Csikszentmihalyi, M., & LeFevre, J. (1989). Optimal experience in work and leisure. *Journal of Personality and Social Psychology, 56*, 815–822.

Fillingim, R., & Blumenthal, J. (1992). Does aerobic exercise reduce stress responses? In J. Turner, A. Sherwood, & K. Light (Eds.), *Individual differences in cardiovascular response to stress* (pp. 203–214). New York: Plenum Press.

Haskell, W. (1987). Overview: Health benefits of exercise. In J. Matarazzo, J. Weiss, J. Heard, & N. Miller (Eds.), *Behavioral health: A handbook of health enhancement and disease prevention* (pp. 409–423). New York: Wiley-Interscience.

Heiss, G. (1988). *Living well with chronic illness*. Fort Bragg, CA: Q.E.D. Press.

Jacobson, E. (1938). *Progressive relaxation* (2nd ed.). Chicago: University of Chicago Press.

Kabat-Zinn, J., Lipworth, L., & Burney, R. (1985). The clinical use of mindfulness meditation for the self regulation of chronic pain. *Journal of Behavioral Medicine, 8*, 163–190.

Lazarus, R. (1981). The stress and coping paradigm. In C. Eisendorfer, D. Cohen, A. Kleinman, & P. Maxim (Eds.), *Conceptual models for psychotherapy* (pp. 70–93). New York: Spectrum.

Lazarus, R., & Folkman, S. (1984). *Stress, appraisal, and coping*. New York: Springer-Verlag.

Lehrer, P., & Woolfolk, R. (1993). Specific effects of stress management techniques. In P. Lehrer & R. Woolfolk (Eds.), *Principles and practice of stress management* (2nd ed., pp. 481–520). New York: Guilford Press.

Linden, W. (1990). *Autogenic training: A clinical guide*. New York: Guilford Press.

Linkowski, D., & Dunn, M. (1974). Self-concept and acceptance of disability. *Rehabilitation Counseling Bulletin, 16*, 28–32.

Maranto, C. (1993). Music therapy and stress management. In P. Lehrer & R. Woolfolk (Eds.), *Principles and practice of stress management* (2nd ed., pp. 407–442). New York: Guilford Press.

Mansourian, B. (1992). Introduction. In A. Davies & B. Mansourian (Eds.), *Research strategies health* (pp. 1–12). Lewiston, NY: Hogrefe & Huber (on behalf of the World Health Organization).

McNair, D., Lorr, N., & Droppelman, L. (1971). *Profile of mood states*. San Diego, CA: Educational and Industrial Testing Service.

Meichenbaum, D. (1993). Stress inoculation training: A 20-year update. In P. Lehrer & R. Woolfolk (Eds.), *Principles and practice of stress management* (2nd ed., pp. 373–406). New York: Guilford Press.

Moos, R. (1979). *Coping with physical illness*. New York: Plenum.

Moos, R. (1992). *Coping response inventory adult form manual*. Palo Alto, CA: Center for Health Care Evaluation, Stanford University Press.

Morgan, W. (1985). Affective beneficence of vigorous activity. *Medicine and Science in Sports and Exercise, 17*, 94–100.

Ornstein, R., & Sobel, D. (1990). *Healthy pleasures*. New York: Addison-Wesley.

Patel, C. (1993). Yoga-based therapy. In P. Lehrer & R. Woolfolk (Eds.) *Principles and practice of stress management* (2nd ed., pp. 53–88). New York: Guilford Press.

Patrick, G. (1984). The effects of wheelchair competition on self-concept and acceptance of disability in novice athletes. *Therapeutic Recreation Journal, 20*(4), 61–71.

Penman, D., Bloom, J., Fotopoulos, S., Cook, M., Holland, J., Gates. C., Flamer, D., Murawski, B., Ross, R., Brandt, U., Muenz, L., & Pee, D. (1986). The impact of mastectomy on self-concept and social function: A combined cross-sectional and longitudinal study with comparison groups. *Woman and Health, 11*(3/4), 101–130.

Santiago, M., Coyle, C., & Kinney, W. (1993). Aerobic exercise effect on individuals with physical disabilities. *Archives of Physical Medicine & Rehabilitaton, 74*, 1192–1198.

Schriver, M., & Cutler-Riddick, C. (1988). Effects of watching aquariums on elders' stress. *Anthrozoos, 9*(1), 44–48.

Seligman, M. (1992). *Learned optimism.* New York: Alfred A. Knopf.

Selye, H. (1974). *Stress without distress.* Philadelphia: J.B. Lippincott.

Spielberger, C., Gorsuch, R., & Luchene, R. (1970). *STAI manual for the State-Trait Anxiety Inventory.* Palo Alto, CA: Consulting Psychologists Press.

Van Doornen, L., & DeGeus, E. (1989). Aerobic fitness and the cardiovascular response to stress. *Psychophysiology, 26*, 127–131.

Vinokur, A., Threatt, B., Caplan, R., & Zimmerman, B. (1989). Physical and psychosocial functioning and adjustment to breast cancer. *Journal of Social and Clinical Psychology, 63*, 394–305.

Walton, S. (1990). Stress management training. *International Journal of Intercultural Relations, 14*, 507–527.

Wankel, L., & Berger, B. (1990). The psychological and social benefits of sport and physical activity. *Journal of Leisure Research, 22*, 167–182.

Watson, M. (1983). Psychosocial intervention with cancer patients: A review. *Psychology in Medicine, 13*, 839–846.

Witt, P., & Ellis, G. (1987). *The Leisure Diagnostic Battery users manual.* State College, PA: Venture Publishing.

Wright, B. (1960). *Physical disability: A psychological approach.* New York: Harper & Row.

chapter 21

The Energy Paradigm
A New Model for Health Care

Roberta B. Trieschmann

Thomas Kuhn, in his classic book, *The Structure of Scientific Revolutions* (1970), indicated that paradigms (models) play a powerful role in determining which issues become legitimate questions for research in any given field and which methodologies are considered acceptable for studying a problem. In health care, the dominant paradigm—the medical model—states that the body is a physical mechanism that can be studied and understood using the methods of the physical sciences. The implicit assumption is that quantitative measurement of physiological function will be sufficient to diagnose the cause of sickness and likewise that treatment can be accomplished at a strictly physical level. Subjective data, emotional reactions, and psychological concepts are viewed as contaminating variables at best or irrelevant at worst. These subjective factors need to be controlled (i.e., excluded) so that they do not hinder progress in the medical sciences.

The evidence is growing, however, that emotional reactions and psychological processes are not irrelevant; rather, they are integral to the homeostasis and healthy functioning of the human body. Hans Selye (1976) pioneered the study of stress, described the physiology of the stress response, and showed how long-term stress produced numerous physical disorders, such as ulcers, arthritis, hypertension, and other disorders. Since the mid-1970s, the psychobiology of stress and its effect on the immune system have become part of a major research endeavor called psychoneuroimmunology. We now know that emotional reactions have a direct and immediate physiological correlate in the human body; Chapter 17 documents this process. Unfortunately, the health care system as a whole is not structured to use these results to assist people to feel better and to reduce their stress because these data do not fit into the medical model of human function. Although a patient may be referred to a psychologist for treatment, the medical paradigm, which gives primacy to physical treatments of the body, remains intact. Psychological services are not considered integral to the recovery of the person but are viewed as an adjunct service that can easily be eliminated if funding is limited or if a schedule conflict prevails.

Unfortunately, the medical paradigm is based on the concept of reductionism, which fractionates the human body into its component parts for study and treatment. This strictly physical approach ignores the systems interactions of the various physical parts because there is no coherent philosophy of health that unites all human functioning at the core of this model. The mind, the feelings, and the soul are extraneous to the focus of the medical system, although all good medical practitioners have never ignored these aspects in their patient care.

THE EVOLUTION OF A MEDICAL PARADIGM

The medical paradigm has prevailed for only a couple of centuries. Prior to this, a religious paradigm of physical function dominated in which health and wellness were viewed within a grander cosmic scheme that included God, nature, and each human's relationship to nature and God. Illness was often viewed as punishment from God. The Church was the locus of most education, and most books were hand-copied by monks in monasteries. Scientific investigation was dependent upon Church support. Any interpretation that interfered with the Church's teachings was banned. In this climate superstition and misinformation were difficult to challenge, and scientific explorations were often deemed dangerous to the Church's authority.

To free science from the church, René Descartes devised an ingenious solution that set the stage for the scientific revolution of the last 300 years. He proposed to separate the body of man from God. He suggested that the body, much like a clock or machine, could be understood as a complex physical mechanism and studied through physical principles, using mathematics as the major method of describing the results of investigations. Thus, the body would be the province of science, whereas the mind and the soul would belong to the Church. In reality, he knew that body and mind could not be separated, but his proposal of the body-mind split became an intellectual contrivance that allowed for a division of power intellectually between the Church and science.

Isaac Newton developed the laws of gravity and expanded the idea of applying physical measurements to material objects, the planets, and eventually to all of the universe. Mathematics would be the language of this new science; subjective data were suspect. If it could not be measured physically, then it was presumed not to exist. Francis Bacon elaborated on these concepts and developed the scientific method that emphasized standardized procedures, control of extraneous variables (viewed as errors), quantitative measurement, and reproducibility of results.

In essence, this political solution worked. The paradigm of Western science investigation was based upon the concept of reductionism; analysis of something into its component parts will produce greater understanding of how it worked. Quantification of data became a cornerstone of the scientific methodology, as did reproducibility of the results through control of extraneous variables and standardized procedures of investigation. Objective, quantifiable data were thus the means to achieve the goal of control over nature in order to influence it in the direction desired by humans.

The physical sciences prospered under this approach and the industrial revolution fueled the belief that this paradigm guaranteed success, ensuring the well-being of humankind. Well-being was synonymous with material comfort and wealth, however, and it was presumed that the Church would take care of the soul. The medical sciences followed this model, as did the science of psychology.

PSYCHOPHYSIOLOGY AND CLINICAL PSYCHOLOGY

Originally the fields of psychology and philosophy were one. Some individuals, however, chose to view the mind as open to the same mode of investigation as the hard sciences, using quantitative measurement techniques. Thus, psychophysiological studies initially characterized the new field of psychology, as the sensory inputs to the brain were measured and described. When it came to behavior, however, there was a further split into two camps. One group followed Freud, and the field of psychoanalysis was born, while the other followed Watson, and the field of behaviorism was created. The latter field emphasized reductionism and quantification of measures and evolved into the field of experimental psychology. The former field of psychoanalysis created a theory of human behavior and a specific methodology for treating behavioral problems. Many disagreed, however, with certain aspects of psychoanalytic theory and moved beyond it to create other theories of personality functioning and other treatment techniques, primarily psychotherapy. The field of clinical psychology descended from this latter branch of psychology's evolution.

The modern clinical psychologist (since the 1950s) has become a hybrid of these branches of psychology in an attempt to create the clinician-scientist. Increasingly, these clinicians stress the need for quantitative measures of human behavior (primarily through psychological tests) and a large variety of intervention strategies that provide qualitative and quantitative measures of results. Psychotherapy and meditation are examples of the former, and biofeedback and classic behavior therapy are examples of the latter. Thus, the field of psychology has been trying to respond to the actual needs of the general population while trying to maintain credibility within the professional community in which the medical and Western science model dominate.

Since the 1950s, the field of medicine has produced a wealth of data on body function, invented phenomenal technology to diagnose and treat illness, and developed a series of powerful chemicals to influence body function with the goal of removing the symptoms of illness—ideally curing all disease. Descartes' intellectual convenience of 300 years ago, however, gradually evolved into the assumption that mind and body *were* separate. And the requirement that all data must be physically quantifiable and objective reinforced the belief that it was not important if it could not be measured. Unfortunately, these intellectual assumptions and the methodology of Western science have created an unrealistic view of life by providing a distorted perception of the nature of .the world and the nature of human beings.

THE ROLE OF PSYCHONEUROIMMUNOLOGY AND ALTERNATIVE MEDICINE

Since the 1970s, however, the separation between mind and body has been challenged by data from the field of psychoneuroimmunology. As chapters in the earlier part of this section indicate, emotional reactions have direct and immediate consequences at the cellular level, influence body states, and lead to organ system dysfunction. Simultaneously, the American public is increasingly disenchanted with traditional medical interventions that are perceived to be invasive and often more destructive than helpful. Thus, the field of alternative medicine is gaining favor with an increasing number of Americans who are seeking such treatments and paying for services out of pocket. These interventions include meditation, acupuncture, massage, rolfing, jin shin jyutsu, reiki, tai chi, yoga, qi gong, naturopathy, homeopathy, and the use of vitamins and herbs, to name just a few. The aversion to invasive and destructive interventions is fueling a movement for natural healing alternatives that are gentle and health promoting. A core theme of these alternative strategies is that they link mind and soul to body and health.

Many of these interventions from the field of alternative medicine succeed in making people feel much better, at least for a while. But results depend upon the number of treatments, the ability of the practitioner, and ultimately the willingness of the person to make the lifestyle changes necessary to alter the factors that led to the malaise initially. These treatments usually are delivered by a practitioner who integrates the mind and emotions with the body which accounts for the positive reception by the American public. But again, the specific treatment approach to the problem is often unifocal and in many cases still emphasizes physical interventions to the person.

Nevertheless, the medical paradigm that well-being results from a strictly physical approach to health problems is crumbling. It is time for a new paradigm to take its place. Kuhn (1970) indicates that the operational paradigm of any scientific area will be strongly defended and adhered to until the sheer weight of evidence that cannot be handled by the old paradigm leads to the introduction of a new paradigm that accounts for the conflicting data. Such a paradigm does exist. It is called the energy paradigm.

THE ENERGY PARADIGM: THE NEXT LOGICAL STEP

The energy paradigm integrates the body, mind, emotions, and soul into a philosophy of health and wellness that reconnects people to nature. This has been the core of Oriental philosophy and medicine for 5000 years (Reid, 1994). In this paradigm, energy is the foundation of all functioning in the world. The universe *is* energy, and all physical material, including living beings, are *products* of that energy. Although the exterior appearance and even the internal structure of all matter may be different, the basis in energy is the unifying concept. Thus, all parts of the universe are linked and consequently interdependent. There are rhythms to the universe and to the flow of energy that promote life, account for change, and involve natural cycles that repeat themselves. Birth, growth, death, decay, rebirth, the diurnal cycle, and seasonal changes are all examples of the natural rhythms of the universe.

The energy paradigm also states that there is a natural harmony and balance among all types of matter if they are not altered by the actions of humans. This natural harmony and balance leads to peace, happiness, health, and well-being when one is in alignment with the natural rhythms of the universe. People's health is inextricably linked to the health of the environment as well as to the health of all living creatures.

The field of physics deals with the concept of energy, and Einstein's equation, $E = mc^2$, that energy equals matter times the speed of light, has been taught in high school for years. Our entire Western civilization is based upon the use of electrical energy, fossil fuel energy, and nuclear energy, but human energy is not mentioned in the field of medicine except in terms of fatigue (the decline of energy) as a symptom of illness. Consequently, energy and its role in human physical functioning are not considered to be important in the West. Yet what is the source of the heartbeat?

What is it that causes a sperm and egg to unite? What causes the fertilized ovum to divide and multiply to produce an embryo, then a fetus, and then an infant? What prompts the birth process signaled by contractions of the uterus? What is the difference between a live body and a corpse? The answer to all of these questions is the universal life force, which we call energy. Quantum physics has been dealing with the concept of energy as the basis for universal functioning for almost a century and has concluded that the laws of Newtonian physics do not apply at the quantum (energy) or systems level. Yet human beings are systems, and the attempts to understand this system by using the principles of Newtonian science have reached their limit. Thus, the stage has been set for medical science to follow the lead of quantum physics, just as medical science originally followed the lead of Newtonian physics.

Clearly the human body is a very complex system, but our medical paradigm seldom looks at the systems aspects of human function. Rather, it remains preoccupied with increasingly smaller units of physiological function in isolation from the world in which the organism lives. In contrast, the energy paradigm is based on the concept of a universal system that includes all planets, all parts of the planet earth, all who live on it, and all aspects of these living creatures, body, mind, emotions, and soul.

Any disturbance to the harmony and balance of energy in the system leads to repercussions within the entire system. Within the energy model, a major disruption to the balance of energy in the human system is emotional reaction. All emotional reactions involve an activation of the sympathetic nervous system, and a resolution of this emotion with a return to balance is fostered by the parasympathetic nervous system. Thus, calm, ease, peace, and feeling good are natural and normal human states. This is the state of balance, harmony, homeostasis. Emotional disturbance and reactions are destructive to the human system because they drain energy. When an emotional reaction occurs, attention should be paid to restoring the energy balance and to replenishing the energy that has been drained. If emotional disturbance continues for an extended period of time, the energy in the human system will remain out of balance. Essentially energy will gradually be diminished because replenishment of the energy is not occurring while the system remains out of balance. Over a period of time, a continued state of energy imbalance will eventually lead to dysfunctions at the physical level. As a signal of energy imbalance, physical symptoms occur, such as headaches, sleep disturbances, pain, allergies, infections, and eventually immune system disturbances and organ system failures. Major medical illnesses, such as cancer, heart disease, and arthritis, may occur after many years of energy imbalance (Reid, 1994).

The cycle of healthy versus nonhealthy states can be shown as follows:

Health:

Emotional calm → balanced energy → happiness → optimal physical function → emotional calm

Unhealthy:

Emotional arousal → unbalanced energy → unhappiness → physical symptoms → emotional arousal

In this system, energy balance is achieved through control of emotional reactions so as to maintain a state of calmness and peace across the day. Health, happiness, and contentment are the outcome, and energy is available for productive and creative efforts of all kinds.

Within this paradigm, a person is born with a certain amount of energy, called prenatal energy, acquired from the parents. Over the lifetime one is expending this energy, either quickly or slowly, depending upon the lifestyle of the individual. Energy depletion occurs as the result of emotional arousal and inattention to the natural rhythms of the body (in harmony with the rhythms of the universe) so that energy is not replenished through a proper and healthy lifestyle. Many years of living in an aroused emotional state (stressed state) and nonreplenishment of expended energy sets the stage for problems at the physical level.

The early warning signs are fatigue, headache, disturbed sleep, muscle tension, and aches and pains. Treatment of these symptoms with caffeine, pain pills, and relaxants only masks the symptoms and allows one to avoid looking at the real problem, a disordered lifestyle and unhealthy approach to emotions. Consequently, the energy imbalance continues, as does the energy depletion, which leads to the next stage—more serious physical disorders, such as immune system disturbances, cancer, and heart disease.

At the point that body system problems appear, the energy imbalance has existed for many years. Unfortunately, the diagnostic procedures of the medical model look strictly at the physical level and totally ignore the real cause, disordered patterns of energy within the human system. Treatments are focused strictly at the physical level as well and do not address the energy problem either.

TREATING ENERGY IMBALANCES

The real solution to the problem is to replenish the energy and to restore the balance of energy within the system. Although one gets a supply of prenatal energy from one's parents, one can access the universal supply of prenatal energy to replenish oneself through meditation, through a variety of qi gong and tai chi exercises, but most completely through Shen Qi, and advanced form of qi gong developed by the Chinese Qi Gong Master, Aiping Wang.

In Shen Qi training, the student becomes reacquainted with the feel of the natural rhythms of the universe within the body, learns to sense the energy flow in daily life, to become nonreactive to emotionally provocative stimuli, to eliminate those influences in life that drain energy, and to access prenatal universal energy to replenish the body supply that had been depleted in previous years of stress-filled life. During the course of training, the superficial symptoms of stress wane first, and eventually the more serious symptoms of bodily dysfunction wane as well. Lifestyle change, however, is essential because emotional reactions to the stress-filled lifestyle actually lead to the energy imbalance in the first place.

Consequently, within the energy paradigm, relief in physical symptoms requires alteration of emotional reactions and behavior. In contrast to the medical paradigm, a clear mind, happy emotions, and a peaceful soul are the *cause* of physical health, not the result of physical health. Likewise, a cluttered mind, a disturbed emotional state, and an unhappy soul are the cause of physical sickness, not the result of physical sickness. The goal now is to teach this new method of lifestyle management to prevent and alter body dysfunctions.

A review of the work of Hans Selye, particularly his book, *The Stress of Life* (1976), reveals that this scientist, who devoted his life to analyzing the physiology of stress, essentially arrived at the same conclusions just described in the context of an energy paradigm. As a physiologist his focus was primarily at the physical level, yet the last sections of his book espouse a similar philosophy as presented here. Mihaly Csikszentmihalyi has written two works that espouse similar points, *Flow: The Psychology of Optimal Experience* (1990) and *The Evolving Self: A Psychology for the Third Millennium* (1993). Happiness, he believes, is the key to psychological health and physical health and is necessary to resolve the social disasters of the late 20th century. Happiness is contingent, however, not on finding optimal external circumstances, but in gaining control over one's mind in order to shape one's reaction to external events rather than being bludgeoned by them.

COPING WITH STRESS IN DAILY LIFE

The psychology and self-help sections of all bookstores are replete with volumes that offer advice and strategies to cope with general and specific types of stressors in daily life. To dismiss such material as "pop psychology" ignores the tremendous need of the public for help in feeling better and the recognition that material success does not provide happiness. People are yearning for answers to the basic questions of the meaning of life and finding that traditional health care professionals and churches do not always provide satisfying assistance. These books do provide some assistance, but do not serve as an adequate substitute for the learning that occurs as the student of a great teacher. Yoga teachers, Zen Buddhist roshis, and Tibetan Buddhist lamas and tulkus are teaching in the West and do provide powerful training that improves a person's overall ability to handle stress in daily life. These approaches do not, however, teach the student specifically to become emotionally unresponsive to provocative external stimuli. Thus, Shen Qi is the only *system* of training that actually teaches an individual to do this each hour, every day, every year, while participating fully in the activities of daily life.

HELPING WOMEN WITH DISABILITIES

The external events of daily existence are increasingly stressful for everyone. However, for women with physical disabilities, the stress is much greater because of the dual minority status of being a woman and having a disability (Deegan & Brooks, 1985; Fine & Asch, 1988). Other chapters in this book outline the nature of these stressors, and other chapters document the types of health problems that women with disabilities are facing. In a previous work (1987), I emphasized the role that stress plays in accelerating the aging process in people with disabilities. However, research is still very limited with regard to this issue. Perhaps the combined efforts of the professionals who contributed to this book will encourage further study in the field of stress management after disability onset.

Within the medical paradigm, where the mind-body split prevails, the stress of women with disabilities is primarily the province of the psychologist. The resulting physical problems are the province of the medical professionals. Yet the energy paradigm states that many of the medical problems since the onset of the disability are strongly influenced by the psychological state of the woman with the disability. Thus, we need to reverse the traditional emphasis in our medical system so as to give increased priority to research and treatment of stress issues in this population of women. The stressors, the role of emotions in producing physical symptoms, and strategies to alter emotional reactions to stressors must be emphasized in future research.

CONCLUSIONS

We are in a transitional stage in health care research. The shift from the medical paradigm to the energy paradigm *is occurring*, and the future of the National Institutes of Health (NIH) and the medical research centers of prominence today hinge upon recognizing this trend and, with an open mind, learning about the role of energy in preventing sickness and maintaining health. The establishment of an Office of Alternative Medicine at NIH is a promising first step, as is the design of this text to include an emphasis on qualitative as well as quantitative input.

An old Chinese proverb says, "The frog in the well knows nothing of the great ocean." This is a time for unity of diverse points of view. This is a time for collegial action rather than a division into hostile camps, each one casting vituperation upon the other. Alternative medicine is here to stay and is growing exponentially. The understanding of the energy paradigm will provide the conceptual unification of a variety of these approaches. Indeed, this insight will actually strengthen the ability of many health care practitioners to assist people in remaining healthy and to heal themselves of already existing problems. Applying the principles of the energy paradigm will infuse traditional Western medicine with new life and a methodology to actually achieve the goal of curing the many disorders that plague human beings. Furthermore, understanding the energy paradigm will give new inspiration and vitality to the many dedicated professionals who have always dedicated their lives to helping others.

REFERENCES

Csikszentmihalyi, M. (1990). *Flow: The psychology of optimal experience*. New York: Harper Perennial.

Csikszentmihalyi, M. (1993). *The evolving self: A psychology for the third millennium*. New York: Harper Perennial.

Deegan, M.J., & Brooks, N.A. (Eds.). (1985). *Women and disability: The double handicap*. New Brunswick, NJ: Transaction Books.

Fine, M., & Asch, A. (1988). *Women with disabilities: Essays in psychology, culture, and politics*. Philadelphia: Temple University Press.

Kuhn, T. (1970). *The structure of scientific revolutions* (2nd ed.). Chicago: University of Chicago Press.

Reid, D. (1994). *The complete book of Chinese health and healing*. Boston: Shambhala.

Selye, H. (1976). *The stress of life*. New York: McGraw-Hill.

Trieschmann, R. (1987). *Aging with a disability*. New York: Demos.

MANAGING BLADDER AND BOWEL FUNCTION

Danuta M. Krotoski and Carol J. Bennett

The ability to control one's basic bodily functions is crucial for maintaining independence, self-esteem, work, and personal relationships. Many disabling conditions, such as spina bifida, cerebral palsy, and spinal cord injury, can lead to compromised bladder and bowel function. Current interventions, although alleviating some of the problems, may lead to new complications. Permanent or intermittent catheterization of the bladder, for instance, can lead to increased incidence of urinary tract infection, which at one time was one of the leading causes of death following spinal cord injury.

This section focuses on this important issue by first considering limitations in bowel and bladder functioning in the context of daily living and then exploring the impact of this dysfunction on a woman's view of herself and her relationships with others. Perduta-Fulginiti (Chapter 22) captures the importance of both societal and medical factors in enabling women to gain greater control of their lives. She identifies the problems caused by the lack of effective and safe devices for women and the difficulties in accessing toileting facilities in relation to both a work and an intimate environment.

Razi, Young, and Bennett (Chapter 23) describe the anatomy and physiology of urinary voiding, thus providing a basis on which to understand the changes that may occur as a consequence of injury or disability. Furthermore, this information serves as a background for the following chapters that provide information on evaluation of function in the urinary tract as well as current and future methods for improving bladder management. Chancellor (Chapter 24) and Lloyd (Chapter 26) describe new methods for assessing the status of the urinary tract that serve as bases for identifying the most appropriate management methods, and Young and

Brewer (Chapter 25) address the issue of urinary tract infections and describe studies they have undertaken using new catheter tips that have significantly reduced infections in women. Because, under some conditions, pressure that builds in the bladder can result in kidney damage and lead to life-threatening conditions, it is important to be able to accurately evaluate functioning of the tract at all levels and to identify the most effective ways of intervening.

An exciting new development described by Creasey (Chapter 29) is a new device, based on functional electrical stimulation, that allows the individual to control bladder emptying by activating a switch on a radio-transmitter that controls delivery of electrical impulses to the sacral nerves. For those for whom such a device may not be an option, other new treatment options are presented by Bennett, Razi, and Young (Chapter 27). These include new pharmacological approaches and development of new materials, such as collagen, that when injected into the bladder sphincter increase sphincter elasticity and thus provide better voiding control.

A description of toileting devices that are currently available for women with compromised bowel and bladder function is provided by Pires (Chapter 28). From her discussion it is clear that research is needed to develop more useful and cosmetically pleasing devices and that architectural and environmental changes must also be considered.

In looking to the future, the authors focus on a number of priority areas that need the attention of the research community. One of the highest priorities must be to focus on the way women respond to reduced control over bowel and bladder voiding and on how this affects their self-esteem and their interactions with others. One area of particular interest is finding methods to reduce the impact of bladder and bowel dysfunction on sexual interactions. Such studies should look at the psychological factors that affect the woman with a disability and her partner as well as issues associated with devices or physiological responses.

Another important priority must be the development of adaptive devices and equipment to enable women to be more secure, have greater mobility, and lead even healthier lifestyles. Although there are effective devices for males with disabilities, as of the mid-1990s few are available for women. Because the presence of indwelling catheters can lead to infection and may, over the long term, cause urethral erosion and other complications, research and development of effective external devices for women are critical.

Much discussion has centered on the development of multicenter studies to evaluate the role of neural prostheses in neurogenic bladder and bowel dysfunction. Multicenter comparisons of bladder management, particularly utilizing different catheterization management methods in comparison with the use of reflex voiding, is another important need. Further studies should focus on methods to reduce bladder hyperreflexia and the buildup of high pressure in the bladder by developing more effective pharmacological, mechanical, surgical, or electrical interventions.

Urinary tract infections are an important cause of morbidity for many women with disabilities, particularly those with spinal cord injury. It is important to determine whether changes that occur as a consequence of having a neurogenic bladder may make the woman more susceptible to infection. As discussed in the section on stress, high levels of stress compromise immune function and indeed may be an important factor in this population.

Finally, as discussed in an earlier section, much research needs to be done to ensure that women with disabilities have successful and uncomplicated pregnancies. Further research is needed on the impact of pregnancy on bladder management in women with disabilities.

chapter 22

Impact of Bladder and Bowel Dysfunction on Sexuality and Self-Esteem

P. Sonya Perduta-Fulginiti

Neurogenic bowel and bladder management, with its associated physical and functional management concerns, is only one factor within a cascade of events that affect the self-concept of a woman with a physical disability. This chapter focuses on a woman's self-esteem and her ability to view herself as a sexual person as they relate to neurogenic bowel and bladder dysfunction. Because there is virtually no documented quantitative research on the impact of bowel and bladder dysfunction on self-esteem and sexuality, the points discussed in this chapter can serve as potential topics for medical, psychosocial, and sociopolitical research.

SELF-CONCEPT

A woman's self-concept, or how she views herself as an individual within her specific social milieu, is based on the interrelated concepts of gender identity, body image, sexuality, and self-esteem. Gender identity is determined by how individuals define themselves within the context of maleness or femaleness. Another aspect of self-concept is the way individuals perceive their own bodies in comparison to the norms of their unique culture. In U.S. society, feminine normalcy is based on being tall, lean, and physiologically perfect. With the numerous body variations associated with physical disabilities, such as spasticity, paralysis, or scoliosis, for example, women with disabilities must cope with this clash of societal norms and their own individual reality on a daily basis.

Sexuality, which is also a component of a woman's self-concept, is the overall expression of her physical, functional, and psychosocial sexual characteristics over the life span. How a woman with a physical disability expresses her sexuality is dependent upon when she acquired her disability, the severity of the disability, how she was raised as a child, and how she now expresses those experiences as an adult.

For a woman with a congenitally acquired disability, such as spina bifida, she may never have been considered a sexual being by her parents and may never have learned (or was never expected) to portray herself according to the American ideal of womanhood. She may then act and be perceived as childlike. Alternatively, a woman who acquired her disability as an adult may continue to perceive herself and portray herself as an adult, sexual person. A woman's concept of her worth affects her self-concept. If she perceives herself as being worthy, she will have value in her own eyes and will therefore have a better self-concept. The esteem she receives from others, such as colleagues, family, and friends, also influences her assessment of her self-worth. An inability to control bladder and bowel function may act to compound the general perception of decreased value that society places on women with physical disabilities.

TOILET-TRAINING HISTORY

Little information is available regarding the toilet-training experiences of children with neurogenic bladder and bowel dysfunction. Toilet-training experiences can vary greatly among children. Incontinence is sometimes the occasion for belittlement, reprimands, and punishment; other times it is of little concern to caregivers. Also, incontinence of urine may elicit a different form of response compared with incontinence of feces. For some individuals, incontinence of urine and feces is perceived to be a natural part of this transitionary process. Thus, success at toilet training is achieved in different ways—through positive reinforcement or sometimes punishment.

For a woman who develops a neurogenic bladder and bowel, the similarities between her experiences in rehabilitation and her childhood toilet-training experiences can be dramatic and have a profound impact on her. The combination shower/commode chair or raised toilet seat with grab bars for toileting may not be perceived as being that different from the self-supporting or toilet-adapted potty chair and thus impact on the woman's feelings of independence and sexuality. As she learns to acquire greater control over her bowel and bladder functions, a woman must cope with many emotions during the transitionary process where she may be incontinent of both urine and feces. These emotions may involve negative responses that could negatively affect her ability to cope and affect her ability to maintain a positive self-image.

Women with neurogenic bladder and bowel may need to cope with incontinence for the remainder of their lives. Their coping mechanisms may be based, either consciously or subconsciously, on memories of their past experiences with toilet training and how society views individuals who are incontinent. Regardless of whether these past memories hold negative or positive feelings, the addition of societal pressures for maintaining the "norm" and the way in which these pressures can influence a person's self-worth and sexuality are important factors that need to be characterized.

NEUROGENIC BOWEL AND BLADDER MANAGEMENT

The various regimes associated with management of neurogenic bowel and bladder can affect a woman's self-esteem and sexuality and will be influenced by her type of disability, independence/dependence levels, equipment needs, length of disability with resultant aging issues, and physical access issues.

Type of Disability

The type of disability often affects the levels of continence, thus influencing the choice of bowel and bladder programs. For example, a woman with a spinal cord injury (SCI) may consistently utilize a program of intermittent catheterization (IC) every 6 hours. Her bowel program may be performed every other day in the evenings, in which she uses only digital stimulation. She may have remained consistently successful for the past 5 years. On the other hand, a woman with multiple sclerosis (MS) may have difficulty managing her neurogenic bowel and bladder because her functional abilities are fluctuating. For a short period of time, she may be in total control of her elimination without any incontinence. Unexpectedly, one morning she may wake up and be incontinent of urine before she gets out of bed. She may also experience difficulty in emptying her bowels. How does this vacillation in bowel and bladder function, compared with a permanent dysfunctional status, affect how a woman perceives herself? Does permanence, progression, or inconsistency of neurological conditions with resultant neurogenic bladder and bowel dysfunction mirror a consistency or fluctuation in feelings of self-worth and sexuality?

Independence/Dependence

The degree to which a woman is able to manage her own bladder and bowel programs can have a tremendous impact on the way she perceives herself. The experience of a woman with a high-level SCI who requires another individual to intermittently catheterize her every 4–6 hours and to insert a suppository and provide rectal digital stimulation on a daily basis is quite different from that of a woman whose disability allows her to be independent in these functions. For any woman with a physical disability that prevents her from performing her own toileting, it is necessary to assess how having another person empty her bladder and her bowel makes her feel about herself as a woman. These are very intimate acts that are carried out in privacy by most people. Are coping mechanisms needed to maintain a sense of self during these invasive acts—if not in the long term, then perhaps initially? Does preparation for these activities, such as undressing and full genital exposure, affect a woman's perception of herself as a sexual being?

Equipment Needs

Women who have neurogenic bladders may utilize IC, external stimulation techniques, indwelling catheters, or urinary diversions for their management program. For some of these programs, specific pieces of equipment are needed, as discussed in greater detail in Chapter 28. This equipment must be purchased and transported during typical daily routines. Depending on her disability, the woman may have difficulty carrying this equipment or may not be able to have an adequate supply on hand to meet her needs. She must be concerned about how and in what she will carry these items, where she will find accessible bathrooms, and how she will deal with collection devices. She will have to deal with the fact that equipment, such as leg bags, may become apparent to those around her and thus may influence her self-concept and how she is viewed by others.

If a woman with a neurogenic bladder chooses to employ a noninvasive form of bladder emptying, incontinence padding may be a necessity in order to ensure that clothing, wheelchair cushions, and furniture remain dry. To what degree does the presence of diapering materials affect a woman's self-esteem? Does she need to wear diapering materials because accessible public bathrooms are not readily available? How does she dispose of soiled diapering materials in a way that does not draw attention to her bladder management program?

Traveling with the equipment needed for both bowel and bladder management programs can be cumbersome. Additional baggage may be needed to transport supplies. Considering the difficulties that may be associated with carrying any baggage, compromises may again need to be made regarding what will be taken on business trips and vacations. The need for large equipment, such as a shower/commode chair, may curtail any travel plans. Requesting this type of equipment from hotels/motels may cause some emotional discomfort, perhaps initially.

Finally, the cost of this equipment must be considered. Is this type of equipment covered by the person's health insurance plan? If not, does the woman then need to make compromises in her personal and social life to set aside the financial resources to purchase these essential supplies? When one must compromise personal needs and social activities on a continual basis, how does that affect self-esteem?

Length of Disability

A woman's perception of herself may vary, depending on the length of time she has had her disability and the related bowel and bladder dysfunction. For those women with acute SCI or those having recently lost bowel and bladder function due to a neurological disease process, their priority may be to get their bowel and bladder programs regimented so as not to be incontinent. This initial loss of bladder and bowel control may be devastating to a woman's self-esteem and could lead to reduced sexual activity. For women who have had acquired disabilities for 15 years or more, determining when and where they can find an accessible bathroom may be the major issue in their plans for the day. Their long-term methods of neurogenic bowel and bladder elimination have now become their "norm" and integrated over time into their self-concept. The degrees to which initial compared with long-term management of neurogenic bowel and bladder dysfunction can influence self-esteem, sexuality, and sexual activity is clearly a matter for research.

Aging Issues

Women are living longer with their disabilities, introducing a series of important issues for which we do not have answers. Little is known about the long-term effects of bowel and bladder medications and their simultaneous effects on related organ neurophysiological functioning. Furthermore, in persons with SCI, neurogenic bowel and bladder function appears to change over time, although the changes are not uniform within this population (Whiteneck, 1993).

Bowel management may change as the woman ages. Some individuals have a decrease in bowel transit time, while others have an increase in transit time. A change in motility, expulsion, and total emptying may become a major concern for someone whose morning prework routine consisted of a 20- to 30-minute bowel program that now may take 1½ hours. Bouts of fecal incontinence may become more frequent than usual. These changes in function may cause an uncertainty with already established bowel programs and can severely limit daily life activities and reduce the quality of life.

Another potential change may be the need for IC and the use of medications for bladder emptying in women who had for many years used external stimulation methods. Possible progression to indwelling catheters, bladder augmentation, or urinary diversions to maintain bladder and kidney health may be a reality for some women with disabilities. These changes in bladder management, along with a newly acquired need for equipment and medications, may change the way the woman views herself and may lead to a significant change in her self-esteem and personal relationships.

Changes that occur in the musculoskeletal system as a consequence of aging with a disability may also compromise a woman's ability to continue her present independent bladder and bowel programs. Shoulder, arm, and wrist injuries, incurred by years of weightbearing on joints not intended for that purpose, can severely deter the ability to transfer onto the toilet seat, to insert a suppository, or to perform self-catheterization. In addition to current information on changes in bowel and bladder function in women with SCI, there is a critical need for research on the needs of women with other disabilities such as MS, juvenile diabetes, and spina bifida. Comparisons of data collected on the coping mechanisms and the physiological and functional changes associated with aging with various disabilities would provide the medical and the disability communities with important insights for choosing the most appropriate management strategies.

Physical Access Issues

The issue of architectural accessibility plays a vital role in the management of one's bladder and bowels, as discussed in Chapter 28. In the majority of cases, women with disabilities have bathrooms in their homes that are physically accessible to suit their functional abilities. Outside the home, everyone, including persons with disabilities, need public bathrooms that can be accessed easily as they travel, shop for groceries and clothing, and participate in sports and all of life's other activities. For women with mobility impairments that require accessible bathrooms, functioning within the community can become especially burdensome. Architecturally inaccessible buildings limit the women's ability to participate in all aspects of community life. This in turn can negatively affect their self-esteem.

Women who require accessible bathrooms may plan their day's activities around accessible locations with such bathrooms and the availability of personal assistants, if necessary. The work involved in this planning can be quite extensive. No one has measured the energy requirements, the frustrations, and the impact of these stresses on the lives of women with disabilities, their family members, and friends. Not all accessible buildings have accessible bathrooms, and not all described accessible bathrooms are actually universally accessible. There are many restaurants, movie theaters, vacation hotels, and shops that have accessible entrances, but do not have universally accessible public restrooms.

Imagine being a woman with a disability who uses a wheelchair for mobility. You are completing a business trip and are in an unfamiliar city. You and your colleagues spot a restaurant with "Handicapped Parking" and a ramp entering the building. You decide to eat there and to discuss the results of your business meeting. After the meal, you locate the bathroom and, much to your dismay, it is not wheelchair accessible. There can be multiple reasons for bathroom inaccessibility. One may be that the door to the bathroom is only 29 inches wide, too narrow for a wheelchair. Another may be that, although there are grab bars in one of the stalls, the stall is still too narrow to accommodate a wheelchair. Or, the stall may be wide enough to accommodate the wheelchair but not deep enough to allow for safe transfer onto the toilet seat or closure of the stall door. Finally, the stall may be wide enough, but the toilet seat may be too low. Bathrooms are sometimes up or down any number of stairs in a building without an elevator or wheelchair lift or on the other end of the building. Gaining access to such a bathroom may require the help of maintenance staff with a special elevator key. The staff member may then need to accompany the woman and wait while she uses the restroom.

Another unpleasant scenario occurs when people without disabilities use stalls designated for persons with disabilities. By doing so, they leave women with disabilities with no other options. Imagine being a woman in a wheelchair who needs to empty her bladder. You enter the restroom only to find a person without a wheelchair in the accessible stall and five empty narrow stalls. As you wait, knowing that you have no voluntary control of your bladder, you realize that you will become incontinent because of a lack of awareness on the part of the individual.

When the option to utilize restrooms does not exist, or when a woman becomes incontinent, how does she interact with her friends, family members, or business colleagues? How do circumstances like these affect a women's self-esteem or sexuality? Social interaction, romantic encounters, and business meetings are likely to end abruptly and these social interactions, dates, and business liaisons may not occur again.

Perhaps a woman with a disability is at work when she attempts to utilize the restroom, only to find an able-bodied person occupying the accessible stall. If incontinence is a possibility in her daily life, she may be prepared by routinely carrying a change of clothes with her. How does she feel when she arrives at work in one outfit and then returns from the bathroom in another? Does the knowledge of her bladder incontinence affect how her peers view her? Without a change of clothing, this woman would need to go home. Is this acceptable to her employer? When does this become unacceptable? Does her employer know about her bladder problems? Would the potential issue of bladder incontinence need to be discussed with her employer?

This lack of universally accessible bathrooms and sensitivity suggests that the needs of a person with a disability are not generally considered. From those establishments that have accessible parking and entrances but no accessible bathroom, the message is to come in and spend your money here, but not to expect to use the bathroom. The need to travel to other floors of buildings and to other buildings altogether, while able-bodied persons have convenient access, clearly states that the needs of the woman with a disability are not valued. Obviously, such messages can lower the self-esteem of women with disabilities. Research should address how they cope with these issues on a daily basis and how much these issues affect their feelings of self-worth.

SEXUAL FUNCTION

Neurogenic bowel and bladder dysfunction can have a significant impact on sexual activity, potentially reducing spontaneity by increasing pre-sex preparation related to the practicalities of what to do with drainage equipment and how to deal with the potential for incontinence. A woman's functional abilities, comfort level with sexual activity, and skill in managing these issues can influence sexual expression.

Partners

With regard to the acceptance of or adaptation to neurogenic bowel or bladder issues, there is a belief that the establishment of sexual relationships between two persons with disabilities is easier than a relationship between an able-bodied partner and a woman with a disability. The basic premise of this concept is that partners with disabilities have similar bowel and bladder management concerns. In some cases, the presence of urinary drainage bags, similar bowel programs, and the chance for incontinence may decrease the anxiety associated with the discussion and acceptance of these intimate issues.

Similarities in bladder and bowel management techniques, however, are only one aspect of the complexities associated in establishing intimate relationships. Men with disabilities who have neurogenic bladder/bowel issues may have different concerns with causes of incontinence than a woman with a disability. Are men with disabilities aware of the bladder and bowel management issues of women with disabilities, and vice versa? If a man or a woman with a disability is having difficulty coping with his or her own bladder and bowel management, he or she may not be able to cope with a potential partner's issues at all.

If a woman with a disability becomes involved in a relationship with an able-bodied partner, when do the issues of elimination become a topic for discussion? Perhaps the able-bodied partner has no prior knowledge of any of these types of concerns. How will this knowledge affect the relationship? If the woman has a previous history of relationship terminations once this knowledge becomes evident, these experiences may prevent her from becoming sexual with partners or may prevent the establishment of relationships altogether. These can certainly influence how she perceives herself as a woman and as a sexual being.

Spontaneity

For women with disabilities who have neurogenic bladder and bowels, spontaneity with sexual activity may not be possible. For those women who use external stimulation or IC for bladder emptying and a bowel program for bowel evacuation, any initiation of sexual activity close to their regimented emptying schedules may result in incontinence. This is a distinct possibility because sexual excitement, intercourse, and orgasm increase the reflex activity within the sacral plexus of the spinal cord. This increase in sacral reflex activity can also trigger bladder and bowel emptying.

Women who use incontinence padding for protection, who have an indwelling catheter, or who use an ostomy bag may feel uncomfortable with their presence during foreplay activities. Imagine a woman with a disability who is sitting on the couch watching a movie with her partner. Suddenly, the mood becomes amorous with necking and fondling of body parts. The partner's hands begin moving lower, when she remembers her bladder needs to be catheterized, or her almost full ostomy bag or her indwelling catheter with urine-filled leg bag that she is wearing need to be emptied. How will she react? Her reactions may be quite different, depending upon whether she has had past intimate experiences or no intimate experiences with this partner. Does this partner know that she uses these elimination management techniques? If foreplay is halted in order to deal with these issues, will it resume afterwards?

Pre-Sex Preparation

As detailed in the aforementioned scenario, women with neurogenic bowels and bladders must prepare for sexual activity to prevent the development of any compromising situations. When a sudden amorous mood develops, a woman who uses incontinence padding may need to excuse herself so that she can remove the padding. Initiation of sexual activity close to any bladder- or drainage bag-emptying schedule will prompt the need to perform these tasks prior to continuation of these activities.

Women who use external stimulation for their bladder management may not totally empty their bladders with each triggering episode, so possible urinary incontinence may occur with sexual activity. In an informal unpublished survey of 24 women who have neurogenic bladders as a consequence of SCI, 14 reported urinary incontinence with sexual activity. Therefore, it is important that planning for incontinence occurs (Perduta-Fulginiti, 1991). Strategies such as the placement of waterproof padding over the mattress, the storage of towels or other absorbent materials within reach, and the briefing of one's partner may be necessary.

Sexual activity close to the scheduled bowel evacuation time may have to be postponed altogether to prevent incontinence of bowel contents, especially if the woman has a sensitive or irritable bowel or a rectum full of stool. It is important that the woman check her rectum prior to any sexual activity to determine if bowel incontinence may occur with sexual stimulation. If stool is found within the rectum, emptying the bowel prior to sexual activity may not guarantee bowel continence during sexual activity.

In some cases, sexual stimulation following recent completion of a bowel program may only promote further evacuation of bowel contents. Eight women in the aforementioned informal survey stated they have had bowel incontinence during sexual activity. Considering these findings, a woman with a disability may then choose to forgo sex at this time or to please her partner without achieving full sexual self-gratification.

Certain types of sexual positions or sexual activities may need to be restricted due to neurogenic bowel and bladder dysfunction. If urinary incontinence is a distinct possibility, the woman may feel uncomfortable having her partner perform cunnilingus. Anal intercourse may not be an acceptable option any longer for the woman with an irritable or overly sensitive bowel. As noted earlier, sexual arousal and continued sexual stimulation may be temporarily postponed or curtailed altogether because of neurogenic bowel and bladder management issues. The need for cognitive and practical planning before sexual activity can be initiated or continued may be the reality of living with a neurogenic bowel or bladder. If sexual desire outweighs the possibility of incontinence, preventing oneself from achieving full sexual gratification or preparing for inevitable incontinence may be necessary. The elimination of certain sexual activities from a woman's sexual repertoire may cause feelings of dissatisfaction or sexual frustration.

Urinary and Bowel Appliances

Women with disabilities who have neurogenic bladders may generally use any of the following urinary appliances: straight, Foley, and suprapubic catheters; urostomy equipment; and leg and bedside drainage bags. Sexual activity for these women presents some challenges, specifically with regard to the presence of indwelling catheters, the urinary drainage equipment, and the urostomy bags. Suggestions to empty ostomy bags, to tape catheters to the abdomen or thighs (Bregman, 1975), and to use tubing extensions for drainage bags are commonplace. These approaches allow sexual activity to occur without urinary incontinence and traumatic dislodging of any appliances. Ostomy bags can also be covered with decorative fabric, if desired.

For the woman with a neurogenic bowel, the presence of an ostomy bag may be the only bowel appliance that influences sexual activity. Depending upon the type of ostomy, such as ileostomy, colostomy, or sigmoidostomy, the presence and contents of the bag may be time-limited or a constant feature. Prior to sexual activity, removal of a sigmoidostomy bag may be done only in specific regimented bowel programs. This will allow for greater flexibility in sexual positioning. Emptying the contents of the ostomy bag can prevent incontinence. Again, a woman might choose to cover this type of ostomy bag.

Actual Incontinence

The emotions portrayed during the preventative and preparative techniques for incontinence with sexual activity can be dramatically different from those experienced during or after the actual act of urinary or fecal incontinence. What feelings are expressed when a woman realizes she has urinated on her partner during orgasm? How does she feel when her partner explains that sexual activity must end because of bowel incontinence? What are the reactions of the partner?

In the informal study of 24 women with SCI, bladder incontinence was usually cleaned up and sexual activity resumed, whereas bowel incontinence was considered to have a more negative effect on the resumption of sexual activity (Perduta-Fulginiti, 1991). One woman stated the need to weep following her first episode of bowel incontinence during sex with her partner. She also became hesitant to initiate and participate in sexual activity close to her bowel program schedule and worried about bowel incontinence with similar sexual positions. Clearly, her sexuality and self-esteem were affected by this event. Further studies of incontinence during sexual activity are needed to determine how self-esteem and sexuality are altered and what coping mechanisms are successful in maintaining a positive self-concept.

CONCLUSIONS

Undoubtedly, neurogenic bowel and bladder dysfunction can affect the self-esteem and sexuality of women with physical disabilities in relation to social, psychological, and physical management issues. It is imperative to understand that the impact of bowel and bladder dysfunction is only one small aspect of the complex biopsychosocial ramifications that persons with disabilities must face on a daily basis. Other physiological issues that persons with neurogenic bowel and bladder dysfunction may be concerned with are motor paralysis, loss of sensation, skin problems, joint contractures, spasticity, respiratory impairment, and circulatory compromise. These issues can also lower their self-esteem and interest in sexuality.

The frequent lack of community architectural accessibility can magnify these toileting challenges. When public places do not provide adequate facilities, the message is clear: People with disabilities are not welcome; they must enter through the back door; they cannot travel without assistance from the able-bodied; they must use special transportation; and they must not expect to empty their bladders outside of their own homes. In this sense, people with disabilities are not considered part of "normal" society. Adherence to disability stereotypes keeps persons with disabilities out of the mainstream of American society. The negative beliefs that people with disabilities are ill, ignorant, without emotion, asexual, pitiful, and incapable of employment are perpetuated daily through personal interactions and through both the private and public sectors of the media.

People with disabilities must cope with this daily battering of their self-concepts from physiological, psychological, and social perspectives. It is only through valid quantitative research that these issues can be clearly documented and their resolutions identified. As part of these studies, the impact of bladder and bowel dysfunction and other physical complications of disability must be carefully researched. Research is needed to determine what coping mechanisms are successful in promoting self-esteem and thereby encouraging persons with disabilities to contribute as members of our society. In addition, sociopolitical research must be initiated to identify how society can assist in dispelling the myths and negative beliefs of persons with disabilities. Perhaps with time, better education, and the increased visibility of persons with disabilities participating in the common life pursuits of employment, education, relationships, and parenting, our society will learn to value the needs and skills of all persons with disabilities.

REFERENCES

Bregman, S. (1975). *Sexuality and the spinal cord injured woman.* Minneapolis: Sister Kinney Institute.

Perduta-Fulginiti, S. (1991). *Sexual function of women with spinal cord injury.* Unpublished informal survey.

Whiteneck, G. (Ed.). (1993). *Aging with spinal cord injury.* New York: Demos Publications.

chapter 23

Anatomy and Pathophysiology of Voiding Dysfunction

Salman S. Razi, Mary N. Young, and Carol J. Bennett

ANATOMY OF THE FEMALE BLADDER AND URETHRA

The bladder is a hollow muscular reservoir that serves to store and periodically release urine. Anatomically, the bladder is composed of a tetrahedron-shaped body and a smooth triangular-shaped base called the trigone. The female urethra is approximately 4 cm in length and 6 mm in diameter, extending from the bladder neck to the external urethral meatus. Studies have shown that the bladder neck predominately provides coaptation, or continence. Two sphincters that assist in providing continence have been identified: a smooth muscle internal sphincter and a striated urogenital external sphincter (Figure 1). A true anatomical sphincter does not exist at the bladder neck or within the urethra; however, a physiological, functional internal sphincter consisting of smooth muscle, collagen, elastic fibers, and vascular tissue is present. The smooth muscle sphincter is composed of a dominant inner longitudinal layer and a thin outer circular layer that traverses nearly the entire length of the urethra. Collagen is the main structural component of the urethra and, as mentioned, is also found within the internal sphincter. Collagen is important for passive closure of the urethra (Hickey, Phillips, & Hukins, 1982).

As in men, the striated external urethral sphincter in women is anatomically present and encircles the smooth muscle sphincter. In addition, there is a separate periurethral striated musculature whose activity is recorded when electromyograms (EMGs) are performed as part of a urodynamic study. These striated muscles are thought to be innervated by the somatic nerve, which is thought to have a pelvic component.

Continence is maintained when urethral tone or pressure exceeds intravesical pressure. Increased urethral tone is provided by both smooth and

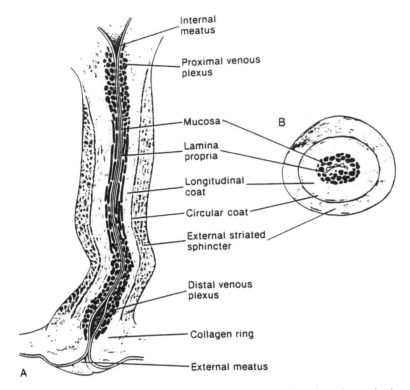

Figure 1. Anatomy of the female urethra. A: Anatomy of the female urethra—longitudinal view. B: Anatomy of the female urethra—cross-sectional view. (From Hinman, F., Jr. [1993]. Female genital tract and urethra. In F. Hinman, Jr. [Ed.], *Atlas of urosurgical anatomy* [p. 404]. Philadelphia: W.B. Saunders; reprinted by permission.)

striated muscles of the urethra. The combination of bladder and urethral physiological and anatomical properties provides continence in women.

BLADDER AND URETHRAL INNERVATION

The bladder and urethra are innervated by both the autonomic and somatic nervous systems (Figure 2). These systems work in conjunction with each other to facilitate normal bladder filling and emptying while maintaining continence.

The autonomic nervous system is subdivided into the parasympathetic and sympathetic nervous system. The parasympathetic afferent nerves originate from sacral (S) spinal cord levels 2, 3, and 4. They are preganglionic fibers in the ventral nerve roots and coalesce to form the pelvic (splanchnic) nerve. The cholinergic nerve endings stimulate detrusor contraction and bladder emptying.

The sympathetic nerves originate from the interior medial lateral nuclei, from thoracic (T) 12 to lumbar (L) 2 segments of the spinal cord, and

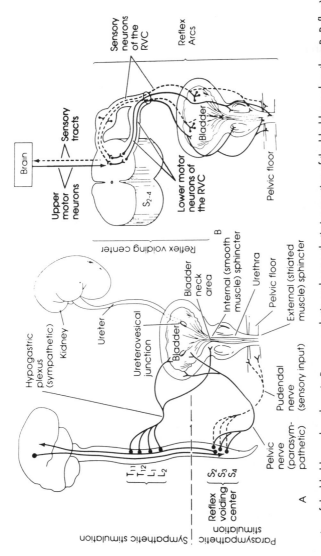

Figure 2. Innervation of the bladder and urethra. A: Parasympathetic and sympathetic innervation of the bladder and urethra. B: Reflex Voiding Center (RVC). A closer look. (From Zejdlik, C.P. [1992]. Maintaining urinary function. In C.P. Zejdlik [Ed.]. *Management of spinal cord injury* [2nd ed., p. 355]. Boston: Jones and Bartlett; reprinted by permission.)

301

coalesce to form the hypogastric nerve. The sympathetic nerve is adrenergic and primarily supplies the bladder base and urethra, holding the bladder neck closed during the bladder filling phase and providing continence. The innervation to the bladder dome is mainly cholinergic, whereas the tone to the bladder neck and urethra is mainly a result of adrenergic input.

Females do not have an anatomically defined striated external sphincter; however, intermural and extrinsic striated muscles surround the urethra, providing the urethral tone necessary to maintain continence. This striated muscle is under somatic control and is innervated by the pudendal nerve. Some research suggests that involvement of the pelvic nerve and other unnamed tributaries may also contribute somatic innervation to the striated muscle of the female urethra.

VOIDING SEQUENCE

Bladder filling and urine storage occurs via sympathetic facilitation and parasympathetic inhibition. During this stage, cholinergic nerve effects are diminished, allowing the bladder to fill under low intravesical pressure. At the same time, adrenergic fibers are stimulated, providing bladder neck closure and allowing filling without leakage of urine (Figure 3). Under normal circumstances with increased abdominal pressure such as sneezing or coughing, the bladder neck should remain closed and urinary continence should be maintained.

When micturition occurs, sensory input travels from the bladder via afferent fibers to sacral segments 2, 3, and 4 of the spinal cord and continues in the spinothalamic tract to the micturition center in the brain. The micturition center controls the autonomic system until innervation from the pudendal nerve voluntarily relaxes the external (striated muscle) sphincter. The sympathetic arm of the autonomic system is then inhibited, allowing for bladder neck opening, while the parasympathetic nervous system is facilitated, resulting in an increase in detrusor pressure and bladder emptying. Bladder emptying, therefore, involves a coordinated contraction of the bladder smooth muscle with decreased resistance at the bladder neck (internal smooth muscle sphincter) and external (striated muscle) sphincter.

VOIDING DYSFUNCTION IN SELECT NEUROLOGICAL CONDITIONS
Lesions Above the Brain Stem

Cerebral vascular accident (CVA), or stroke, is a significant cause of morbidity and mortality in the United States and Europe. There are various etiologies that can potentiate this disease and concomitantly result in voiding dysfunction. Acute urinary retention may occur immediately follow-

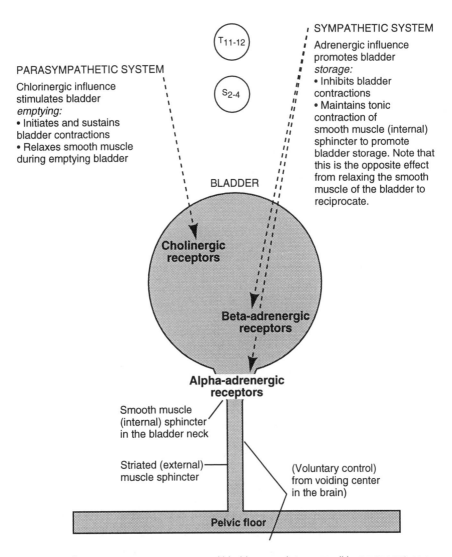

PARASYMPATHETIC SYSTEM

Chlorinergic influence
stimulates bladder
emptying:
• Initiates and sustains
bladder contractions
• Relaxes smooth muscle
during emptying bladder

T$_{11-12}$

S$_{2-4}$

SYMPATHETIC SYSTEM

Adrenergic influence
promotes bladder
storage:
• Inhibits bladder
contractions
• Maintains tonic
contraction of
smooth muscle (internal)
sphincter to promote
bladder storage. Note that
this is the opposite effect
from relaxing the smooth
muscle of the bladder to
reciprocate.

BLADDER

Cholinergic receptors

Beta-adrenergic receptors

Alpha-adrenergic receptors

Smooth muscle
(internal) sphincter
in the bladder neck

Striated (external)
muscle sphincter

(Voluntary control)
from voiding center
in the brain)

Pelvic floor

Figure 3.   The autonomic nervous system and bladder control. (From Zejdlik, C.P. [1992]. Main-taining urinary function. In C.P. Zejdlik [Ed.], *Management of spinal cord injury* [2nd ed., p. 377]. Boston: Jones and Bartlett; reprinted by permission.)

ing the initial accident. A fixed deficit usually manifests over the next few weeks to months, and during this time bladder dysfunction becomes apparent. The bladder typically becomes hyperactive, a condition known as detrusor hyperreflexia. Sensation in individuals who have this condition is usually intact, and as the bladder begins to contract involuntarily, an attempt is made to voluntarily control leakage via forceful contraction of the external (striated) sphincter. Thus, a pseudocoordination defect between bladder and external sphincter develops. This is known as pseudodyssynergia (Wein & Barrett, 1982) and most commonly results in urgency with urge incontinence.

CVA usually afflicts older individuals, and urological conditions ranging from prostatic outlet obstruction to stress incontinence may be preexistent (Mundy & Blaivas, 1984). Bladder dysfunction after a stroke may partially be the result of a preexistent urological abnormality; therefore, treatment modalities focused solely on detrusor hyperreflexia could potentially be more detrimental than beneficial.

Parkinson's disease is another entity whose origin lies above the brain stem, causing urological disability. This disease primarily affects the pigmented neurons of the substantia nigra. The age of onset is typically between 45 and 65 years, and voiding dysfunction occurs in 25%–75% of patients with Parkinson's disease. Symptoms experienced are usually frequency, urgency, incontinence, and nocturia. The bladder develops high pressures and uninhibited contractions (detrusor hyperreflexia) with concomitant poor sphincter or urethral relaxation, resulting in urge incontinence (Pavlakis et al., 1983).

Lesions Below the Brain Stem

Spinal cord injury can be grouped into suprasacral (upper motor neuron) and sacral (lower motor neuron) spinal cord injury. Both levels of injury can be caused by a variety of etiologies. Suprasacral lesions (those occurring above T12/L1) result in a high-pressure, hyperactive bladder (Figure 4). In individuals with spinal cord injury, unlike the pseudodyssynergia that develops in CVA patients, the external sphincter may contract involuntarily and therefore the bladder and external sphincter exhibit true dyssynergia. Lack of perineal sensation and bladder hyperactivity can result in frequent incontinence and voiding without awareness.

Sacral spinal lesions (lesions at or below T12/L1) result in a low-pressure, areflexic, or flaccid bladder that fails to empty properly (Figure 5). Rather than being incontinent, these individuals often cannot void. The internal smooth muscle sphincter is competent but nonrelaxing, while the external sphincter experiences diminished tone (McGuire, 1984).

Multiple sclerosis (MS) is one of the most common neurological diseases resulting in voiding dysfunction (Blaivas, 1985). This disease is characterized by focal neural demyelination and results in impairment of nerve conduction. This disease does not afflict individuals in a similar fashion. Approximately 10% of undiagnosed MS patients initially present with urological difficulties. Up to 90% can develop hyperreflexia bladders (Blaivas, 1985; McGuire, 1984; Mundy & Blaivas, 1984), and 65% of these individuals have striated sphincter dyssynergia. Bladder areflexia has also been

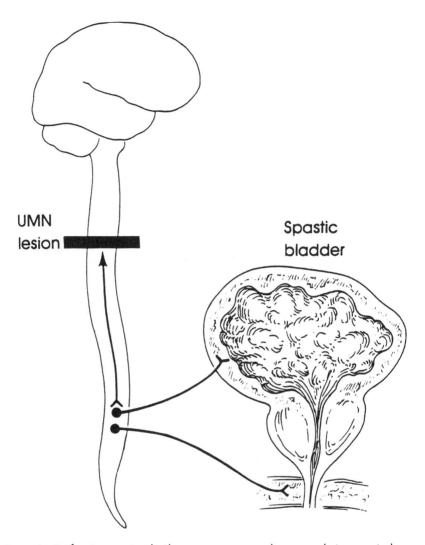

UMN lesion

Spastic bladder

Figure 4. Dysfunction associated with upper motor neuron damage results in a spastic detrusor. (From Zejdlik, C.P. [1992]. Maintaining urinary function. In C.P. Zejdlik [Ed.], *Management of spinal cord injury* [2nd ed., p. 356]. Boston: Jones and Bartlett; reprinted by permission.)

reported in up to 40% of individuals; however, a majority of these progress to bladder hyperreflexia. Blavais and Barbalais (1984) identified particular risk factors for the development of voiding dysfunction in MS patients, including indwelling catheters, detrusor sphincter dyssynergia in men, and decreased compliance, often yielding intravesical pressures greater than 40 cm of water. Careful follow-up, including the routine upper tract evaluation, urinalysis, and urodynamic testing, is essential to avoid sustained

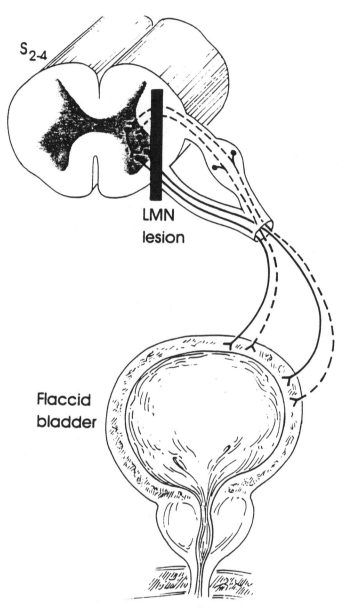

S$_{2-4}$

LMN
lesion

Flaccid
bladder

Figure 5. Dysfunction associated with lower motor neuron damage results in a flaccid detrusor. (From Zejdlik, C.P. [1992]. Maintaining urinary function. In C.P. Zejdlik [Ed.], *Management of spinal cord injury* [2nd ed., p. 357]. Boston: Jones and Bartlett; reprinted by permission.)

elevated intravesical pressures and potential subsequent urological damage to the kidneys.

CONCLUSIONS

This chapter has focused on the anatomy and innervation of the bladder and urethra in women, the normal voiding sequence, and some specific changes in voiding patterns that are associated with select neurological conditions. This background provides a foundation for addressing methodologies designed to improve bladder function in women with disabilities.

REFERENCES

Blaivas, J.G. (1985). Nontraumatic voiding dysfunction in the adult: II. Multiple sclerosis and diabetes mellitus. *AUA Update, Series, Lesson 12, Volume 4*.

Blaivas, J.G., & Barbalais, G.A. (1984). Detrusor external sphincter dyssynergia in men with multiple sclerosis: An ominous urologic condition. *Journal of Urology, 131*, 94.

Hickey, D.S., Phillips, J.L., & Hukins, D.W. (1982). Arrangement of collagen fibrils and muscle fibers in the female urethra and their implications for control of micturition. *British Journal of Urology, 54*(5), 556–561.

Hinman, F., Jr. (1993). Female genital tract and urethra. In F. Hinman, Jr. (Ed.), *Atlas of urosurgical anatomy* (pp. 389–408). Philadelphia: W.B. Saunders.

McGuire, E.J. (1984). Clinical evaluation and treatment of neurogenic vesical dysfunction. In J. Libertion (Ed.), *International perspectives in urology* (Vol. 2, pp. 1–15). Baltimore: Williams & Wilkins.

Mundy, A.R., & Blaivas, J.G. (1984). Non-traumatic neurologic disorders. In A.R. Mundy, T.P. Stephenson, & A.J. Wein (Eds.), *Urodynamics: Principles, practice, and applications* (pp. 278–287). New York: Churchill-Livingston.

Pavlakis, A.J., Siroky, M.B., Goldstein, I., & Krane, R.J. (1983). Neurologic findings in Parkinson's disease. *Journal of Urology, 129*, 80.

Wein, A.J., & Barrett, D.M. (1982). Etiologic possibilities for increased pelvic floor electromyography activity during bladder filling. *Journal of Urology, 127*, 949.

Zejdlik, C.P. (1992). Maintaining urinary function. In C.P. Zejdlik (Ed.), *Management of spinal cord injury* (2nd ed., pp. 353–396). Boston: Jones and Bartlett.

SUGGESTED READINGS

Barrett, D.M., & Wein, A.J. (1991). Voiding dysfunction: Diagnosis, classification and management. In J.Y. Gillenwater, J.T. Grayhack, S.S. Howards, & J.W. Duckett (Eds.), *Adult and pediatric urology* (2nd ed., pp. 1001–1099). St. Louis: C.V. Mosby.

Wein, A.J. (1992). Neuromuscular dysfunction in the lower urinary tract. In P.C. Walsh, A.B. Retik, T.A. Stamey, & E.D. Vaughn Jr. (Eds.), *Campbell's urology* (6th ed., pp. 573–613). Philadelphia: W.B. Saunders.

chapter 24

Bladder Dysfunction
Evaluation and Outcome

Michael B. Chancellor

An important aspect of improving the health of women with physical disabilities is proper bladder management. Before we can determine the best bladder management for a particular woman, proper evaluation must be undertaken. The cornerstone for accurate diagnosis of neurogenic bladder dysfunction in women is urodynamic testing. Urodynamic evaluation can help to determine negative outcomes and provide guidance for the most effective bladder management. This chapter discusses the techniques of urodynamic testing, patterns of bladder dysfunction after neurological diseases or impairments, and prediction of long-term complications as part of goals for setting a research agenda for the late 1990s.

PROPER URODYNAMIC TESTING

Empirical therapy for dysfunctions of voiding based solely on urinary symptoms is never a wise approach. The reason for this is that many of the voiding symptoms secondary to various neurological impairments are similar. Furthermore, symptoms secondary to neurological diseases are similar to symptoms secondary to other common urological conditions, such as a pelvic floor dysfunction and prolapse in women and benign prostatic hyperplasia and prostate cancer in men (Chancellor & Blaivas, 1992; Chancellor & Rivas, 1993).

Urodynamic study is currently the only functional test for the urinary tract. The purpose of urodynamic evaluation is to determine and classify the type of voiding dysfunction and to recognize risk factors, such as detrusor-external sphincter dyssynergia (DESD) and decreased bladder compliance. Parameters of importance for urodynamics include capacity of urinary storage, urethral closing function, and bladder and urethral micturition responses.

The term urodynamics describes a number of complementary tests of varying degrees of complexity that can be performed individually or in combination, depending on the clinical circumstance. Urodynamic evaluation varies from a simple bedside "eyeball" cystometry to sophisticated multichannel video-urodynamic studies (Table 1). Some individuals may need only a baseline screening study, such as residual urine volume measurement, while others may require more extensive testing. Study selection will depend upon the nature of the person's problem and available resources (Hinman, 1979; Ouslander, Greengold, & Chen, 1987; Wein & Barrett, 1988).

During the urodynamic investigation, it is imperative to reproduce the voiding symptoms (Blaivas, 1988; Sonda, Kogan, Koff, & Diokno, 1983). When a woman with physical disability complains of urinary incontinence, the initial goal of the evaluation should be to reproduce the incontinence and to use this information to determine its cause. A physician and/or nurse experienced in urodynamics should perform and observe the study. Interpreting a paper tracing of a previously performed urodynamic study by a technician should be avoided.

Table 1. Evaluation techniques

History and physical

Neurological examination
   Anal tone and control
   Bulbocavernosus reflex
   Perianal sensation

Urinanalysis and culture

Upper urinary tract evaluation
   Intravenous pyelogram
   Renal ultrasound
   Radioisotope renogram

Incontinence pad test and voiding diary

Urodynamic studies
   "Eyeball" cystometrogram
   Electronic cystometrogram
   Uroflow
   Residual urine (catheterization vs. ultrasound measurement)
   Urethral pressure profile
   Sphincter electromyography
   Multichannel studies: Subtracted intraabdominal pressure to obtain true detrusor pressure
   Video-urodynamics
   Pharmacological testing: bethanechol supersensitivity test

Voiding cystourethrogram

Cystourethroscopy

Advances in urodynamics have led to a significant improvement in the understanding of the normal and abnormal function of the bladder and urethra. At the same time, it is now easier than ever to select the most appropriate therapy that addresses the underlying pathology in individuals with established or progressive upper tract disease (McGuire, Bennett, Konnak, Sonda, & Savastano, 1981).

PATTERNS OF BLADDER DYSFUNCTION

The bladder and urethra can respond to a neurological disease in only a limited number of ways. This principle is critical in the evaluation and care of women with disabilities. Neurological lesions produce either a loss of function or a release of function. Loss of function is exemplified by paralysis of the bladder as a consequence of lower motor neuron lesions, whereas release of function is exemplified by detrusor overactivity in suprasacral spinal cord injury.

Individuals with suprasacral spinal cord lesions, such as spinal cord injury (SCI) and multiple sclerosis (MS), are prone to developing detrusor hyperreflexia and detrusor-external sphincter dyssynergia (Blaivas, 1982; Chancellor & Blaivas, 1991; Fam & Yalla, 1988). In DESD, there is inappropriate contraction of the striated urethral musculature during involuntary detrusor contractions (Blaivas, 1982). Because the bladder is contracting against a closed sphincter, the resulting detrusor high pressures can cause vesicoureteral reflux. There is a 50% or greater chance of developing urological complications within 5 years of diagnosis of DESD (Blaivas & Barbalias, 1984; Borges & Hackler, 1982; Fam & Yalla, 1988; Lloyd, 1986; Tribe, 1963). The incidence of urological complications with DESD is lower in women than men because of lower sphincter outlet resistance.

Persons with lumbosacral lesions such as cauda equina injury and myelodysplasia are more likely to develop a flaccid bladder, defined as detrusor areflexia by the International Continence Society (Abrams, Blaivas, Stanton, & Andersen, 1988; Blaivas, 1982, 1988; McGuire, Woodside, Borden, & Weiss, 1981). It is essential to standardize the terminology associated with urodynamics to allow the accurate exchange and comparison of information among physicians, health care providers, and consumers. The official terminology suggested by the International Continence Society provides such an established framework, whereby clinicians and consumers from around the world with interest in urodynamics can speak the same language (Abrams et al., 1988).

INITIAL ASSESSMENT

The initial urodynamic assessment should include a comprehensive history and physical examination. In women, the gynecological and menstrual history is important in determining pelvic floor function. The pelvic exam may reveal vaginal atrophy, urethral hypermobility, and pelvic floor relaxation. Routine laboratory tests, including urinalysis and culture and serum creatinine, should be obtained. An elevated serum creatinine may herald changes in the upper tract as a consequence in increased urethral pressure in an otherwise asymptomatic patient.

Diagnosis of neurogenic bladder dysfunction should not be based on symptoms alone. The bladder is an "unreliable witness" because of considerable overlap between urgency and stress incontinence symptoms, and also between urgency and obstructive symptoms (Chancellor & Rivas, 1993). A thorough urodynamic is the gold standard (Blaivas, 1982; Blaivas & Olsson, 1988; Kaplan, Chancellor, & Blaivas, 1991).

The following tools are used to assess urodynamic function in women with disabilities.

Voiding Diary

A simple and inexpensive technique we use routinely with many women with voiding dysfunction and/or urinary incontinence is the voiding diary (Larsson, Abrams, & Victor, 1991). Women who come to our clinic are instructed to record time and volume of all oral fluid intake and time and volume of all urination for a consecutive period of 24 hours. They are also instructed to record time and estimate amount (small, medium, large) of any incontinence episode and what they were doing to cause the incontinence (Figure 1). It is important, however, to not base therapy solely on the voiding diary. The voiding diary can sometimes be unreliable because voiding habits may differ over time and individuals may exhibit variable compliance.

Pad Test

In women who complain of urinary incontinence, objective quantification of urine lost is helpful for rational therapy. The perineal pad testing has gained popularity as an objective test for this purpose. The pad test is easy to conduct and interpret and provides useful information in the evaluation of patients with incontinence (Sutherst, Brown, & Shower, 1981). The total amount of urine lost during the test period is determined by weighing the absorbent pads.

Uroflow

The urinary flow reflects the net outcome of bladder contractility and outlet resistance. The presence of bladder outlet obstruction leads to a decrease in flow rate and elevation of detrusor pressure. It was originally hoped, as electronic uroflow meters were perfected, that the uroflow would predict bladder outlet obstruction. Unfortunately, a reduction in flow rate is not specific for outlet obstruction. A reduction in flow rate can be caused by

Bladder Diary:
Name:_____ Date:_____

Time	Amount of liquid you drink	Volume of urination	Volume of catheterization	Urine leakage (small, medium, large)
6: 00 AM				
7: 00 AM				
8: 00 AM				
9: 00 AM				
10: 00 AM				
11: 00 AM				
12: 00 Noon				
1: 00 PM				
2: 00 PM				
3: 00 PM				
4: 00 PM				
5: 00 PM				
6: 00 PM				
7: 00 PM				
8: 00 PM				
9: 00 PM				
10: 00 PM				
11: 00 PM				
12: 00 Midnight				
1: 00 AM				
2: 00 AM				
3: 00 AM				
4: 00 AM				
5: 00 AM				

Figure 1. Bladder voiding diary.

either obstruction or impaired bladder contractility or a combination of both (Chancellor, Kaplen, Axelrod, & Blaivas, 1991). Therefore, uroflow by itself cannot exclusively diagnose obstruction and has little role in the diagnosis of bladder dysfunction in women with physical disabilities.

Cystometry

The cystometrogram (CMG) has been considered the "reflex hammer" of the urologist. The type of information the examiner wishes to learn from a urodynamic study may determine the type and level of sophistication needed. Information that is required for appropriate urodynamic evaluation can be gathered from a thorough CMG. This information includes bladder compliance, sensation, capacity, and contractions. Compliance is assessed by determining the change in volume divided by the change in pressure. This important parameter is calculated by dividing the volume change by the change in detrusor pressure, expressed as ml/cm H_2O. The shape of the CMG curve is influenced by the rate of bladder filling. A fast-filling CMG may elicit an artificially low bladder compliance that may not be reproduced by the rate of the patient's urinary production (Coolsaet, 1985).

The first step in performing a proper CMG evaluation is the insertion of a small catheter without using a balloon at the bladder neck. The CMG may be performed using liquid or gas. Although CO_2 gas CMG has the advantage of being quick and clean, it has several major disadvantages:

1. Filling the bladder with gas is much less physiological than filling it with fluid.
2. A very fast filling rate can alter bladder compliance.
3. Because of gas compressibility, subtle pressure changes may be missed.
4. CO_2 dissolution forms carbonic acid and may be irritating.
5. Because there is no fluid, incontinence simply cannot be measured.
6. A voiding study is therefore not possible.

The use of liquid medium for all urodynamic testing is strongly encouraged. Liquid infusant for CMG can be sterile water, saline, or radiographic contrast (Cass, Ward, & Markland, 1970; Gleason, Bottaccine, & Reilly, 1977; Jorgensen, Lose, & Andersen, 1988; Merrill, Bradley, & Markland, 1972).

A variety of urodynamic catheters are available. Single-, double-, and triple-lumen catheters all have their proponents. Transducer-tipped catheters are also used; however, they are fragile and expensive. The diameter of the catheter itself can have an effect and alter the voiding phase of a urodynamic study. It is generally agreed that catheters of 10 French or less in diameter do not cause significant obstruction during the micturitional phase of the study. Good results can also be obtained with a two-catheter technique where one is for filling and the other is connected to a pressure transducer. After the bladder is filled to capacity, the filling catheter is removed, leaving a very small pressure catheter that disturbs micturition less. An indwelling catheter with the balloon should be avoided while performing the urodynamic study. With the balloon inflated, gathering data on incontinence, micturition, voiding pressure, and pressure/flow is impossible.

Intravesical pressure is the sum of the pressure generated by the bladder (detrusor pressure) and the forces exerted on the bladder by the intraperitoneal contents (intra-abdominal pressure). A more accurate measurement of the actual pressure generated by the detrusor muscle is the detrusor pressure (Pdet) obtained by subtracting the intra-abdominal pressure from the total intravesical pressure.

$$\text{Detrusor pressure (Pdet)} = \text{Vesical pressure (Pves)}$$
$$- \text{Intraabdominal pressure (Pabd)}.$$

Multichannel urodynamics enables the detection of detrusor contractions that might otherwise be masked by the effects of abdominal pressure on the intravesical pressure tracing (Figure 2).

Video-Urodynamics

Video-urodynamics (fluoroscopy) adds an anatomical dimension to the urodynamic study that is complementary to the pressure study. One key advantage of video-urodynamic study is that it can correlate the location of outlet obstruction and other pathology with multichannel bladder and urethral pressure studies (Bates & Corney, 1971; Blaivas & Fisher, 1981). The second key advantage of video-urodynamic utilization is in diagnosis of incontinence (Miller, 1971). Although careful history, physical examination, and CMG can often elucidate incontinence, fluoroscopy can "clinch" the diagnosis. Video-urodynamics helps identify bladder neck and urethral incompetence and can confirm rotational descent of the bladder neck and urethra in women during stress maneuvers. The major disadvantage of this method of video-urodynamics is the costly investment in equipment (Figure 3), not always possible for smaller medical groups.

Video-urodynamics is performed by filling the bladder with radiographic contrast solution and performing intermittent fluoroscopic imaging. The presence of ureteric reflux, bladder trabeculation, or diverticular formation is noted and the intravesical pressure response to filling recorded. In the presence of involuntary detrusor contractions, the bladder neck may be seen to open and leakage is evident. Filling is continued until the individual undergoing the procedures expresses an urgent desire to void; at that stage, the maximum tolerated volume is recorded and the filling catheter is removed (Schafer, 1990).

Urethral Pressure Profile

The urethral pressure profile (UPP) is a graphic representation of intraluminal pressure along the length of the urethra. It is performed by slow retraction of the catheter at a usual rate of 1–40 cm/min. The functional urethral profile length is represented by the length of the anatomical urethra along which the urethral pressure exceeds the intravesical pressure. The urethral pressure is measured at regular intervals and recorded as a function of distance (Brown & Wickham, 1969; Edwards & Malvern, 1974; Harrison & Constable, 1970). Errors due to tubing compliance and resistance

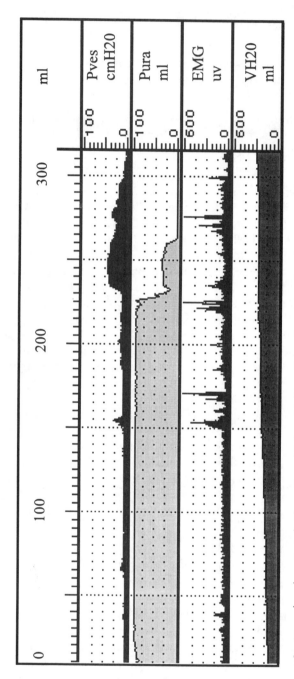

Figure 2. Normal urodynamic study. The patient voided at a bladder volume of 235 ml, with voiding pressure of 45 cm H_2O and simultaneous relaxation of the external sphincter as represented by a drop in Pura. Pves: bladder pressure; Pura: urethral pressure at the level of the external sphincter; EMG: electromyelogram; VH_2O: volume of fluid instilled into the bladder.

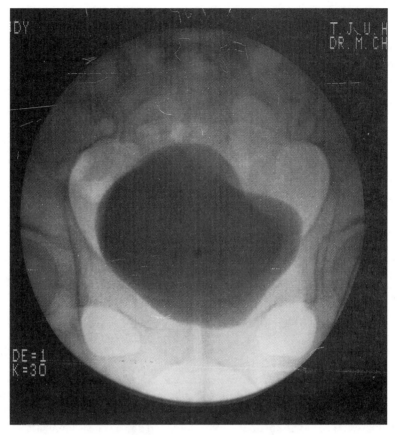

Figure 3. Normal female bladder during video-urodynamic with smooth wall bladder, closed bladder neck, and no vesicoureteral reflux.

may cause an artificially high pressure to be recorded. Moreover, infusion techniques have a relatively slow response to increasing pressures (Abrams, & Feneley, 1978).

Mechanisms must exist to maintain the urethral pressure at higher levels than the intravesical pressure in order for people not to develop stress urinary incontinence. During exercise, the intravesical pressure may increase to 200 cm H_2O. It is generally thought that the transmission of pressure to the intra-abdominal proximal urethra is an important mechanism for ensuring continence (Figure 4) (Constantinou, Faysal, Rother, & Govan, 1981; Massey, Anderson, & Abrams, 1987). Although both maximum urethral closure pressure and functional urethral length tend to be lower in persons with genuine stress incontinence, so much overlap exists in individuals without this problem that they cannot be used as reliable

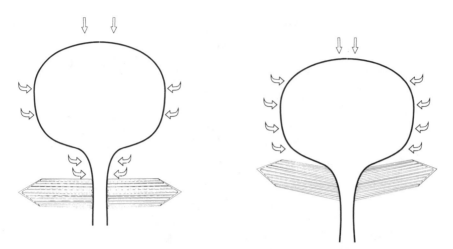

Figure 4. Illustration of pelvic floor and urinary sphincter mechanism of maintaining urinary continence. The drawing on the left illustrates a normal anatomical relationship with simultaneous transmission of intraabdominal pressure to both the bladder and proximal urethra. On the right, the musculofascial support is weakened with descent of the bladder neck and proximal urethra. There is unequal transmission of intraabdominal pressure, and stress incontinence ensues. (From Chancellor, M.B., & Blaivas, J.G. [1994]. Physiology of the lower urinary tract. In E.J. McGuire & E.D. Kursh [Eds.], *Female urology* [pp. 39–57]. Philadelphia: J.B. Lippincott; reprinted by permission.)

indicators (Asmussen & Ulmsten, 1976; Van Geelen, 1983). Static profiles, therefore, provide little useful information, but in the context of a full urodynamic test may provide additional parameters toward the appropriate diagnosis (Anderson, Shepherd, & Feneley, 1983). The diagnostic yield from urethral profilometry can be increased by the addition of dynamic factors such as posture change, the Valsalva maneuver, voluntary squeeze, and coughing (Griffiths, Van Mastrigt, & Bosch, 1989).

When urethral pressure is measured without fluoroscopic control, it is impossible to determine the exact site of the anatomical bladder neck. Thus, when the proximal urethra is nonfunctional, the first rise in pressure occurs not at the site of the bladder neck, but in the more distal urethra. Subsequently, one may conclude erroneously that it represents a bladder neck obstruction.

Electromyography

Pelvic floor and urinary sphincter electromyography (EMG) measures the electrical activity of the sphincter muscle. The beginning of a voluntary detrusor contraction is marked by relaxation of the external urethral sphincter. When this happens, the sphincter EMG becomes electrically silent and the maximum urethral pressure drops dramatically. Sphincter relaxation persists throughout the detrusor contraction, and at the end of voiding electromyographic activity resumes.

Surface pad electrodes are commonly used rather than needle electrodes during urodynamic study because they are painless and easy to apply. Surface electrodes are placed on the skin overlying the muscle of the superficial anal sphincter to pick up motor unity activity produced by various muscles in its vicinity. Anal plug electrodes measure the activity of the superficial anal sphincter through the rectal mucosa. Similarly, two concentric rings can be mounted on a urethral catheter. Using this device, direct measurement from the external urethral sphincter can be made. Although in theory this type of EMG should be accurate, in practice good recordings from the sphincter are difficult to achieve and many artifacts are seen. Needle electrodes employing wire, monopolar, bipolar, or concentric electrodes are the most accurate method for recording the EMG activity of the external sphincter. When EMG is not available, simultaneous measurement of bladder and urethral pressure under fluoroscopic monitoring is useful in diagnosing DESD in SCI patients.

Continuous Ambulatory Urodynamic Studies

Bladder overactivity may be difficult to detect during conventional urodynamic studies. In the course of a day, when a woman is distracted by her activity, she may have a sudden reflex detrusor contraction that she cannot stop and she develops an urge incontinence. However, during a urodynamic study with a catheter in place, the person's attention is focused and the pelvic floor is tightened. In the artificial circumstance of the urodynamic laboratory, the person may be able to prevent or abort any involuntary detrusor contractions. Recent studies have shown that continuous ambulatory bladder monitoring is a more sensitive method than the conventional urodynamics method at detecting detrusor overactivity (O'Donnell & Marshall, 1988; van Waalwijk van Doorn, Remmere, & Janknegt, 1991; Webb, Griffiths, Ramsden, & Neal, 1990). Continuous urodynamic monitoring was found to be technically satisfactory and acceptable in 85% or more cases. Passerubu-Glazel, Cisterino, Artibani, and Pagano (1992) found ambulatory urodynamic to be 25%–33% better than conventional urodynamics in making diagnoses in children with neurogenic dysfunction.

Classification of Stress Incontinence

Normally, urine (and radiographic contrast) is retained in the bladder by the sphincteric action of the proximal urethra and bladder neck. Thus, no radiographic contrast is seen in the urethra unless the patient is voluntarily voiding or is incontinent. The base of the bladder is usually flat and located at or just above the symphysis pubis. When the sphincter fails in its function, radiographic contrast is seen in the urethra without a detrusor contraction (Blaivas, 1983). This condition of stress incontinence may be classified from Type 0 to Type III. Type 0–II represent urethral hypermobility, and Type III implies intrinsic sphincter deficiency. When classifying stress incontinence in women with disabilities, one should remember that there may be changes in the pelvic floor as a consequence of reduced mobility.

Type 0 For this level the individual has a history of stress incontinence, but incontinence is not reproduced during the examination. The bladder neck and urethra descend during cough or strain on fluoroscopy and the urethra opens, but there is no leakage. Maximal urethral closure pressure is normal. The person probably prevents incontinence by momentarily contracting the external urethral sphincter.

Type I There is a minimum descent of the bladder neck and urethra during stress, with visible urinary leakage. The individual exhibits normal maximum urethral closure pressure and no cystocele or herniation of the bladder.

Type II There is an obvious cystourethrocoele present with visible urinary leakage during stress. Normal maximum urethral closure pressure is present.

Type III The bladder neck opens during bladder filling without detrusor contraction. Type III stress urinary incontinence is also called intrinsic sphincter deficiency. Visible urinary leakage is seen with minimal or no stress. The variable vesical neck and urethral descent (often none at all) and the maximal urethral closure pressure are very low. This condition occurs almost always because of failed previous surgery (McGuire, 1980; McGuire, Lytton, Kohorn, & Pepe, 1980) or a neurological lesion involving the thoracolumbar and sacral outflow (Barbalias & Blaivas, 1983; Blaivas & Olsson, 1988).

Snook and Swash (1984) reported abnormalities of pelvic floor innervation in women with urinary incontinence after childbirth and suggested a neurological etiology to stress incontinence. From a therapeutic standpoint, it has been suggested that Type III stress incontinence does not fare as well after the usual urethropexy operations and that an operation such as the pubovaginal sling or periurethral bulking agent injection is more appropriate (Blaivas & Olsson, 1988; McGuire, 1980; McGuire, Bennett, Konnak, Sonda, & Savastano, 1987) (Figure 5).

PATTERNS OF BLADDER DYSFUNCTION AFTER NEUROLOGICAL INJURY

Various classifications have been proposed to describe voiding dysfunction after neurological injury. However, most classification schemes assume that voiding dysfunction is predictable based on the level of spinal injury and disease. Specifically, dysfunction at levels above the sacral spinal cord

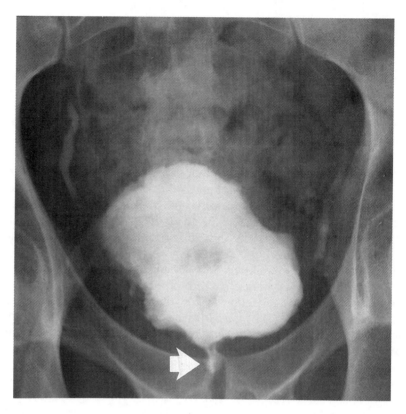

Figure 5. Type III stress urinary incontinence with intrinsic sphincter deficiency and opened bladder neck (arrow).

results in an upper motor neuron lesion and a hyperreflexic bladder, whereas dysfunction involving either the sacral spinal cord or the cauda equina will result in a lower motor neuron lesion and bladder flaccidity (Blaivas, 1982; Wein & Barrett, 1988).

However, individuals with multiple injuries, incomplete injuries, and nontraumatic spinal cord diseases may have mixed voiding dysfunction. There are reports in the literature that detrusor areflexia may occur with upper motor neuron lesions (Arnold, Fukui, Anthony, & Utley, 1984; Light, Faganel, & Beric, 1985). Arnold and co-workers (1984) reported detrusor areflexia in two individuals, one who had a complete cervical C5 lesion and the other with an incomplete thoracic lesion, who had detrusor areflexia (Blaivas, 1982). Light and associates (1985) described 13 persons with suprasacral SCI detrusor areflexia. These individuals could be classified into two groups: the first with subclinical lumbosacral injury and a second who developed detrusor contractions at 16.6 months after the injury.

It should be noted that, in the second group, detrusor contractions occurred at a later date than the return of somatic reflex activity.

Detrusor areflexia may occur with upper motor neuron lesions, presumably due to a coexistent clinical or subclinical sacral spinal cord lesion. Two other possibilities that may account for a diagnosis of detrusor areflexia in persons with presumed suprasacral spinal cord lesions are a failure to fill the bladder to a large enough volume to provoke a reflex detrusor contraction on the urodynamic study and initial bladder overdistention resulting in an acontractile bladder.

We have analyzed the results of urodynamic evaluation in 489 persons with spinal cord lesion and ascertained the relationship between bladder function patterns and a neurological deficit (Kaplan, Chancellor, & Blaivas, 1991). The bladder and sphincter behavior of 284 patients with traumatic SCI are depicted for cervical, thoracic, lumbar, and sacral levels of injury (Figure 6). Approximately 40% were women, with an even ratio of distribution among the different levels of injury. Of 104 individuals with cervical SCI, 15% had detrusor areflexia. The remaining 88 individuals (85%) had involuntary detrusor contractions; 57 of 88 (65%) had detrusor-external sphincter dyssynergia. All of the 87 persons with thoracic SCI had detrusor hyperreflexia; 78 of 87 (90%) had DESD. Individuals with lumbar spinal injury exhibited the most mixed urodynamic patterns: 40% had detrusor areflexia, and 60% had detrusor hyperreflexia (half with DESD and half without). Individuals with sacral SCI were the only group with normal urodynamic studies (12%).

Detrusor areflexia was present in 64%; 54 patients had low bladder compliance, 43 of 54 (80%) had detrusor areflexia, and 76% had sacral injury. Studies have shown the development of an "adrenergic" overgrowth in the bladder in cats with lower motor neuron injury that may contribute to increased tone within the bladder (Sundin & Dahlstrom, 1973). This finding may have clinical relevance, for it would suggest in patients with detrusor areflexia and low bladder compliance that supplementing intermittent catheterization with anticholinergic agents may improve bladder compliance. It was interesting to note that of the individuals who developed poor compliance (51/489) in association with non–sacral cord injury (11/51), all had myelopathy for at least 4 years. Normal initial bladder compliance does not mean that the person will always have a low-pressure "safe" bladder.

Based on our survey, three general urodynamic patterns of bladder dysfunction can be characterized:

1. Detrusor hyperreflexia with synergistic external sphincter function: This pattern is seen in persons with brain injury and incomplete and nontraumatic spinal injury. Management of detrusor hyperreflexia is generally with anticholinergics.

Cervical Traumatic SCI: 104 Patients

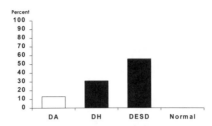

Thoracic Traumatic SCI: 87 Patients

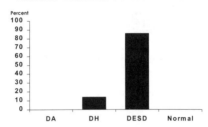

Lumbar Traumatic SCI: 61 Patients

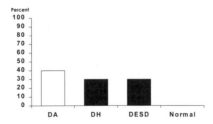

Sacral Traumatic SCI: 32 Patients

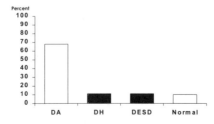

Figure 6. (A) Cervical traumatic SCI: 104 patients, (B) thoracic traumatic SCI: 87 patients, (C) lumbar traumatic SCI: 61 patients, (D) sacral traumatic SCI: 32 patients. DA: detrusor areflexia; DH: detrusor hyperreflexia; DESD: detrusor hyperreflexia with detrusor-external sphincter dyssynergia.

2. Detrusor hyperreflexia with detrusor-external sphincter dyssynergia: This pattern is seen mostly in complete thoracic and cervical SCI. Intermittent catheterization with anticholinergic agents is necessary (Figures 7 and 8).
3. Detrusor areflexia: This pattern is seen in persons with sacral and many lumbar-level injuries. Management with intermittent catheterization may require anticholinergics and bladder augmentation if compliance is poor (Figure 9).

Comparative Urological Outcome

A controversial and key issue in the long-term management of women with physical disabilities is bladder management by indwelling versus intermittent catheterization. McGuire and Savastano (1986) compared 35 women with SCI and followed them for 2–12 years. A total of 13 were treated with indwelling catheters, and 22 were treated with intermittent catheterization. Of the women with indwelling catheters, 46% required urethral reconstruction, 54% developed pyelonephritis, 92% developed febrile urinary tract infections, and 100% developed bladder calculi. This contrasted with the results seen in the intermittent catheterization group, where none of the women had urethral damage, none developed pyelonephritis, 32% developed febrile urinary tract infections, and no women had bladder calculi.

Despite these impressive superior statistics with intermittent catheterization, up to 70% of women with physical disabilities are still managed with indwelling catheters (Jackson & DeVivo, 1992). There are a number of reasons for choosing indwelling catheters. The most common reasons for choosing indwelling catheters include 1) it involves less work, needing to be changed only once a month versus four to eight times daily; 2) it is difficult for some women with mobility impairments disabilities to perform self-catheterization; and 3) urinary leakage between catheterization is often unresponsive to anticholinergics. It will take innovative research and solutions to help women with physical disabilities avoid long-term indwelling catheters.

Continent Catheterizable Abdominal Stoma

Finally, quality of life issues prompted us to offer a continent urinary diversion to women with physical disabilities with a end-stage neurogenic bladder and a destroyed urethra caused by chronically indwelling urethral catheters (details are provided in Chapter 27). Preoperative evaluation and urodynamic studies in a preliminary series of three women revealed a bladder capacity of less than 100 ml, bilateral vesicoureteral reflux, recurrent febrile urinary tract infections, an incompetent urethral sphincter, and incontinence around an indwelling catheter in all three. Although highly

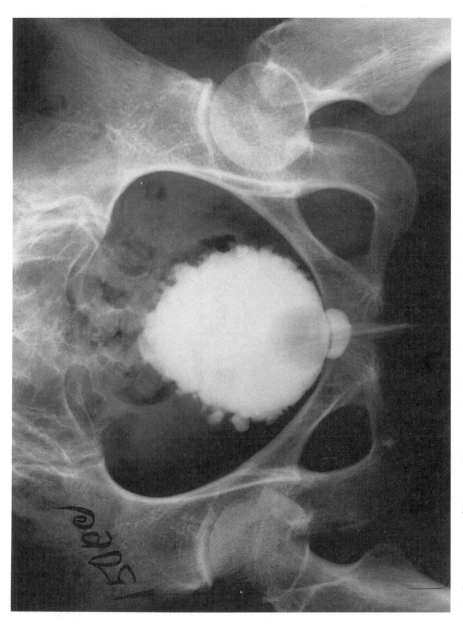

Figure 7. Voiding cystogram of 34-year-old woman with C5-quadriplegia with DESD. The bladder is small and trabeculated. During a reflex detrusor contraction the internal sphincter (bladder neck) was open, but no contrast is seen across the external striated sphincter.

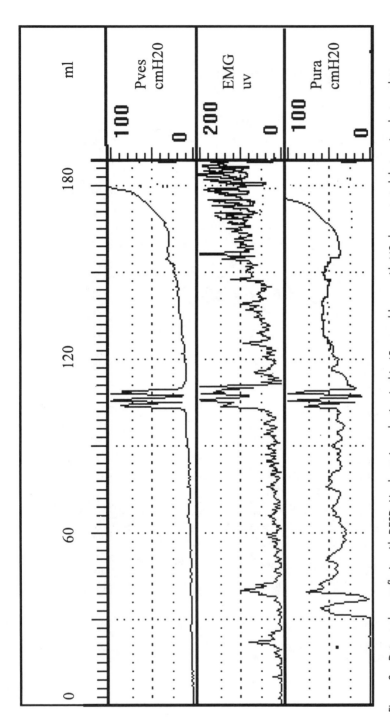

Figure 8. Detrusor hyperreflexia with DESD. Urodynamic evaluation in this 45-year-old man with MS demonstrated that an involuntary detrusor contraction occurred at 180 ml with voiding pressure above 100 cm H_2O and increased activity of sphincter EMG and maximum urethral pressure at the level of the external sphincter. Pves: bladder pressure; EMG: electromyelogram; Pura: urethral pressure at the level of the external sphincter. (From Chancellor, M.B., & Blaivas, J.G. [1993]. Multiple sclerosis. *Problems in Urology, 7,* 15–33; reprinted by permission.)

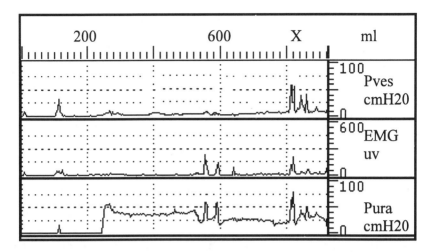

Figure 9. Detrusor areflexia in a 54-year-old woman with MS complaining of frequency and dribbling incontinence. Her residual urine volume was 450 ml, and her bladder filling pressure was less than 10 cm H$_2$O to 800 ml without voluntary or involuntary detrusor contractions. She did not leak urine with coughs between 500–600 ml (x). Pves: bladder pressure; EMG: electromyelogram; Pura: urethral pressure at the level of the external sphincter. (From Chancellor, M.B., & Blaivas, J.G. [1993]. Multiple sclerosis. *Problems in Urology, 7,* 15–33; reprinted by permission.)

motivated, these women were unable to perform urethral self-catheterization. Each was opposed to having an incontinent abdominal urinary stoma (Moreno et al., in press).

The urinary reservoir was created from 30 cm of detubularized right colon. The continent mechanism utilized an intussuscepted and imbricated ileocecal valve. The umbilicus was chosen as the urostomy site because of cosmetic appearance and easy catheterization for a woman who has minimal dexterity. Follow-up ranged from 18 to 30 months. Symptomatic autonomic dysreflexia and urinary tract infection decreased postoperatively in all women. Of the two women who were sexually active, the frequency of activity increased from 8 to 15 episodes/month in one and from 3 to 4 episodes/month in the other. They both reported improved sexual enjoyment. Body image was improved and urological management satisfaction increased in all three women.

In conclusion, continent urinary diversion in selected women is a reasonable alterative to indwelling catheterization and ileal diversion. The umbilical stoma provides an excellent cosmetic result that can be catheterized easily with minimal dexterity. Continent urinary diversion in women provided improved self-image and sexuality.

New Pharmacological Approach

Anticholinergic drugs presently available are only partially effective in the hyperactive neurogenic bladder. In addition, there are significant undesirable side effects that cause some individuals to stop the medication. New agents that can effectively treat the hyperactive bladder to prevent urinary incontinence between self-catheterization are greatly needed. Capsaicin, the pungent ingredient found in red peppers, is a neurotoxic compound that causes initial excitation, then desensitization, of unmyelinated sensory neurons. Capsaicin is capable of depleting sensory afferent of noxious neuropeptides, including substance P. The potential clinical implications of using this agent to pharmacologically defunctionalized bladder sensory afferent is exciting (Maggi, 1992). Such an action would be ideal for the treatment of detrusor hyperreflexia and sensory urgency.

There is also a change in the nerve fibers that serve the micturition reflex after neurological injury. de Groat et al. (1990) described the normal neural control switch in which, when the bladder fills up, the afferent pathway travels via myelinated afferent fibers into the spinal cord. After a spinal cord injury, the normal afferent is interrupted, and afferent signals can travel via unmyelinated C fibers (Figures 10 and 11). These unmyelinated C fibers' pathway is blocked by the drug capsaicin. Intravesical capsaicin has been shown to inhibit detrusor hyperreflexia in a group of patients with MS (Fowler, Jewkes, McDonald, Lynn, & de Groat, 1992). The patients who responded to the treatment enjoyed improvement for several months, and no significant complications occurred. Although potential problems exist with the mode of drug administration and undesirable sequelae of the initial excitatory effects, this is an interesting concept that

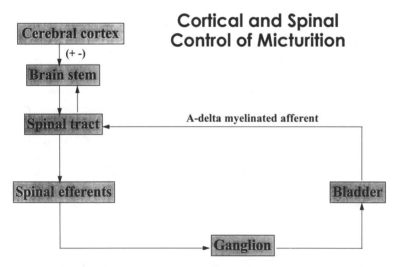

Figure 10. Diagram of the central reflex pathways that regulate micturition in the cat. In an animal with an intact neuraxis, micturition is initiated by a supraspinal reflex pathway passing through a center in the brain stem. The pathways are triggered by myelinated afferent connected to tension receptors in the bladder wall. (Adapted from de Groat et al., 1990; used with permission.)

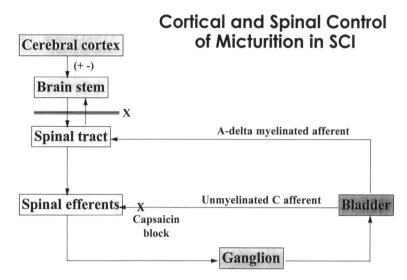

Figure 11. Diagram of the central reflex pathways that regulate micturition in spinal animals, connections between the brain stem and the sacral spinal cord are interrupted (X), and micturition is initially blocked. However, in chronic spinal cord injury, a spinal reflex mechanism emerges that is triggered by unmyelinated (C-fiber) vesical afferent. The C-fiber reflex pathways are usually weak or undetectable in animals with an intact nervous system. Capsaicin (20–30 mg/kg, subcutaneously administered) blocks the C-fiber reflex in chronic spinal cat, but does not block micturition reflexes in intact cats. (Adapted from de Groat et al., 1990; used with permission.)

holds promise of future avenues of drug treatment (Craft & Porreca, 1992; Maggi, 1991; Maggi et al., 1989; de Groat et al., 1990).

CONCLUSIONS

Advances in urodynamics and especially video-urodynamics (fluoroscopy) allow us to accurately evaluate voiding dysfunction and have led to a significant improvement in the understanding of the normal and abnormal function of the bladder and sphincter. Urodynamics has allowed us to prospectively identify individuals at risk for upper tract deterioration. Clinicians should be wary of predicting bladder dysfunction based solely on the neurological level of injury and empirical treatment.

REFERENCES

Abrams, P.H., Blaivas, J.G., Stanton, S.L., & Andersen, J.T. (1988). Standardisation of lower urinary tract function. *Neurourology & Urodynamics, 7,* 403.

Abrams, P.H., & Feneley, R.C.L. (1978). The significance of the symptoms associated with bladder outlet obstruction. *Urology International, 33,* 171.

Anderson, R.S., Shepherd, A.M., & Feneley, R.C.L. (1983). Microtransducer urethral profile methodology: Variations caused by transducer orientation. *Journal of Urology, 130,* 727.

Arnold, E.P., Fukui, J., Anthony, A., & Utley, W.L.F. (1984). Bladder function following spinal cord injury: A urodynamic analysis of the outcome. *British Journal of Urology, 56,* 172.

Asmussen, M., & Ulmsten, U. (1976). Simultaneous urethrocystometry and urethral pressure profile measurement with a new technique. *Acta Obstetrica Gynecologica Scandinavica, 54,* 385.

Barbalias, G.A., & Blaivas, J.G. (1983). Neurologic implications of the pathologically open bladder neck. *Journal of Urology, 129,* 780.

Bates, C.P., & Corney, L.E. (1971). Synchronous cine/pressure/flow cytography: A method of routine urodynamic investigation. *British Journal of Radiology, 44,* 44.

Blaivas, J.G. (1982). The neurophysiology of micturition: A clinical study of 550 patients. *Journal of Urology, 127,* 958–963.

Blaivas, J.G. (1983). Classification of stress urinary incontinence. *Neurourology & Urodynamics, 2,* 103.

Blaivas, J.G. (1988). Techniques of evaluation. In S.V. Yalla, E.J. McGuire, A. Elbadawi, & J.G. Blaivas (Eds.), *Neurourology and urodynamics: Principles and practice* (pp. 155–198). New York: Macmillan.

Blaivas, J.G., & Fisher, D.M. (1981). Combined radiographic and urodynamic monitoring: Advances in techniques. *Journal of Urology, 125,* 693.

Blaivas, J.G., & Barbalias, G.A. (1984). Detrusor-external sphincter dyssynergia in men with multiple sclerosis: An ominous urologic condition. *Journal of Urology, 131,* 94.

Blaivas, J.G., & Olsson, C.A. (1988). Stress incontinence: Classification and surgical approach. *Journal of Urology, 139,* 727.

Borges, P., & Hackler, R.H. (1982). The urologic status of the Vietnam War paraplegic: A 15 year prospective follow-up. *Journal of Urology, 127,* 710.

Brown, M., & Wickham, J.E.A. (1969). The urethral pressure profile. *British Journal of Urology, 41,* 211–217.

Cass, A.S., Ward, B.D., & Markland, C. (1970). Comparison of slow and rapid fill cystometry using liquid and air. *Journal of Urology, 104,* 104.

Chancellor, M.B., & Blaivas, J.G. (1991). Diagnostic evaluation of incontinence in patients with neurological disorders. *Comprehensive Therapy, 17,* 37–43.

Chancellor, M.B., & Blaivas, J.G. (1992). Unstable bladder and anatomic defects. In H.J. Bushsbaum & J.D. Schmidt (Eds.), *Gynecologic and obstetric urology* (3rd ed.) (pp. 371–400). Philadelphia: W.B. Saunders.

Chancellor, M.B., & Blaivas, J.G. (1993). Multiple sclerosis. *Problems in Urology, 7,* 15–33.

Chancellor, M.B., & Blaivas, J.G. (1994). Physiology of the lower urinary tract. In E.J. McGuire & E.D. Kursh (Eds.), *Female urology* (pp. 39–57). Philadelphia: J.B. Lippincott.

Chancellor, M.B., Kaplan, S.A., Axelord, D., & Blaivas, J.G. (1991). Bladder outlet obstruction versus impaired detrusor contractility: Role of uroflow. *Journal of Urology, 145,* 810–812.

Chancellor, M.B., & Rivas, D.A. (1993). The American Urological Association symptom index for women with voiding symptoms: Lack of index specificity for benign prostate hyperplasia. *Journal of Urology, 150,* 1706–1709.

Constantinou, C.E., Faysal, M.H., Rother, L., & Govan, D.E. (1981). The impact of bladder neck suspension on the mode of distribution of abdominal pressure along the female urethra. In N.R. Zinner & A.M. Sterling (Eds.), *Female urethra* (pp. 121–132). New York: Alan R. Liss.

Coolsaet, B.R. (1985). Bladder compliance and detrusor activity during the collection phase. *Neurourology & Urodynamics, 4*, 263–273.

Craft, R.M., & Porreca, F. (1992). Treatment parameters of desensitization to capsaicin. *Life Sciences, 51*, 1767–1775.

de Groat, W.C., Kawatani, M., Hisamitsu, T., Cheng, C.L,, Ma, C.P., Thor, K., Steers, W., & Roppolo, J.R. (1990). Mechanism underlying the recovery of urinary bladder function following spinal cord injury. *Journal of the Autonomic Nervous System, 30*(Suppl.), 571–577.

Edwards, L., & Malvern, J. (1974). The urethral pressure profile: Theoretical consideration and clinical applications. *British Journal of Urology, 46*, 325.

Fam, B., & Yalla, S.V. (1988). Vesicourethral dysfunction in spinal cord injury and its management. *Seminars in Neurology, 8*, 150–155.

Fowler, C.J., Jewkes, D., McDonald, W.I., Lynn, B., & de Groat, W.C. (1992). Intravesical capsaicin for neurogenic bladder dysfunction. *Lancet, 339*, 1239.

Gleason, D.M., Bottaccine, M.R., & Reilly, R.J. (1977). Comparison of cystometrograms and urethral profiles with gas and water media. *Urology, 9*, 155.

Griffiths, D., Van Mastrigt, R., & Bosch, R. (1989). Quantification of urethral resistance to bladder function during voiding with special reference to the effects of prostate size reduction on urethral obstruction due to benign prostatic hyperplasia. *Neurourology & Urodynamics, 8*, 17–27.

Harrison, N.W., & Constable, A.R. (1970). Urethral pressure measurement: A modified technique. *British Journal of Urology, 42*, 229.

Hinman, F., Jr. (1979). Urodynamic testing: Alternatives to electronics. *Journal of Urology, 121*, 643.

Jackson, A., & DeVivo, M. (1992). Long-term urological follow-up in females with spinal cord injuries. *Archives of Physical Medicine & Rehabilitation, 73*, 1029.

Jorgensen, L., Lose, G., & Andersen, J.T. (1988). Cystometry: H_2O or CO_2 as filling medium? A literature survey of the influence of the filling media on the qualitative and the quantitative cystometric parameters. *Neurology & Urodynamics, 7*, 343.

Kaplan, S.A., Chancellor, M.B., & Blaivas, J.G. (1991). Bladder and sphincter behavior in patients with spinal cord lesions. *Journal of Urology, 146*, 113–117.

Larsson, G., Abrams, P., & Victor, A. (1991). The frequency/volume chart in detrusor instability. *Neurourology & Urodynamics, 10*, 533–543.

Light, J.K., Faganel, J., & Beric, A. (1985). Detrusor areflexia in suprasacral spinal cord injuries. *Journal of Urology, 134*, 295.

Lloyd, K. (1986). New trends in urologic management of spinal cord injured patients. *Central Nervous System Trauma, 3*, 1.

Maggi, C.A. (1991). Capsaicin and primary afferent neurons: From basic science to human therapy? *Journal of the Antononic Neurovous System, 33*, 1.

Maggi, C.A. (1992). Therapeutic potential of capsaicin like molecules: Studies in animals and humans. *Life Science, 51*, 1777–1781.

Maggi, C.A., Barbank, G., Santicoli, P., Beneforte, P., Misuri, D., Meli, A., & Turini, D. (1989). Cystometric evidence that capsaicin sensitive nerves modulate the afferent branch of micturition reflex on humans. *Journal of Urology, 142*, 150.

Massey, J.A., Anderson, R.S., & Abrams, P. (1987). Mechanisms of continence during raised intra-abdominal pressure. *British Journal of Urology, 60*, 529–631.

McGuire, E.J., Woodside, J.R., Borden, T.A., & Weiss, R.M. (1981). The prognostic significance of urodynamic testing in myelodysplastic patients. *Journal of Urology, 125*, 205.

McGuire, E.J., & Savastano, J.A. (1986). Comparative urological outcome in women with spinal cord injury. *Journal of Urology, 135,* 730–731.

McGuire, E.M. (1980). Urodynamic findings in patients after failure of stress incontinence operations. In N.R. Zinner & A.M. Sterling (Eds.), *Female incontinence* (pp. 351–360). New York: Alan R. Liss.

McGuire, E.M., Lytton, B., Kohorn, E.I., & Pepe, V. (1980). Value of urodynamic testing in stress urinary incontinence. *Journal of Urology, 124,* 256.

McGuire, E.M., Bennett, C.J., Konnak, J.A., Sonda, L.P., & Savastano, J.A. (1987). Experience with pubovaginal slings for urinary incontinence at University of Michigan. *Journal of Urology, 138,* 525.

Merrill, D.C., Bradley, W.E., & Markland, C. (1972). Air cystometry II: A clinical evaluation of normal adults. *Journal of Urology, 108,* 85.

Miller, E.R. (1971). Combined monitoring for the study of continence and voiding. In F.J. Hinman, Jr. (Ed.), *Hydrodynamics of micturition* (pp. 5–17). Springfield, IL: Charles C. Thomas.

Moreno, J.G., Chancellor, M.C., Karasick, S., King, S., Abdill, C.A., & Rivas, D.A. (1994). Improved quality of life and sexuality with continent urinary diversion in quadriplegic women with umbilical stoma. *Archives of Physical Medicine & Rehabilitation, 75,* 758–762.

O'Donnell, P.D., & Marshall, M. (1988). Telemetric ambulatory urinary incontinence detection in the elderly. *Journal of Ambulatory Monitoring, 1,* 23.

Ouslander, J.G., Greengold, B., & Chen, W. (1987). Complications of chronic indwelling urethral catheters among male nursing home patients: A prospective study. *Journal of Urology, 138,* 1191.

Passerubu-Glazel, G., Cisterino, A., Artibani, W., & Pagano, F. (1992). Ambulatory urodynamics: Preliminary experience with vesicourethral holter in children. *Scandinavian Journal of Urology & Nephrology, 141*(Suppl.), 87–92.

Schafer, W. (1990). Principles and clinical application of advanced urodynamic analysis of voiding function. *Urology Clinics of North America, 17,* 553–566.

Snook, S.J., & Swash, M. (1984). Abnormalities of the innervation of the urethral striated sphincter musculature in incontinence. *British Journal of Urology, 56,* 401–405.

Sonda, L.P., Kogan, B.A., Koff, S.A., & Diokno, A.C. (1983). Neurologic disease masquerading as genitourinary abnormality: The role of urodynamics in diagnosis. *Journal of Urology, 129,* 1175–1178.

Sundin, T., & Dahlstrom, A. (1973). The sympathetic innervation of the urinary bladder denervation at the spinal root level: An experimental study in cats. *Scandinavian Journal of Urology & Nephrology, 7,* 131.

Sutherst, J., Brown, M., & Shower, M. (1981). Assessing the severity of urinary incontinence in women by wearing perineal pads. *Lancet, 1,* 1128–1130.

Tribe, G.R. (1963). Causes of death in the early and late stages of paraplegia. *Paraplegia, 1,* 19–47.

Van Geelen, J.M. (1983). The urethral pressure profile in continent women. *Thesis Schriks' Drukkerij,* Asten, 1–25.

van Waalwijk van Doorn, E.S.L., Remmere, A., & Janknegt, R.A. (1991). Extramural ambulatory urodynamic monitoring during natural filling and normal daily activities: Evaluation of 100 patients. *Journal of Urology, 146,* 124–131.

Webb, R.J., Griffiths, C.J., Ramsden, P.D., & Neal, D.E. (1990). Measurement of voiding pressures on ambulatory monitoring: Comparison with conventional cystometry. *British Journal of Urology, 65,* 152–154.

Wein, A.J., & Barrett, D.M. (1988). *Voiding function and dysfunction: A logical and practical approach* (pp. 143–178). Chicago: Year Book Medical Publisher.

chapter 25

Urinary Tract Infections in Females with Spinal Cord Injuries

Mary N. Young and Jan M.H. Brewer

According to the *Chart Book on Disability in the United States* (Kraus & Stoddard, 1989), there are approximately 13.5 million Americans who have physically severe functional limitations; of these, 8.9 million are women. Severe limitations in function are categorized under seeing, hearing, lifting, walking, and the degree to which affected individuals are bedridden. Multiple sclerosis (MS) and paralysis are the most limiting of the chronic conditions.

Many women with physical disabilities have neurogenic bladders or urinary incontinence that places them at increased risk for urinary tract infection (UTI). Stamey and Sexton (1975) estimated that 10%–20% of all women have UTI at some point in their lives. They concluded that, although serious morbidity and loss of renal function were rare, the cost in terms of patient discomfort, anxiety, and medical expense was substantial. Stamey and Sexton demonstrated that colonization of the vaginal and urethral mucosa preceded the occurrence of bacteria in the urine, and the main contributor to susceptibility was colonization of the vaginal vestibule with fecal *Enterobacteria*. They further stated that women resistant to UTI rarely experienced colonization of their vaginal vestibule and possessed a specific vaginal antibody against their own fecal *Escherichia coli*, whereas women susceptible to UTI had no such vaginal antibody. Fowler (1986) reported that *E. coli* are responsible for 75% of UTI in adult women. He agreed with Stamey and Sexton (1975) that the presence of bacteria in the urine of infected women was preceded by colonization of the vaginal and urethral mucosa with the infecting organism. The women represented in both

This work is supported in part by the National Institutes of Health, Grant HD30536.

these studies were women without disabilities who had normal urinary function. The data become more significant for people with disabilities when there is neurogenic bladder dysfunction associated with elevated filling and voiding pressures and incontinence, which greatly increases the risk for UTI.

Colonization of the distal urethra in male patients with spinal cord injury (SCI) is well documented. Montgomerie and Morrow (1980) and Gilmore, Schick, Young, and Montgomerie (1992) studied the colonization of *Pseudomonas* and *Klebsiella* in the perineum and urethra in males with SCI. These studies, almost exclusively on male patients, showed considerably more urethral colonization in men wearing external catheters; however, this group did not show a higher incidence of UTI. O'Neil, Jenkins, and Wells (1982) showed that colonization of the female urethra occurs in the first 1.5 cm of the urethra, and they developed a catheter kit with a urethral introducer tip to bypass the colonized portion of the urethra during catheterization. These studies were also done on women without disabilities.

Few studies have looked specifically at both urethral colonization and UTI in women with disabilities. The few studies that have been done have focused primarily on women with SCI. Compounding matters, women represent a minority of persons with SCI, and few studies address their unique concerns. The National Institute on Disability and Rehabilitation Research (NIDRR) Consensus Statement (1992) on UTI concluded that data collected from male studies should not be extrapolated to female management principles.

URINARY TRACT INFECTIONS AND INTERMITTENT CATHETERIZATION

The NIDRR Consensus Statement (1992) listed the risk factors for UTI in the SCI population as overdistended bladder, vesicoureteral reflux, high-pressure voiding, large postvoid residuals, presence of stones in the urinary tract, and outlet obstruction. Although the risk for infection is reduced with intermittent catheterization, the risk for UTI still exists. For both female and male hospitalized patients, this results in increased morbidity, loss of therapy time, increased length of hospital stay, and increased costs for rehabilitation.

A review of the literature also establishes numerous risk factors for increased UTIs in persons with SCI. McGuire and Savastano (1983) reported that, although one third of the individuals in their study maintained on long-term intermittent catheterization remained free of UTI, the remaining two thirds had chronic or recurring bacteriuria. Lloyd, Kuhlemeier, Fine, and Stover (1986) reported that 80% of patients voiding reflexively had chronic or recurrent bacteriuria.

Bennett, Young, and Darrington (1995) demonstrated that not only is the incidence of UTI higher in females on intermittent catheterization, but the pathogens differ as well. The predominant organisms in males are *Pseudomonas* and *Klebsiella*, whereas in women they are *E. coli* and *Enterococcus*. The infection rate was reduced 30% over a 3-year period using a catheter system developed by the Medical Market Group (MMGO) of Atlanta, Georgia. In this system, the catheter is enclosed in a plastic sleeve and contains a urethral introducer tip that bypasses the first 1.5 cm colonized portion of the urethra rather than the conventional closed method system without the introducer tip. Even though the MMGO catheter system reduced the overall infection by 30%, women continued to maintain a higher infection rate than their male counterparts (9 females with 17 infections compared with 45 males with 58 infections over the same time period and frequency of intermittent catheterization). The incidence of *E. coli* infection in women was reduced from 84% to 53% using the MMGO system, although in the male population the incidence was only 18% ($p < .02$). Pearman, Bailey, and Riley (1991) also reported a higher occurrence of UTI in females with SCI on intermittent catheterization. Other studies have also shown a reduction in UTI in both men and women with SCI in the hospital setting using the MMGO catheter system. For instance, 80% of the control group using a sterile system with a straight catheter had more than one infection per admission in comparison to the group using the MMGO kit that had 44.4% infection per admission (Charbonneau-Smith, 1993). Pang-Wright and Dasalla (1990) also demonstrated a lower incidence of UTI using the MMGO but could not establish a significant difference because of a small sample size.

ROLE OF INCONTINENCE AND URINARY TRACT INFECTIONS

The higher incidence of UTIs in women may be related to the proximity of bowel/stool contamination and may be linked to the patient's bowel management program; there is a large amount of fecal contamination of the perineum in women who are incontinent. In our ongoing research, we hypothesized that women who have their bowel program on the commode should have less contamination of the perineum and thereby reduce their infection rate on intermittent catheterization. Unpublished baseline data on urethral colonization of persons who were on intermittent catheterization and were bowel incontinent showed that 4 of 7 women had *E. coli* colonization in their urethra, whereas 5 of the 7 were colonized with *Enterococcus*. In 15 female staff volunteers who were continent, 7 of 15 were colonized with *Enterococcus*, whereas 4 of the 15 were colonized with *E. coli*. Although half of the female staff had urethral colonization, none reported symptoms of UTI; all of the women with SCI had UTIs. We are currently attemping to determine whether the UTI rate in women with SCI is directly related to bowel incontinence and urethral colonization by comparing those who perform their bowel program in bed with those who perform this program on the commode.

No studies were found in the literature that addressed the question of fecal contamination and the risk of UTI in women with disabilities. A study of 99 male patients in a Veterans Administration (VA) nursing home care unit reported that the incidence of UTI in men with bowel incontinence was 70% compared with 25% in bowel-continent men (Lara, Troop, & Beadleson-Baird, 1990).

UTIs can also adversely influence urinary continence in women. Many women report they become wet between catheterizations when they develop a UTI; they are otherwise dry. Other women with disabilities who do not have neurogenic bladders and are continent may develop urge incontinence with a UTI and become functionally incontinent because access to bathroom facilities is limited. Because an acceptable external collection device does not exist for women, many women with neurogenic, stress, or functional incontinence are maintained on indwelling catheters with the resultant complications.

PROFESSIONAL BELIEF SYSTEMS AND URINARY TRACT INFECTIONS

The bladder management method prescribed for many women with SCI is the use of long-term indwelling catheters. This method has been associated with numerous complications. These include vesicoureteral reflux, urethral incompetence and leakage, hydronephrosis, autonomic dysreflexia, bladder calculi, renal calculi, labial erosion, and carcinoma of the bladder (Esrig, McEvoy, & Bennett, 1992; Trop & Bennett, 1992). Two nonsurgical alternatives to an indwelling catheter are reflex voiding while wearing incontinence padding or intermittent catheterization (IC) with or without anticholinergic therapy. Despite the acknowledged complications associated with the use of indwelling catheters, this method remains the primary or only bladder management option for many women. The lack of availability of a suitable external incontinence device and the inability of tetraplegic women to perform intermittent catheterization are the usual reasons given for this choice. A study by Bennett, Young, Adkins, and Diaz (1995) compared bladder management outcomes between three groups of women on different bladder management programs. The study clearly showed that IC with anticholinergic therapy was the best method of management.

Many women who are tetraplegic with limited hand function have reduced chances of being successful at urethral intermittent catheterization. Other factors may influence the patient's success with IC, such as patient motivation, lifestyle, standard of living, and the availability of financial resources for attendant care. Our own study demonstrated that some individuals with good hand function have chosen to remain on indwelling catheters, while others with limited hand function have chosen IC using adaptive devices.

Other studies also reflect the difficulties just described. Joiner and Lindan (1982) reported that 7 of 24 women returned to indwelling catheters because of problems encountered with dysreflexia, reduced ability to catheterize due to obesity, architectural barriers, and the lack of suitable clothing that enabled easy access for IC. Barnes, Shaw, Timoney, and Tsokos (1993) reported that 50% of the women discharged home on IC returned to indwelling catheters, reporting as the major reason for failure persistent incontinence despite anticholinergic therapy. However, there is concern regarding returning women to indwelling catheters solely as a consequence of leakage between ICs. Indeed, 90% of women on indwelling catheters have leakage around the catheter and have frequent urethral erosion (Bennett et al., 1995; McGuire & Savastano, 1986).

Although Jackson and DeVivo (1992) did not show significant differences in complication outcomes between women on indwelling catheters and men voiding by reflex on external catheterization, Bennett et al. (1994) showed a higher complication rate for women on catheters than women voiding reflexly and wearing padding. The issue of voiding with a persistently elevated detrusor pressure exists; however, wetness and the abhorrence of wearing padding remain the major reasons women returned to indwelling catheters. Secondary problems such as *Candida* skin rashes and pressure ulcers are common. Therapy should be modified to maintain dryness in women between catheterizations by using concurrent drug therapy with tricyclic antidepressants and anticholinergic agents. Alternatively, bladder augmentation should be considered to reduce intravesical pressures in an effort to maintain a catheter-free state.

Acceptable surgical alternatives to indwelling catheters and padding exist for women with limited hand function, but more research is needed on women with disabilities. Educational materials need to be developed and made available to women with disabilities to help them make informed decisions about their bladder management program. In addition, more attention needs to be paid to collaborative practices utilizing occupational therapists for assistive devices and innovative clothing options to help women obtain and maintain independence in catheterization.

Another area in which consensus has not been established is the definition and treatment of UTIs. An uncomplicated UTI is usually described as an afebrile infection in a patient with a structurally and functionally normal urinary tract. The organisms are usually susceptible to and eradicated by a short course of oral antibiotics. A complicated UTI would be described as an infection in a patient with pyelonephritis and/or a urinary tract with a structural or functional abnormality that would reduce the efficacy of antimicrobial therapy. These infections are often resistant to many antibiotics. For many women with neurogenic bladder dysfunction, UTI would be categorized as complicated.

Lapides (1974) believed that host resistance was the most important factor in preventing lower UTIs and that the presence of microorganisms in the bladder played a secondary role. He argued that a change in bladder mucosa must take place for the infecting organisms to produce a clinical UTI. He advocated clean-technique IC, provided the bladder was maintained at low pressure (below 40 cm H_2O) and the patient catheterized frequently enough to prevent overdistention. The consensus report on UTI in SCI (NIDRR, 1992) listed symptomatic UTI as leucocytes in the urine, discomfort or pain over the kidneys, onset of urinary incontinence, fever, increased spasticity, autonomic hyperreflexia, cloudy urine with increased odor, malaise, lethargy, or sense of unease. Expanding on these findings, Stover, Lloyd, Waites, and Jackson (1989) stated that there was no consensus on the significance UTI played in the overall management in patients with neurogenic bladder dysfunction. Because there are wide differences between practitioners over what is considered a clinical or symptomatic UTI and when or if they should be treated, more clinical research needs to be conducted in the areas of prevention and treatment.

CONCLUSIONS

Most studies on UTI on women with disabilities are done on women with SCI, so there is a need for research to focus on other disabilities to assess their risk factors for UTI. Extrapolated data from SCI patients should not be applied to women with other disabilities, although some correlations for risk factors can be made. Further studies should include a more broad-based population with disabilities. More research and data need to be collected from multiple centers and the outcomes presented from a broad range across rehabilitation to remove institutional belief systems and bias. Ultimately, management intervention can be directed from outcome research to give women more guidance to make informed decisions about their bladder management options.

REFERENCES

Barnes, D.J., Shaw, P.J.R., Timoney, A.J., & Tsokos, N. (1993). Management of the neuropathic bladder by suprapubic catheterization. *British Journal of Urology*, 72, 169–172.

Bennett, C.J., Young, M.N., Adkins, R., & Diaz, F. (1995). Comparison of bladder management complication outcomes in female spinal cord injured patients. *Journal of Urology*, 153, 1458–1460.

Bennett, C.J., Young, M.N., & Darrington, H. (1995). Difference in UTI in male and female spinal cord injured patients on IC. *Paraplegia, 33*, 69–72.

Charbonneau-Smith, R. (1993). No-touch catheterization and infection rates in a select spinal cord injured population. *Rehabilitation Nursing, 18*(5), 296–299.

Esrig, D., McEvoy, K., & Bennett, C.J. (1992). Bladder cancers in the spinal-cord injury patients with long-term catheterization: A casual relationship. *Seminars in Urology, 10*, 102–108.

Fowler, J.E. (1986). Urinary tract infections in women. *Urology Clinics of North America, 13*(4), 673–683.

Gilmore, D.S., Schick, D.G., Young, M.N., & Montgomerie, J.Z. (1992). Effect of external urinary collection system on colonization and urinary tract infections with *Pseudomonas* and *Klebsiella* in men with spinal cord injury. *Journal of American Paraplegia Society, 15*(3), 206–208.

Jackson, A.B., & DeVivo, M. (1992). Urological long-term followup in women with spinal cord injuries. *Archives of Physical Medicine & Rehabilitation, 76*, 1029–1032.

Joiner, E., & Lindan, R. (1982). Experience with self intermittent catheterization for women with neurogenic dysfunction of the bladder. *Paraplegia, 20*, 147–153.

Kraus, L.E., & Stoddard, S. (1989). *Chartbook on Disabilities in the United States.* Washington, DC: U.S. National Institute on Disability and Rehabilitation Research.

Lapides, J. (1974). Neurogenic bladder, principles of treatment. *Urology Clinics of North America, 1*, 81–97.

Lara, L., Troop, P.R, & Beadleson-Baird, M. (1990). The risk of urinary tract infection in bowel incontinent men. *Journal of Gerontology Nursing, 16*(5), 24–26.

Lloyd, L.K., Kuhlemeier, K.V., Fine, P.R., & Stover, S.L. (1986). Initial bladder management in spinal cord injury: Does it make a difference? *Journal of Urology, 135*, 523–527.

McGuire, E.J., & Savastano, J. (1983). Long-term followup of spinal cord injury patients managed by intermittent catheterization. *Journal of Urology, 129*, 775–776.

McGuire, E.J., & Savastano, J. (1986). Comparative urological outcomes in women with spinal cord injury. *Journal of Urology, 135*, 730–731.

Montgomerie, J.Z., & Morrow, J.W. (1980). Long-term pseudomonas colonization. *American Journal of Epidemiology, 112*(4), 508–517.

National Institute on Disability and Rehabilitation Research (NIDRR) Consensus Statement. (1992). The prevention and management of urinary tract infections among people with spinal cord injuries. *Journal of American Paraplegia Society, 15*(3), 194–207.

O'Neil, A.G.B., Jenkins, D.T., & Wells, J.I. (1982). A new catheter for the female patient. *Australia New Zealand Journal of Obstetrics Gynaecology, 22*, 151–152.

Pang-Wright, B., & Dasalla, E. (1990, September). A descriptive study utilizing two different intermittent catheterization techniques in SCI clients in an acute rehab facility [abstract]. Educational Conference, American Association of Spinal Cord Injury Nurses, Las Vegas, NV.

Pearman, J.W., Bailey, M., & Riley, L.P. (1991). Bladder installations of Trisdine compared with catheter introducer for reduction of bacteriuria during intermittent catheterization of patients with acute spinal cord trauma. *British Journal of Urology, 67*, 483–490.

Stamey, T.A., & Sexton, C.C. (1975). The role of vaginal colonization with *Enterobacteriaceae* in recurrent urinary infections. *Journal of Urology, 113*, 214–217.

Stover, S.L., Lloyd, L.K., Waites, K.B., & Jackson, A.B. (1989). Urinary tract infection in spinal cord injury. *Archives of Physical Medicine & Rehabilitation*, *70*, 47–54.

Trop, C.S., & Bennett, C.J. (1992). Complications of long-term indwelling Foley catheters in female patients with neurogenic bladders. *Seminars in Urology, 10*, 115–120.

chapter 26

Assessment of Complications of Neurogenic Bladder Dysfunction

L. Keith Lloyd

Although bladder dysfunction is extremely common in females, secondary upper tract abnormalities are fairly uncommon. The issues related to neurogenic bladder dysfunction in women require further study. At our center at the University of Alabama, we have been following a group of women with spinal cord injury (SCI) with secondary bladder and bowel dysfunction. These women generally have the most severe alterations of bladder function and are at the greatest risk of developing upper urinary tract disorders as a result of that bladder dysfunction.

Approximately 20% of the individuals with SCI in this country are female. Women with SCI are a clear-cut minority, suggesting that the small number of female patients seen at many centers has been partly responsible for the lack of research in this area (Stover & Fine, 1986).

Data from the National Spinal Cord Injury Statistical Center allow us to form a demographic profile of women with SCI. The mean age at injury is 29 years and is essentially the same for men and women. Given this young age at onset of disability, this condition requires treatment over a relatively long period of time. If we assume normal life expectancy for females to be approximately 77 years, then a woman with this disability will live with impaired bladder function for a period of 40–50 years. During this time, long-term follow-up will be required, including management of complications that may arise as a result of the bladder dysfunction.

Of all women with SCI, approximately half have complete SCI and half have incomplete injuries. Furthermore, approximately half have sustained injuries that result in quadriplegia and half have disabilities that result in paraplegia (Stover & Fine, 1986). The level and completeness of injury will determine, in part, the person's overall rehabilitation potential and ability to manage different types of bladder management programs.

Table 1. Bladder management options in females

Voiding
  Strain-assisted
  Pharmacological assisted
  Normal
Intermittent catheterization
Indwelling catheter
Suprapubic catheter
Urinary diversion
  Conduit
  Continent diversion

Bladder dysfunction may cause either urinary incontinence, urinary retention, or a combination of the two. The options for managing urinary bladder dysfunction in women are listed in Table 1. There is no universal agreement on the best approach to the management of persons with bladder dysfunction. In general, we prefer that both men and women be free of indwelling catheters, but because of treatment limitations in the past a substantially greater number of women have been treated with long-term indwelling catheters than have males. This has been, in part, related to the impression that women tolerate indwelling catheters much better than do men (Jackson & DeVivo, 1992).

Table 2 presents data from The National Spinal Cord Injury Statistical Center. Among the findings are that 3 years postinjury approximately one third of the respondents remain on indwelling catheters, approximately one third remain on intermittent catheterization, a small number have suprapubic tubes, and about 20% of the patients void either normally, with pharmacological assistance or with Credé maneuvers. Suprapubic catheters generally have been placed only as a result of complications of urethral catheters; thus, it is unusual to require suprapubic catheter placement early after injury (Feneley, 1983).

There are two major goals of bladder management. The first is to have a bladder management program that is socially and functionally acceptable

Table 2. Bladder management in females with SCI 3 years postinjury

Indwelling catheter	34%
Intermittent catheterization	30%
Suprapubic catheter	4%
Voiding	19%

Data from National Spinal Cord Injury Statistical Center (Stover & Fine, 1986).

to the individual. The second is to have a bladder management program that will have minimal impact on the general health of the individual and place her at low risk of developing upper urinary tract dysfunction. If these two goals are achieved, women with urinary dysfunction should remain healthy and happy for a long period of time.

Once neurogenic bladder dysfunction develops and some form of management program is instituted, the woman is at risk for development of bladder or upper urinary tract complications. Urethral erosion, fibrosis of the bladder wall, vesicoureteral reflux, urothelial tumors, and calculi are all complications that may occur over time in women who are treated with long-term indwelling urethral catheters (Lindan, Leffler, & Bodner, 1987; McGuire & Savastano, 1986; Trop & Bennett, 1992). Some of these complications also occur with intermittent catheterization or in individuals who are voiding but have problems with chronic urinary tract infection (UTI) (Joiner & Lindan, 1982; Timoney & Shaw, 1990).

Factors that relate to upper urinary tract dysfunction include sustained elevated pressures within the bladder; development of vesicoureteral reflux, which is perhaps more common in women because of the underlying bladder anatomy; and urinary infection, which is again a more common problem among women than among men. All of these factors may act independently or in combination to have an impact on the upper urinary tract over long years of follow-up (Lloyd, 1986).

Upper urinary tract problems include ureteral or pelvic dilation, resulting in hydronephrosis, renal calculi, pyelonephritis, and renal scarring (Kuhlemeier, Huang, Lloyd, Fine, & Stover, 1985). Although vesicoureteral reflux is not, strictly speaking, a complication of the upper urinary tract, it is listed here because of its major impact in terms of episodes of pyelonephritis and renal scarring (Table 3).

All of these conditions have one principal feature in common—an early manifestation of some impairment of renal tubular function (Price, Kottke, & Olson, 1975). Therefore, if a test exists that measures renal tubular function, health providers should be able to detect changes in the

Table 3. Upper urinary tract dysfunction in neurogenic bladder

Pyelonephritis
Renal calculi
Vesicoureteral reflux
Renal scarring
Hydronephrosis
Ureteral dilatation

upper urinary tract at an early time and consider instituting appropriate changes in the type of bladder management to protect the upper urinary tract. This principle has been the basis of our long-term follow-up program (Lloyd, Dubovsky, Bueschen, & Witten, 1981).

Renal function can be measured crudely by serum creatinine, slightly more accurately by creatinine clearances, or most accurately by carefully performed inulin (glomerular filtration) clearances or para-amino hippurate (tubular secretion) clearances (Kuhlemeier, Huang, Devivo, & Lloyd, 1986; Price, Kottke, & Olson, 1975). Normal glomerular filtration rates range from 100–200 cc/min and tubular secretion, as measured by para-amino hippurate, is roughly 500–600 cc/min. The combination of these two measures is what is termed *effective renal plasma flow* (ERPF) or *total renal function*. As a result of many years of basic science and clinical research by numerous investigators, the methodology for measuring renal function by means of radioisotopes has been developed as a sound clinical methodology for evaluating renal function associated with various conditions (Bueschen & Witten, 1979; Halko, Burke, Sorkin, & Enenstein, 1973; Schlegel & Bakule, 1970; Tauxe, Maher, & Taylor, 1971).

It is important to remember that profound alterations of the upper urinary tract may occur in persons with neurogenic bladder dysfunction in the absence of any symptoms (Lloyd et al., 1981; Lloyd, Kuhlemeier, Fine, McEachran, & Stover, 1987). Furthermore, these changes may occur regardless of the method of bladder management being used. Although these upper urinary tract abnormalities may be more likely to occur with some methods than others, it is imperative that long-term follow-up of all individuals include a systematic method of follow-up for the detection and treatment of urinary tract dysfunction. Neurogenic bladder dysfunction, whether it be due to SCI or other neurological diseases, is generally a lifelong problem and is not a static system. Major alterations and instability are present during the first year following injury, but even 10–15 years postinjury, changes in bladder function occur for which we do not have reliable explanations.

One advantage of the model system of care is that it includes a callback system so that individuals who have had an SCI are specifically called and asked to come in for periodic annual evaluations (Lloyd et al., 1987). Individuals who drift out of this system may not present for a follow-up examination and testing until symptomatology occurs, which could be relatively late in the course of the disease. Those who do become symptomatic generally seek treatment, and it is hoped that appropriate urological investigation would be undertaken at that time. Usually no change in bladder management is necessary, but, depending upon the problem, alterations in bladder management may be appropriate and may result in prevention of further upper tract problems.

A number of methods are available for longitudinal evaluation of the upper urinary tract. The excretory urogram (EXU) or intravenous pyelography (IVP) has been utilized for roughly 75–80 years and is a test with which all clinicians are familiar. It provides good anatomical delineation of the upper urinary tract but provides extremely poor functional information (Hoffman & Greyhack, 1960). The comprehensive renal scintillation procedure (CRSP), discussed later in more detail, is a very sensitive measurement of upper urinary tract ERPF or total function and an excellent method of long-term follow-up of persons with neurogenic bladder dysfunction (Kuhlemeier et al., 1985; Lloyd et al., 1981). Renal ultrasound examination (RUSE) has been utilized in recent years and, again, provides good anatomical display of the upper urinary tract, relatively poor visualization of the ureters, and little information regarding function (Lloyd et al., 1987). Other tests such as magnetic resonance imaging (MRI) or computed tomography (CT) are appropriate in special situations but do not really have a role in routine follow-up of the upper urinary tract (Table 4).

In our ongoing study evaluating the utility of the IVP, the RUSE, and the CRSP, we have been able to compare results but lack follow-up data. We have had significant experience in the past comparing the results of the CRSP and the IVP, and it seems clear that the CRSP is a far more sensitive test for detecting upper urinary tract dysfunction (Lloyd et al., 1981).

The CRSP is an excellent measure of renal function but does not really give worthwhile information regarding anatomy (Schlegel & Bakule, 1970). When the study was initially introduced, physicians, who were used to reviewing IVPs, tried to view the CRSP renal scans in much the same way as they viewed the IVPs. The numerical or functional information provided by the renal function curves, however, is the most important information obtained rather than scintiphotos, which give only a crude display of anatomy. Although the IVP gives superior anatomical evaluation, it is a very poor indicator of renal function and, in our experience, has shown that even very poorly functioning kidneys may look reasonably normal on IVP. Renal ultrasound also displays good anatomical information but poor functional assessment. Several studies have shown the su-

Table 4. Radiologic evaluation of the upper urinary tract

Excretory urography
Renal pyelography
Renal ultrasound
Comprehensive renal scintillation procedure
Computed tomography
Magnetic resonance imaging

periority of RUSE for detecting renal masses, but this is generally not an important issue in follow-up of persons with bladder dysfunction.

Early radiographic changes that may be seen in an asymptomatic individual include stones within the renal collecting system, dilatation of the renal collecting system, and dilation of the ureter.

COMPREHENSIVE RENAL SCINTILLATION PROCEDURES

The CRSP is performed by injecting a radioisotope intravenously and then measuring excretion of that isotope using a wide field view γ-scintillation crystal (Bueschen & Witten, 1979). Following injection of the isotope, counts are obtained over each renal area at 1-minute intervals for 27 minutes. Scintiphotos are taken utilizing 3-minutes of accumulated counts at intervals throughout the study. Time activity curves are generated showing transit of the isotope through the kidneys. Usually most of the isotope is excreted within 27 minutes after injection. A serum sample is obtained at 44 minutes after injection and is utilized to calculate the effective renal plasma flow (Tauxe et al., 1971). Previously, an isotope labeled with ^{131}I-orthoiodohippurate was utilized for the testing procedure. More recently, a new agent labeled with technetium, mercaptoacetylglycerine (Tc Mag 3), has been utilized. Technetium is a high-energy isotope that provides much higher counts and probably increases the accuracy of the study.

As emphasized previously, the ability to generate renal excretion curves is the important feature of this methodology. Following injection of the isotope, counts increase rapidly over the renal areas, permitting the relative blood flow in the two kidneys to be measured during the first 2 minutes following injection. This allows determination of the percent function present in each kidney.

Differential renal function, as described earlier, generally lies between 45% and 55%, although some of our studies of patients with SCI suggest that it may go as low as 42% and still be within a satisfactory range. Peak isotope accumulation should be within 6 minutes following injection; however, if patients are dehydrated, peak times may go up to 12–14 minutes. If the times are symmetrical, this may not be a significant abnormality. Marked delay of transit of isotope through the kidney may be an indicator of obstructive changes. The parameters of a normal CRSP in patients with SCI are shown in Table 5 (Kuhlemeier, McEachran, Lloyd, & Stover, 1984).

COMPARISON OF CRSP AND IVP

A number of years ago, we believed it was important to perform a study where CRSP results were compared to the standard upper tract evaluation

Table 5. Normal values—comprehensive renal scintillation
procedures

Effective renal plasma flow (ERPF)—greater than 400 ml/min
30–35 min return—greater than 66%
Percent relative blood flow each kidney—42%–58%
Peak counts—less than 12 min

Adapted from Kuhlemeier (1984).

utilized at that time, namely the IVP (Lloyd et al., 1981). We performed both studies on a large number of persons with SCI over several years and compared the ability of the two methods to detect upper tract abnormalities. IVPs were rated so that they could be handled statistically and the following grading system utilized: Grade 0 for normal, Grade 1 for mild dilatation of the ureters or collecting system, Grade 2 for moderate dilatation of the ureters or collecting system, and Grade 3 for severe dilatation of the ureters or collecting system. Grade 4 was assigned for an absent of nonfunctioning kidney. The normal parameters for the comprehensive renal scintillation procedure are shown in Table 5. This information was accumulated from a study of renal donors and modified slightly by subsequently evaluating a large number of patients with SCI (Kuhlemeier et al., 1986).

In comparing all of the individuals with SCI, we found a high number of abnormalities both on the IVP and the CRSP. Most of these were fairly mild Grade 1 abnormalities, but a small number of individuals had Grade 2 or Grade 3 abnormalities. A major feature of the study was to show that no significant abnormalities were missed utilizing a CRSP. Furthermore, during subsequent studies we have shown that Grade 1 changes on the IVP are probably not clinically significant. These are as likely to remain stable or revert to normal by 1-year follow-up as they are likely to progress. All of the individuals who had Grade 2 or 3 abnormalities on IVP with a normal CRSP were patients who had been previously treated and who were now stable and remained stable in follow-up. These were usually individuals who had significant medical problems, had undergone treatment for bladder dysfunction, and, at the time of evaluation, were considered stable with satisfactorily functioning urinary tracts. It was felt that renal function had been improved but that the anatomical picture had not yet reverted to normal. As a result of that study and a number of subsequent ones that we performed, we do not believe that any important urographic abnormalities are missed by the CRSP. In fact, our studies have shown that the CRSP is a much more sensitive test of upper urinary tract dysfunction. Our subsequent modification of the parameters of a normal CRSP for the person with SCI has helped decrease the sensitivity slightly while maintaining a satisfactory level of specificity (Kuhlemeier, McEachran, Lloyd, & Stover, 1984; Kuhlemeier, Huang, et al., 1985; Kuhlemeier et al., 1986).

We have seen declining renal function as a result of vesicoureteral reflux without upper tract radiographic changes. In our opinion this has eliminated the need for routine cystograms and these are usually now only obtained in conjunction with video-urodynamic, fluoroscopy studies.

Other significant advantages that are particularly important for women with SCI include the relatively noninvasive nature of the test, lack of allergic reactions; lack of interference from bowel gas or fat, and, hence, no requirement for patient preparation—a significant problem for persons with neurogenic bladder and bowel. These factors make the test much more readily acceptable by persons with SCI, thus increasing the likelihood for follow-up examination. These factors are also important when we plan to recommend annual examinations for the first 5 years after injury and then biannually or triannually. Given the usual young age at injury, this means that a fairly large number of studies would need to be done over the person's lifetime. The aforementioned considerations plus the decreased radiation exposure combine to make this an attractive test for evaluating the upper urinary tract.

Our present routine for follow-up of persons with neurogenic bladder dysfunction is to perform a CRSP and flat plate of the abdomen yearly for 5 years. Video-urodynamic studies are performed mainly during the first year after injury with a follow-up study done at 1 year post-injury. If the individual is stable at that time, then follow-up urodynamic studies are not performed unless triggered by abnormalities on the CRSP or clinical problems. Those who remain stable without clinical problems at 5 years after follow-up then proceed to biannual or triannual examination. If the CRSP is abnormal at follow-up, patients are returned for more careful investigation including a video-urodynamic study, IVP, and possible endoscopy (Lloyd et al., 1987).

During long-term follow-up it is important to remember that ERPF declines normally with age (Kuhlemeier et al., 1986). This correlates to some degree with body mass and physical activity and tends to peak in females in the mid- to late teens and males in approximately the mid-20s. Following these peaks there is a gradual decline over time, but there significant differences remain between ERPF in males and females. This decline in ERPF should be taken into account in evaluations. At the same time, it is also important to recognize that each person serves as his or her own baseline. Changes in the ERPF from year to year can be viewed, therefore, in the context of aging, and individuals return for more intensive evaluation only when greater than normal changes occur. Table 6 shows the normal ERPF values for males and females over time.

PREDICTING UPPER TRACT DYSFUNCTION

Working with individuals who had at least 2 years of follow-up data with IVP and a CRSP, we tried to determine which factors were predictive of

Table 6. Effective renal plasma flow (ERPF) in females by age

Age	Single kidney (ml/min) Spinal cord injured (SCI)	Non-SCI
16–20	310	308
21–30	240	306
31–40	245	304
41–50	200	275
51–60	235	228

the development of significant upper tract abnormalities defined as Grade 2–3 changes on IVP (Lloyd et al., 1987). We evaluated a group of individuals on whom we had collected at least 2 years of data with a maximum of 24 months between the evaluations. Fifteen to twenty variables were selected, and multiple regression analysis was performed. Factors that were found to be significantly predictive of pyelocaliectasis included presence of a kidney stone in any year of follow-up. Presence of a bladder diverticulum was predictive of development of upper tract changes within the next year. This is a relatively advanced bladder abnormality and not a mild change, such as trabeculation. Vesicoureteral reflux in year 1 was predictive of significant abnormality in year 2, and a change in effective renal plasma flow also predicted development of significant pyelographic abnormalities during follow-up. These variables were considered significant predictors for development of upper tract changes and factors that may indicate the need for a change in bladder management. This information will allow us to interact with individuals early, making appropriate changes in bladder management, with the goal of stabilizing or improving renal function.

LONG-TERM FOLLOW-UP

A study was performed at our center evaluating long-term follow-up in females with SCI (Jackson & Devivo, 1992). As noted previously, about 20% of the patients at our center are women, and data were obtained over a 12-year period at the Spain Rehabilitation Center at the University of Alabama. The women were grouped according to the following criteria: discharge data from rehabilitation, evaluations 2–5 years postinjury, 6–9 years postinjury, and greater than 10 years postinjury. Not all of these women had serial evaluations, but each individual had at least some evaluations throughout these time frames. This gave us a cross-sectional evaluation of a population of women with SCI and how they fared up to 16 years following injury.

Indwelling urethral catheters were used for bladder management in approximately 70% of the women. Because of changes in management philosophy, currently only about 30% use indwelling catheters. None of the women in the early years following injury had suprapubic catheters or ileal conduits performed. However, among women more than 10 years postinjury, a few had required suprapubic catheter placement generally because of damage to urethral function from long-term indwelling catheters. The majority, however, were maintained on indwelling catheters for the duration of the study intervals.

The complications evaluated included pyelocaliectasis, bladder calculi, renal calculi, and vesicoureteral reflux and were compared in both men and women. There were no significant differences among the individual complications. However, the total number of complications was found to be significantly much higher in males than in females. Women had more upper tract calculi (15% vs. 11%), although this was not statistically significant. Bladder calculi were approximately equal, and although there were small differences in complication rates between males and females, none of these approached statistical significance except as just noted for the higher number of total complications among males.

There was a slight decline in ERPF in both males and females over time, but this was not substantially different than what might be expected with normal aging. Males generally have higher effective renal plasma flows at peak levels than females, although the levels tend to get closer with aging. This mirrors the situation seen in normal renal transplant donors. Importantly, we found no significant effect on renal function according to the method of bladder management or according to neurological classification in the women followed for 16 years.

The long-term incidence of severe renal complications for females was relatively low, as it was for males. In spite of the fact that most women in this group were on indwelling urethral catheters as the primary mode of bladder management throughout the study, they did not appear to suffer significant upper urinary tract abnormalities. Based on this limited number of individuals with long-term follow-up, renal function appears to be maintained fairly well over time regardless of the method of bladder management.

We are still unsure about what the minimal amount of follow-up urinary evaluation should be in persons with significant neurogenic bladder dysfunction. Clearly, if individuals are having symptomatic episodes, such as recurrent UTI episodes, then careful investigation is needed to determine if a change in bladder management should be made. Individuals who are asymptomatic with stable bladder management need only periodic evaluation, and perhaps after they are stable and asymptomatic this can be performed every few years.

Two major problems in long-term management for both men and women with significant neurogenic bladder dysfunction are UTI and renal calculi (Hall, 1989; Lloyd et al., 1987; Stover, Lloyd, Waites, & Jackson, 1989). Better control of these two conditions are issues that might merit further research. Long-term indwelling catheterization of women remains controversial (Jackson & DeVivo, 1992; Trop & Bennett, 1992). Many believe that this technique should be avoided, but at least during the period of 10- to 15-year follow-up seen in this study at Spain Rehabilitation Center, women with indwelling catheters appear to fare relatively well. Some of the data regarding long-term catheter management and bladder tumors may require follow-up of 20–25 years (Trop & Bennett, 1992).

CONCLUSIONS

An issue of great importance to the woman living with an SCI is quality of life (Billau & Howland, 1991). It is important not to minimize the fact that bladder management is only one aspect of the overall rehabilitation program. The appropriate form of management should be adapted to the individual's rehabilitation status, personal goals, and willingness to assume responsibility for the method of bladder management (Watson, 1983). In this context we should be able to maintain satisfactory levels of renal function and have a method of bladder management with which the individual remains satisfied over long periods of time.

REFERENCES

Billau, B.W., & Howland, D.R. (1991). Self-catheterization for the women with quadriplegia. *American Journal of Occupational Therapy, 45,* 366–369.

Bueschen, A.J., & Witten, D.M. (1979). Radionuclide evaluation of renal function. *Urology Clinics of North America, 6,* 307–314.

Feneley, R.C. (1983). The management of female incontinence by suprapubic catheterization with or without urethral closure. *British Journal of Urology, 55,* 203–207.

Halko, A., Burke, G., Sorkin, A., & Enenstein, J. (1973). Computer-aided statistical analysis of the scintillation camera 131-I-hippuran renogram. *Journal of Nuclear Medicine, 14,* 253–258.

Hall, M.K. (1989). Renal calculi in spinal cord injury patient: Association with reflux, bladder stones and Foley catheter drainage. *Urology, 34,* 126–128.

Hoffman, W.W., & Greyhack, J.T. (1960). The limitations of the intravenous pyelogram as a test of renal function. *Surgery, Gynecology and Obstetrics, 110,* 503–508.

Jackson, A.B., & DeVivo, M. (1992). Urological long-term follow-up in women with spinal cord injuries. *Archives of Physical Medicine and Rehabilitation, 73,* 1029–1035.

Joiner, E., & Lindan, R. (1982). Experience with self intermittent catheterization for women with neurological dysfunctions of the bladder. *Paraplegia, 47,* 147–153.

Kuhlemeier, K.V., Huang, C.T., DeVivo, M.J., & Lloyd, L.K. (1986). Year to year changes in effective renal plasma flow in asymptomatic spinal cord injury patients. *Urology, 28,* 270–274.

Kuhlemeier, K.V., Huang, C.T., Lloyd, L.K., Fine, P.R., & Stover, S.L. (1985). Effective renal plasma flow: Clinical significance after spinal cord injury. *Journal of Urology, 133,* 758–761.

Kuhlemeier, K.V., Lloyd, L.K., & Stover, S.L. (1985). Long-term follow-up renal function after spinal cord injury. *Journal of Urology, 134*, 510–513.

Kuhlemeier, K.V., McEachran, A., Lloyd, L.K., & Stover, S.L. (1984). Renal function after acute and chronic spinal cord injury. *Journal of Urology, 131*, 439–444.

Kuhlemeier, K.V., McEachran, A., Lloyd, L.K., Stover, S.L., & Fine, P.R. (1984). Serum creatinine as an indicator of renal function after spinal cord injury. *Archives of Physical Medicine and Rehabilitation, 65*, 694–698.

Lindan, R., Leffler, E.J., & Bodner, D. (1987). Urological problems in the management of quadriplegic women. *Paraplegia, 25*, 381–385.

Lloyd, L.K. (1986). New trends in urologic management of spinal cord injury patients. *Journal Center for New System for Trauma, 3*, 3–12.

Lloyd, L.K., Dubovsky, E.V., Bueschen, A.J., & Witten, S. (1981). Comprehensive renal scintillation procedures in spinal cord injury: Comparison with excretory urography. *Journal of Urology, 126*, 10–13.

Lloyd, L.K., Kuhlemeier, K.V., Fine, P.R., McEachran, S.B., & Stover, S.L. (1987). Prediction of pyelocaliectasis in follow-up of patients with spinal cord injury. *British Journal of Urolology, 59*, 122–126.

McGuire, E.J., & Savastano, J. (1986). Comparative urological outcome in women with spinal cord injury. *Journal of Urology, 135*, 730–731.

Price, M., Kottke, F.J., & Olson, M.E. (1975). Renal function in patients with spinal cord injury: The eighth year of a ten-year continuing study. *Archives of Physical Medicine and Rehabilitation, 56*, 76–80.

Schlegel, J.U., & Bakule, P.T. (1970). A diagnostic approach in detecting renal and urinary tract disease. *Journal of Urology, 104*, 2–6.

Stover, S.L., & Fine, P.R. (Eds.). (1986). *Spinal cord injury: The facts and figures.* Birmingham: University of Alabama at Birmingham Press.

Stover, S.L., Lloyd, L.K., Waites, K.B., & Jackson, A.B. (1989). Urinary tract infection in spinal cord injury. *Archives of Physical Medicine and Rehabilitation, 70*, 47–54.

Tauxe, W.N., Maher, F.T., & Taylor W.F. (1971). Effective renal plasma flow: Estimation from theoretical volumes of distribution of intravenously injected ^{131}I orthoiodohippurate. *Mayo Clinic Proceedings, 46*, 524–528.

Timoney, A.G., & Shaw, P.J. (1990). Urological outcome in female patients with spinal cord injury: The effectiveness of intermittent catheterization. *Paraplegia, 28*, 556–563.

Trop, C.S., & Bennett, C.J. (1992). Complications from long-term indwelling Foley catheters in female patients with neurogenic bladders. *Seminars in Urology, 10*, 155–120.

Watson, N. (1983). Spinal cord injury in the female. *Paraplegia, 21*, 143–148.

chapter 27

Current Bladder Management Treatment Options for Women with Disabilities

Carol J. Bennett, Salman S. Razi, and Mary N. Young

In developing new effective treatment interventions for bladder dysfunction in women, it is important to be able to identify the pathophysiological mechanisms involved. One of the first steps is to carefully assess patterns of voiding, as explained by Chancellor in Chapter 24. Evaluation of neuropathic voiding dysfunction is best categorized by following the classification established by Wein (Barrett & Wein, 1991). In this system, the bladder is viewed as a capacity vessel, with any changes in function related to failure to store or failure to fill. Failure to store includes problems related to either detrusor hyperactivity, bladders with decreased compliance, sensory urgency, stress incontinence, or nonfunctional bladder necks. Examples of situations in which the bladder demonstrates failure to store then would be those in which the bladder has neurologic, myogenic, psychogenic, or idiopathic dysfunction, as well as those where there is decreased outlet resistance. When determining optimal treatment options for a particular individual, two factors must be considered. One is the social acceptance of the method, particularly as it relates to the individual's ability to function within her community, and the other, as described previously in this section, is the maintenance and/or preservation of the upper tracts and kidneys. For example, from a urological perspective as well as from a social point of view, its preferable not to have a catheter or a stoma. Unfortunately, that is not always feasible.

Medical factors that influence the choice of options when determining optimal bladder management alternatives include the prognosis of the underlying impairment, the woman's degree of hand dexterity, her ability to transfer, her desire to avoid surgery, her fertility status and sexual activity, and her desire to remain appliance free. The most critical factor in choosing long-term management is the woman's own motivation, because that will lead to compliance with the chosen intervention. The urologist must work with the woman to consider all of these factors before establishing a bladder management system. Changing bladder management should be considered if one or more of the following is seen: upper tract deterioration, recurrent urosepsis, lower tract deterioration, or unacceptable incontinence (Table 1). Likewise, severe adverse reaction to medication might prompt alternative treatment consideration.

INCREASING BLADDER STORAGE

To optimize the ability to store an adequate volume of urine, a number of treatment options can be considered. These include noninvasive, timed (or prompted) voiding, which may be useful in situations where there is a component of detrusor instability or, for example, where the areflexic bladder is due to diabetes mellitus. Pharmacological therapy can be very effective, but its usefulness must be weighed against the drug's side effects. Likewise, biofeedback, electrical stimulation, or sacral rhizotomy can be useful in selected cases. Finally, surgical options such as augmentation cystoplasty and continent and incontinent diversion can be utilized when appropriate. The ability to increase urine storage as a result of inadequate outlet resistance is often specific to the individual and may also be specific to the disabling condition. Urine storage can be increased through a variety of techniques such as electrical stimulation and through various surgical alternatives such as bladder suspension. Circumventing the problem with the use of external collection devices or indwelling catheters or pharmacologically with drugs such as desmopressin acetate are also options. Desmopressin acetate is utilized to decrease urine production and may be the optimal treatment in selected cases.

Increasing bladder capacity via medical management has included the use of anticholinergic agents that work by increasing the volume at the first detrusor contraction. Thus, with proper anticholinergic therapy, a blad-

Table 1. Indications for changing bladder management

Upper tract deterioration
Lower urinary tract deterioration
Recurrent urosepsis or urine infection
Poor storage capacity
Inadequate emptying
Poor control
Significant medication side effects
Skin changes secondary to incontinence or collection device
Patient preference

Adapted from Barrett & Wein (1991).

der contraction that occurs at 100 cc of filling may not occur until a volume of 400–500 cc of filling has been reached. In addition, these drugs decrease the amplitude of contraction while increasing bladder capacity. Side effects from anticholinergic medication include dry mouth, tachycardia, and decreased gastric motility. The most commonly experienced side effect, dry mouth, can be quite uncomfortable and may lead to reduced use of this treatment. Conservative options such as chewing gum or sucking on hard candy may ameliorate this condition. Propantheline, administered at 15–30 mg, 3 times daily is an example of this class of drug. Oxybutynin, an antispasmodic muscle relaxant medication with anticholinergic properties, is perhaps the most commonly utilized bladder relaxant. Its side effects are similar to those of the anticholinergic drugs. The normal adult dosing is 5 mg, 3 times daily, but the dosage should be reduced in children and the elderly. Calcium antagonists have been evaluated for use in reducing detrusor hypercontractility. These drugs exhibit both an antimuscarinic effect as well as calcium antagonist effect, which in combination serve to reduce bladder contractility. Terodiline taken at 12.5 mg, 2 or 3 times daily is the recommended dose. Side effects may include hypotension, facial flushing, headache, constipation, nausea, and palpitations.

Antidepressants are also useful in combination with anticholinergic medications to reduce bladder contractions. These drugs both decrease bladder contractility and increase outlet resistance. The dose of imipramine, a commonly used antidepressant, is 25 mg, 4 times daily, with half that dose utilized in the elderly.

Drugs that increase outlet resistance are in the class of medications termed α-agonists. These drugs can result in an elevation of the blood pressure and are therefore contraindicated in those individuals with pre-existing hypertension. For those individuals with urethral dysfunction and mild stress incontinence, however, the agonists can be very effective. Drugs that lower urethral resistance are termed blockers and include phenoxybenzamine and prazosin. Prazosin has been shown to cause blockade in the smooth muscle of both the canine and human urethra (MacGregor & Diokno, 1981) as well as lower outlet resistance. Treatment with prazosin is generally begun in daily divided doses of 2 mg, increasing to a maximum of 10–12 mg in 3 divided doses. Potential side effects include hypotension with resultant lightheadedness, palpitations, and syncope. The occurrence of these side effects can be reduced by initiating therapy at 1 mg then slowly increasing both the dose and frequency of administration.

LONG-TERM INDWELLING CATHETERS

Numerous studies point to the deleterious effects of the long-term use of indwelling catheters in women with neuropathic bladders (Trop & Bennett,

1992). These include infection, bladder calculi, fistulae, urethral erosion, pyelonephritis, vesicoureteral reflux, autonomic dysreflexia, incontinence, decubitus ulcers, and, rarely, bladder carcinoma. They may also contribute to diminished bladder capacity and compliance of the neuropathic bladder. Trop and Bennett (1992) retrospectively evaluated three groups of women based on length of time that they had used an indwelling catheter, those with catheters 4–10 years, 12–20 years, and 21–36 years. Although patients in all categories experienced significant morbidity, the number and severity of the complications increased with length of time with the indwelling catheter. Of the 24 women in the group, 4 who had catheters for 21–36 years developed bladder carcinoma (3 with transitional-cell carcinoma and 1 with squamous cell cancer). Thus, acceptable alternatives to indwelling catheters are necessary. We feel that bladder augmentation or continent diversion are excellent alternatives in carefully selected women. Care must be taken to select the procedure that will 1) protect the upper tracts and 2) provide a low-pressure, large-capacity reservoir. Proper placement of the abdominal stoma or instruction in intermittent catheterization via the urethra is mandatory for long-term patient success with a neobladder.

MANAGEMENT OF STRESS URINE INCONTINENCE

Stress incontinence is the involuntary loss of urine with an increase in intra-abdominal pressure and can be classified on a anatomical basis. It is important to note that changes may occur in the pelvic floor as a consequence of disability. These changes may influence the level of stress incontinence in this group of women, as noted in Chapter 24. Urodynamic evaluation, in particular fluoroscopic video-urodynamic evaluation, aids in defining the bladder urethra relationship and thus assists in predicting optimal surgical treatment. Type 1 and Type 2 stress incontinence are defined according to the degree of urethral mobility and the presence or absence of an associated cystocele. They are amenable to a variety of transvaginal corrective procedures, including the popular needle suspension procedures. Some women, however, experience gross loss of urine during an increase in abdominal pressure. For these women, a suspension procedure would probably be ineffective.

McGuire (1984) first coined the term *Type 3 stress* to identify this group of women who on cystogram or video-urodynamic evaluation have a nonfunctional proximal urethral and bladder neck. These women can be incontinent with a relatively minor increase in their intra-abdominal pressure and will often state that they leak without awareness or provocation. Often, going from the recumbent to the upright position or from the sitting to the standing position is enough to elicit leakage. Those women with neurogenic bladder and proximal urethra dysfunction, or those with prior bladder neck procedures with resultant fibrosis are likely to develop Type 3 incontinence. Whereas both Type 1 and 2 incontinence are associated with some degree of urethral hypermobility, this is not typically seen in Type 3 stress because of the fixed scarred nature of the vesicourethral segment.

Treatment for the nonfunctional urethra/bladder neck, which is more commonly referred to as intrinsic sphincteric deficiency (ISD), involves the use of methods devised to close or coapt the urethra. Collagen was approved by the Food and Drug Administration (FDA) for this purpose. Purified bovine collagen is injected around the urethra at the level of the bladder neck under cystoscopic guidance to provide proximal urethral closure. This surgical technique is noninvasive and is effective in a wide group of people with ISD, including women with Type 3 incontinence. Alternatively, the sling urethrapexy (Figure 1), which utilizes fascia to support the urethra posteriorly, is often utilized for this type of urethral dysfunction. Finally, the artificial urinary sphincter can be used to provide continence. This prosthetic device is approximately 95% effective. Though complications may occur that include erosion, infection, and pain at the implantation site, this is a very effective long-lasting device when well situated.

CONTINENT DIVERSION AND BLADDER AUGMENTATION

Clean intermittent catheterization (CIC), as originally described by Lapides et al. (1976), revolutionized the way in which individuals are able to manage their neuropathic bladder. This technique, along with the ability to safely and efficiently assess function via urodynamics, has had a positive and lasting impact in the maintenance of a "safe" bladder and stable upper tracts (kidneys). Urodynamic advances have allowed us to couple the principles of a "low-pressure reservoir" with CIC, thus reducing the incidence of recurrent urine infection, vesicoureteral reflux, and stone formation. When conservative therapy fails, or if urethral catheterizing is not feasible for technical reasons, alternative procedures should be considered. The ileal loop urinary diversion used to be considered the procedure of choice when an individual presented with an "end-stage bladder." Unfortunately, long-term follow-up of this procedure has shown a high incidence of upper tract deterioration, pyelonephritis, and renal calculi (Cass, Luxenberg, Gelich, & Johnson, 1984). More recently, augmentation enterocystoplasty and continent urine diversion have developed defined niches in long-term bladder management. However, long-term evaluation of this procedure is still needed.

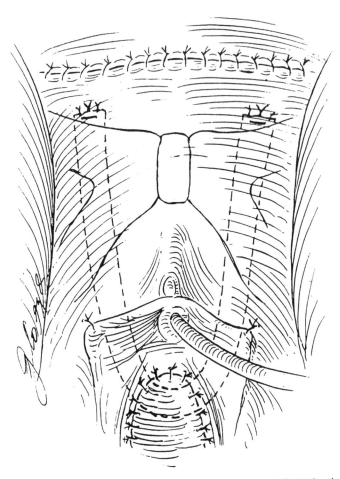

Figure 1. Pubovaginal sling for Type 3 stress incontinence. (From Raz, S. [1992]. *Atlas of transvaginal surgery* [p. 91]. Philadelphia: W.B. Saunders; reprinted by permission.)

AUGMENTATION ENTEROCYSTOPLASTY

The ideal candidate for an augmentation enterocystoplasty would be a person for whom more conservative management approaches have not been successful. The conservative approach includes initiating a course of anticholinergic medication in those persons with elevated filling pressures, as determined by urodynamic assessment (Bennett & Bennett, 1993). Detrusor response to filling and tolerance to the medication are also evaluated. Failure of the medication is indicated by poor detrusor compliance curve with a persistently elevated filling response, and medication intolerance would include prohibitive side effects, including excessive dry mouth, blurred vision, constipation, and gastric upset. Alternative medications should always be tried when first-line anticholinergics fail, because the individual's response can vary considerably from drug to drug. Intractable incontinence, upper tract deterioration, and vesicoureteral reflux in the face of maximal medical therapy are the other indications for augmentation. The preoperative assessment of the individual considered a candidate for these procedures is straightforward and includes a thorough history and physical exam. Upper tract evaluation is essential and can be accomplished with a renal ultrasound or renal scan if there is a question about renal function. Video-urodynamics, as extensively described in Chapter 24, is very useful in assessing detrusor compliance, urethral function, and the presence or absence of vesicoureteral reflux. If catheterization via the stoma is required, a variety of techniques can be employed, including the use of the Mitrofanoff procedure, which utilizes the appendix for the stoma, or the use of an efferent nipple, which utilizes intussuscepted ileum to accomplish this goal (Figures 2 and 3).

If the person undergoing this procedure has compromised hand function, it is critical that, together with the physician, enterostomal therapist, and occupational therapist, she be included in the evaluation and development of the optimal treatment methods. Individuals with limited hand function can learn to catheterize via the urethra or, if necessary, through an abdominal stoma. The surgery must be individualized so that limited hand function does not preclude the use of this procedure. By considering the woman's preferences in stoma placement, along with preoperative training in the techniques of both catheterization setup and intermittent catheterization and the use of adaptive devices when indicated, long-term success with catheterization can be greatly enhanced (Young & McRae, 1991).

CONTINENT DIVERSION

For women with disabilities, continent diversion is most commonly reserved for those individuals who have undergone prior cystectomy. An additional indication for this procedure would be severe urethral dysfunction secondary to a long-term indwelling catheter (Trop & Bennett, 1992). Individuals with this condition are often severely incontinent, despite the presence of a large indwelling catheter. Physical examination usually demonstrates extensive urethral destruction. In addition, associated sacral decubiti may result from long-standing urine contamination and thus require extensive flap reconstruction by a plastic surgeon following the diversion. In those who are willing and able to catheterize a stoma, continent diversion is ideal in that it accomplishes the important goal of providing a low-pressure, large capacity reservoir with a mechanism (either an afferent nipple, or by tunnelling the ureters) designed to prevent reflux and protect

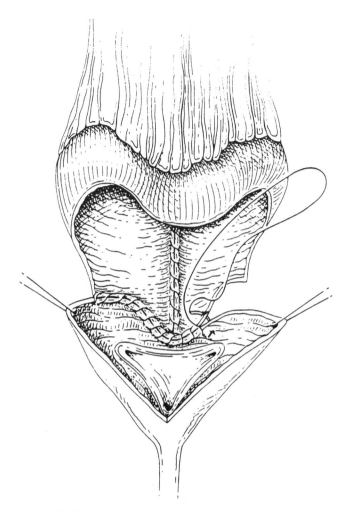

Figure 2. Bivalved bladder with ileal augmentation to increase bladder capacity and decrease bladder pressure.(From Bennett, J.K., Gray, M., Green, B.G., & Foote, J.E. [1992]. Continent diversion and bladder augmentation in spinal cord-injured patients. *Seminars in Urology, 10,* 121; reprinted by permission.)

the upper tracts. The Kock-Pouch urinary diversion, with its afferent nipple that prevents reflux and its efferent nipple that acts as its continence mechanism, is a commonly utilized type of continent diversion (Figure 4).

CONCLUSIONS

Various options are available for improving the management of bladder function for women with disabilities. Our approach has always been to

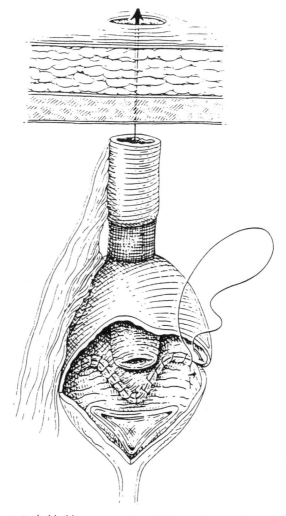

Figure 3. Efferent nipple bladder augmentation which provides a catheterizable stoma. (From Bennett et al. [1992]. Continent diversion and bladder augmentation in spinal cord-injured patients. *Seminars in Urology, 10,* 121; reprinted by permission.)

begin with the least invasive treatment option, which accomplishes the important goal of preserving renal function and preventing infection, while maintaining continence. If these approaches fail, then more elaborate procedures can be considered. The woman's preference as well as her body habitus and lifestyle should always be priorities when designing a bladder management program.

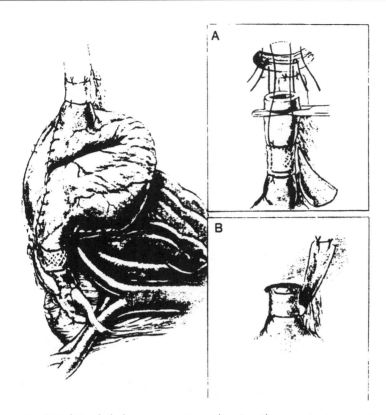

Figure 4. A Kock-Pouch ileal reservoir continent diversion. The upper tracts are protected by nonrefluxing afferent nipple. A: Demonstrates the maturation of efferent nipple. B: Completed efferent nipple abdominal stoma for catheterization. (From Skinner, D., & Lieskovsky, G. [1988]. *Diagnosis and management of genitourinary cancer* [p. 667]. Philadelphia: W.B. Saunders; reprinted by permission.)

REFERENCES

Barrett, D.M., & Wein, A.J. (1991). Voiding dysfunction: Diagnosis, classification and management. In J.Y. Gillenwater, J.T. Grayhack, S.S. Howards, & J.W. Duckett (Eds.), *Adult and pediatric urology.* (2nd ed., pp. 1001–1099). St. Louis: Mosby.

Bennett, C.J., & Bennett, J.K. (1993). Augmentation cystoplasty and urinary diversions in patients with spinal cord injury. *Physical Medicine and Rehabilitation Clinics of North America, 4,* 2.

Bennett, J.K., Gray, M., Green, B.G., & Foote, J.E. (1992). Continent diversion and bladder augmentation in spinal cord-injured patients. *Seminars in Urology, 10,* 121–132.

Cass, A.S., Luxenberg, M., Gelich, P., & Johnson, C.F. (1984). A 22 year follow-up of ileal conduits in children with neurogenic bladder. *Journal of Urology, 132,* 529.

Lapides, J., Diokno, A.C., Gould, F.R., & Lowe, B.S. (1976). Further observations on self-catheterization. *Journal of Urology, 116,* 169–172.

MacGregor, R., & Diokno, A. (1981). The alpha adrenergic blocking action of prazosin hydrochloride on the canine urethra. *Investigative Urology, 18,* 426.

McGuire, E.J. (1984). Clinical evaluation and treatment of neurogenic bladder dysfunction. In J. Libertino (Ed.), *International perspectives in urology.* Baltimore: Williams & Wilkins.

Raz, S. (1992). *Atlas of transvaginal surgery.* Philadelphia: W.B. Saunders.

Skinner, D., & Lieskovsky, G. (1988). *Diagnosis and management of genitourinary cancer.* Philadelphia: W.B. Saunders.

Trop, C.S., & Bennett, C.J. (1992). Complications from long-term indwelling Foley catheter in female patients with neurogenic bladders. *Seminars in Urology, 10,* 2.

Young, M.N., & McRae, K.R. (1991). Self catheterization of continent diversion for patients with quadriplegia. *Progressions, 3,* 3.

chapter 28

Overcoming Functional Limitations

Marilyn Pires

Successful functioning with disabilities requires individual and environmental cooperation. Thus, the ability to exert control over one's bodily functions depends on issues associated with access as well as the level of the person's physical functioning. Overcoming the functional limitations related to bowel and bladder management is paramount among women with disabilities because of issues associated with self-esteem and independence, as discussed in Chapter 22 by Sonya Perduta-Fulginiti. Two different levels of functioning are discussed in this chapter: women with volitional bowel and bladder function who have impaired mobility and women with bowel and bladder dysfunction accompanied by impaired mobility. Although the resulting functional limitations have different etiologies, obtaining personal control of bladder and bowel function is possible using similar practical adaptations.

ACCESS TO TOILETS

Environmental factors can play a critical role in determining a woman's continence. Access to toilets, both in public and in private, is an important consideration for persons with mobility limitations. With the passage of the Americans with Disabilities Act of 1990 (PL 101-336), public facilities are required to be wheelchair accessible. Figure 1 shows guidelines from the Paralyzed Veterans of America (1986) for such facilities. Note that stalls need to be quite large to completely accommodate a wheelchair. Most public restrooms labeled accessible are not deep enough to accommodate a wheelchair. Thus, if a woman is not accompanied by someone who can remove the chair and close the door, she is unable to maintain privacy and exposes herself.

Home toileting facilities also pose a major problem. Because kitchens and bathrooms are the most expensive rooms to remodel, renovations lead-

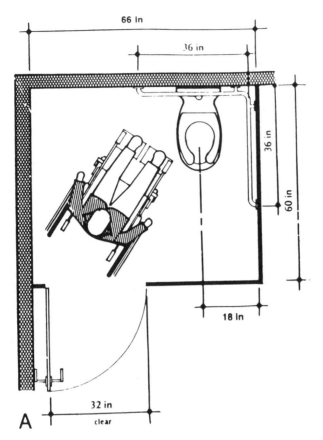

Figure 1. Design guidelines for public toilet stalls, including dimensions. (Courtesy of Paralyzed Veterans of America. [1986]. *Design guidelines qualifying for the tax advantages of Section 102.* Washington, DC: Author.)

ing to completely accessible bathrooms are both difficult and expensive. Most women with disabilities are among those with the lowest income levels; thus, expensive remodeling is often not an option. Additionally, women with disabilities may rent or live in government-supplemented apartments in which such renovations are not always possible.

Toilet Adaptations

Even when accessible bathrooms are available, toilet adaptations require careful consideration. Most elevated full toilets may be the correct height to enable transfers for some persons with mobility impairments. However, elevated toilets become a hindrance rather than a help for persons who must perform bowel management programs. A standard-height toilet with an elevated toilet seat would provide adequate perineal access. There are many different types of elevated toilet seats available, as shown in Figure 2, and the selection should be individualized to meet the needs of the individual. Rehabilitation nurses and other health care professionals should work with each woman to assess her unique toileting needs and to determine the most appropriate adaptive equipment (Pires, 1990).

Commode Chairs Commode chairs are particularly useful for persons with mobility impairments. Commodes are available in a number of different types to accommodate a variety of needs. Seats can be turned for front, rear, right-side, or left-side access, and chairs with removable arms allow greater flexibility to meet individual needs. Women with high spinal cord injury (SCI) or severe functional and mobility limitations can utilize specially designed commode chairs, although these chairs are more practical for bowel evacuation than for urination for this population.

Commode chairs play an important role in the prevention of secondary conditions such as urinary tract infections (UTIs) and pressure ulcers. Although it may seem easier for caregivers to perform bowel programs in bed for persons with severe mobility limitations, such a program is much more likely to lead to contamination of the perineal area and cause a higher rate of urinary tract infection. Using commode chairs for the bowel pro-

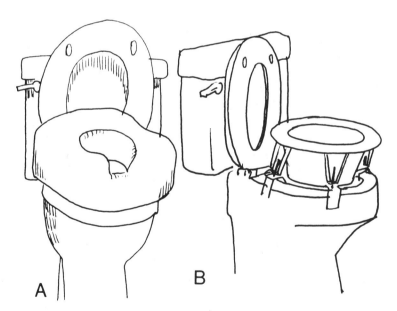

Figure 2. Raised toilet seats are designed with (A) fixed or (B) adjustable height; they can have front, side, or back openings to accommodate wiping or manipulation needed for a bowel program. (From Pires, M. [1990]. Promoting continence for the physically impaired. In K.F. Jeter, N. Faller, & C. Norton [Eds.], *Nursing for continence* [p. 163]. Philadelphia: W.B. Saunders; reprinted by permission.)

gram while the person is in rehabilitation is very important because practices learned in a clinical setting are often internalized as the norm. If rehabilitation facilities are reluctant to complete bowel programs on commode chairs, then individuals and caregivers are less likely to do so at home.

Hand-Held Urinals For persons with volitional bladder control but limited mobility, an alternative is the use of hand-held urinals. For women with physical disabilities who cannot get to a commode or toilet, urination is more difficult than for men who have similar disabilities. The familiar urinal for men has been adapted for women so that its opening can accommodate the entire vulva area. Leakage is often a problem, however (Pires, 1990); the opening should be form fitted. Other female urinals are designed to be used in wheelchairs and consist of a funnel and tubing that drain into a toilet or a collector. Three such devices are illustrated in Figure 3.

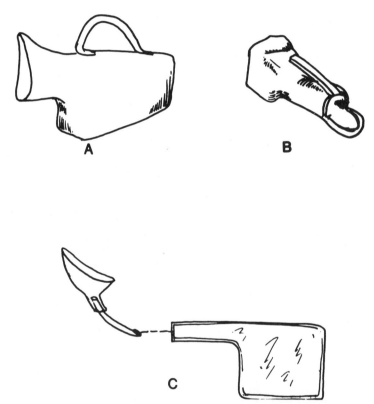

Figure 3. Female hand-held urinals can be of (A) traditional design, (B) specifically designed for use in a wheelchair, or (C) of a funnel design. (From Pires, M. [1990]. Promoting continence for the physically impaired. In K.F. Jeter, N. Faller, & C. Norton [Eds.], *Nursing for continence* [p. 163]. Philadelphia: W.B. Saunders; reprinted by permission.)

Split Wheelchair Cushions   Much research has been directed at the development of cushions that will prevent the formation of pressure ulcers in wheelchair users. Women in wheelchairs might find hand-held urinals easier to use with specially adapted wheelchair cushions cut out to accommodate a urinal (Figure 4). Cushions could be split to accommodate a narrow pan to catch urine without requiring that the woman change her position. These adaptations are particularly useful for those women who have volitional control and fully empty their bladder but cannot get out of the chair or cannot do so rapidly enough.

External Collection Devices   A real need still exists for a suitable female external collection device for women who are incontinent as well as physically immobilized. Adherence of any such device is a problem because of the moist mucous membranes around the female meatus. Such a commercially available device, manufactured by Hollister, is shown in Figure 5 and is reported to have greater success in ambulatory women. There is no successful external collection device for women who are seated in wheelchairs most of the day or who have to scoot on their buttocks to transfer. Industry interest in developing external collection devices for women is limited because the potential market does not support the research development costs. Additionally, women will probably require several types of products applicable to small subgroups, rather than the condom-based external devices that have universal applicability to men.

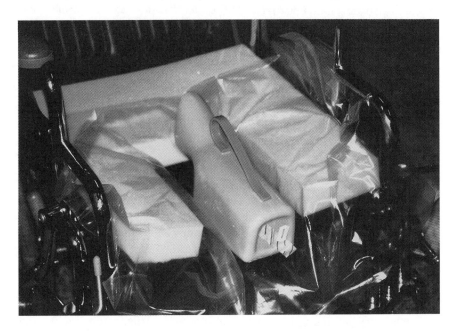

Figure 4.   Wheelchair cushion adapted with a cut-out to accommodate a urinal.

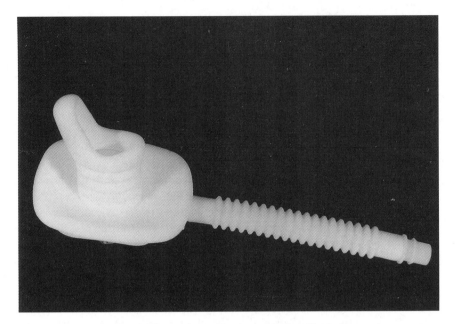

Figure 5. External urinary collection device for women, marketed by Hollister.

The government should be encouraged to play a role in supporting research and development of external collection devices for women and join with industry to market the devices and make them available to women.

Adaptive Clothing Women with impaired mobility can be helped to maintain continence by wearing clothing that allows perineal access. Some clothing adaptations can be made relatively inexpensively. For women who use trousers, one simple adaptation is to replace the whole seam from the front of the garment through the crotch with a Velcro closure that would allow easy access. This modification is probably more functional for men than women but may be useful. Wraparound skirts worn in conjunction with the split cushion just described would allow a woman to void freely without needing to change positions. French knickers allow perineal access by pulling them to one side, although a fair amount of hand function would be needed. Several lines of adaptive garments are available, such as panties with a Velcro crotch opening and removable side panels that facilitate perineal access.

PERINEAL ACCESS

Perineal access for women who rely on catheterization for bladder management is an important issue because it is very difficult for a woman in a sitting position to have access to her perineum. Balance and mobility are needed to undress to perform a self-catheterization. Catheterization on a toilet is optimal if a woman has sufficient mobility.

For women with limited hand function, a labia spreader may be helpful to access her perineum. A number of designs have evolved at various rehabilitation facilities. The Weitlaner retractor with padded tips has been used successfully because it can be maintained in the open position, allowing the labia to stay spread while the woman performs her catheterization (Figure 6).

Because the location of the meatus in females is not as predictable as it is in males, the Lady Cath or Autocath, which may potentially be marketed in the United States by Mentor Inc., was invented by a British gynecologist to assist with gaining access to the meatus for catheterization (Figure 7). When the tip is placed intravaginally, the angle of the catheter is anatomically correct, enabling the woman to easily insert the catheter through the meatus and into the urethra. However, if a woman has sufficient hand function to place the device vaginally, she probably has the hand function to catheterize herself without it. Further development of female catheterization aids should be a research priority.

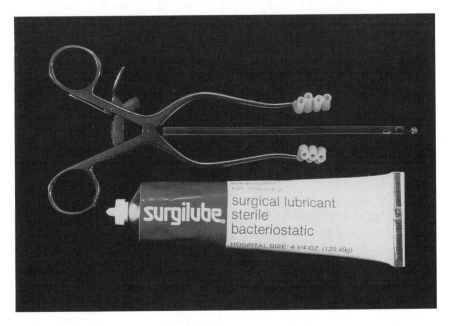

Figure 6. Weitlaner retractor with latex tubing covering the dull tips can be used as a labia spreader. (From Pires, M., & Koontz, R. [1979]. *Weitlaner retractor: An aid to female self-catheterization programs.* Poster presentation of the American Congress of Rehabilitation Annual Meeting, Honolulu, HI; reprinted by permission.)

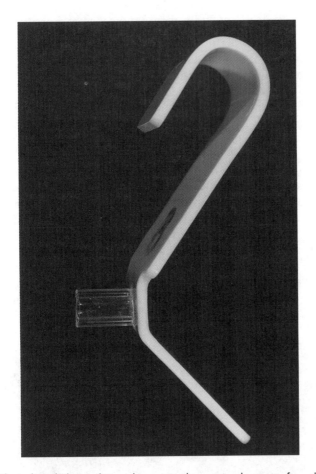

Figure 7. The Lady Cath device, designed to assist with accessing the meatus for catheterization. When properly placed, the tube is at the anatomically correct angle to introduce the catheter through the meatus into the urethra.

PERSONAL AND PROFESSIONAL ATTITUDES AND BLADDER MANAGEMENT TECHNIQUES

Recognizing that a major goal of bladder management programs is to protect the upper urinary tract from damage, researchers have advocated the use of intermittent catheterization (IC) in women with neurogenic dysfunction. Most studies evaluating the efficacy of this method have almost exclusively used male subjects. The data from these studies have been extrapolated to women with little or no supporting research (Cardenas & Mayo, 1987; Jackson & DeVivo, 1992; Stover, Lloyd, Waits, & Jackson, 1989; Young, Bennett, & Diaz, 1994). For most women and their caregivers, adhering to an IC program may require heroic measures. A woman with good upper extremity functioning has several options. Generally for women, the short plastic catheter is better because it is easier to manipulate. Some women have found metal urethral dilating sounds useful in performing self-catheterization. A supply of only two or three sounds is needed. They are cleaned between catheterizations. There have been additional interesting adaptations to create convenience and portability, such as the "E-Z Cath" device (made by Manutec) that facilitates self-catheterization for women in wheelchairs.

For women with limited or no hand function, IC requires resources that are not always available. Availability of personal assistants and the time required to do IC becomes a major concern. Consistency in availability of personal assistants may interfere with the success and safety of an IC program. Furthermore, an IC program may be demanding of family members, leading to restriction of activities, including other employment.

Given these difficulties, bladder management for a woman with bladder dysfunction cannot be considered an isolated event. Rather, it must be an integral part of her overall life management program. An eclectic approach would seem most appropriate. The primary focus should be on the woman, who is central to the bladder management approach. Her overall medical, psychological, social, and vocational goals must be integrated with her bladder management program. Lloyd (1993) recommends a patient-centered approach that recognizes the utility of a variety of bladder management options tailored to the patient's urological and rehabilitation needs. This eclectic approach calls for incorporating a variety of management options, careful long-term follow-up, and flexibility in reassessing the need for alterations in the bladder management program.

CONCLUSIONS

Further research concerning this blended approach requires the study of bladder management alternatives, which have been largely ignored. What can be done to minimize the complications of indwelling catheters? What is the appropriate fluid intake? What concomitant pharmacological management is necessary? What catheter material is optimal? What is the etiology of patulus urethra and how can it be prevented? What is the role of suprapubic catheters in women? Are there catheter-taping techniques that can reduce complications? Is there a complication-free, safe time frame for women with indwelling catheters? Can an algorithm of patient characteristics, time frames, and complications be developed to allow women more bladder management options?

The functional limitations related to bowel and bladder management among women with disabilities represents a research opportunity for women. The challenge for us is to chart these unexplored waters with high-quality, meaningful studies.

REFERENCES

Americans with Disabilities Act of 1990 (ADA), PL 101-336. (July 26, 1990). Title 42, U.S.C. 12101 et seq.: *U.S. Statutes at Large, 104,* 327–378.

Cardenas, D.D., & Mayo, M.E. (1987). Bacteriuria with fever after spinal cord injury. *Archives of Physical Medicine & Rehabilitation, 68,* 291–293.

Jackson, A.B., & DeVivo, M. (1992). Urologic long-term follow-up in women with spinal cord injuries. *Archives of Physical Medicine & Rehabilitation, 72,* 1029–1035.

Lloyd, K.L. (1993). Long-term management of neurogenic bladder: An eclectic approach. *Physical Medicine and Rehabilitation Clinics of North America, 4,* 329–342.

Paralyzed Veterans of America. (1986). *Design guidelines qualifying for the tax advantages of Section 102.* Washington, DC: Author.

Pires, M. (1990). Promoting continence for the physically impaired. In K.F. Jeter, N. Faller, & C. Norton (Eds.), *Nursing for continence* (pp. 157–167). Philadelphia: W.B. Saunders.

Pires, M., & Koontz, R. (1979). *Weitlaner retractor: An aid to self-catheterization programs.* Poster presentation of the American Congress of Rehabilitation Annual Meeting, Honolulu, HI.

Stover, S.L., Lloyd, L.K., Waits, K.B., & Jackson, A.M. (1989). Urinary tract infections in spinal cord injury. *Archives of Physical Medicine & Rehabilitation, 70,* 47–54.

Young, M., Bennett, C., & Diaz, F. (1994). Comparison of bladder management in female SCI patients. *Journal of the American Paraplegic Society, 17,* 100.

chapter 29

Restoration of Bladder and Bowel Function to Women with Spinal Cord Injury

Graham H. Creasey

Women are at a particular disadvantage from impaired bladder and bowel function. The short urethra and the proximity of the external urethral meatus to the anus predispose to urinary infection. This becomes more common if damage to the central nervous system (CNS) causes difficulty in micturition or fecal incontinence. Childbirth and pelvic surgery can contribute to weakened sphincters and pelvic floor, and upper motor neuron damage can result in hyperactive bladder reflexes; these factors lead to urinary incontinence, which is particularly troublesome because of the lack of effective external collection devices for women.

Fortunately, some technical advances now offer significant improvement in function to selected women with neuropathic bladder and bowel. A person with a spinal cord injury (SCI) above the lower part of the spinal cord may well have intact nerves between the sacral segments of the cord and the bladder, bowel, and sexual organs. Although isolated from control by the brain, these nerves can be activated by electrical stimuli to produce function in the organs of the pelvis.

The functions required of the lower urinary tract are to store urine at low pressure, allowing continence, and to expel it completely when desired. Electrical control of these functions requires an understanding of the control of these functions by the nerves and muscles of the pelvis.

Voiding

Voiding is normally produced by contraction of the detrusor muscle in the wall of the bladder, as a result of activity in the parasympathetic nerves originating in the sacral segments of the spinal cord. At the same time the sphincter muscles and the pelvic floor relax, allowing urine to flow at relatively low pressure. Voiding may also be aided by contraction of the abdominal wall and diaphragm.

The anterior roots of the sacral nerves contain neurons to both the bladder wall and the external sphincter. Conventional stimulation of these roots produces contraction of the external sphincter whenever contraction of the detrusor is produced and would normally not be expected to produce voiding. However, it is possible to produce voiding by stimulating the nerves to both muscles intermittently and making use of the fact that the smooth muscle of the bladder contracts and relaxes more slowly than the striated muscle of the external urethral sphincter. If stimulation is applied in bursts lasting a few seconds, with intervals of a few seconds, the sphincter relaxes rapidly between the bursts, while the bladder relaxes more slowly. The pressure in it is maintained sufficiently to produce voiding during these intervals, resulting in an intermittent pattern of voiding. Although this differs from normal human voiding, it resembles the micturition occurring in some animals and can be effective in emptying the bladder.

Continence

Continence is dependent on the sphincter mechanism of the urethra and bladder neck and relaxation of the bladder. The external sphincter is activated by somatic efferent neurons originating in the anterior horn cells of the sacral segments of the cord, whereas sympathetic innervation from the thoracolumbar segments of the cord is probably responsible for tone in the smooth muscle of the internal sphincter and contributes to inhibition of bladder contraction during urine storage.

Incontinence following SCI is commonly caused by hyperactive reflex contractions of the bladder. These reflexes can be abolished by cutting all the sensory nerve roots at S2 and below. This not only improves continence but also increases the compliance of the bladder, so that urine is stored at low pressure. This procedure may thereby reduce the risk of ureteric reflux of urine and of hydronephrosis. In addition, it reduces spasticity of the external urethral sphincter, aiding urine flow rate, and abolishes autonomic dysreflexia triggered from the bladder, bowel, or sexual organs. However, it also abolishes sacral sensation, if present, and this may influence the ability of a person to experience orgasm or reflex erection of the clitoris. The stimulator itself commonly produces erection of the clitoris and increased blood flow to the vagina by activating the sacral parasympathetic fibers (Levin & MacDonagh, 1993). A decision as to whether to cut the sensory roots should therefore be made in consultation with each individual.

SURGICAL TECHNIQUE

An implantable device for applying electrical stimulation as described above has been developed in England by Brindley and has been used in several centers in Europe and the Far East (Brindley, 1991). The implantation of the device requires exposure of the sacral roots by performing a laminectomy of L4–S1 at the base of the spine. The dura mater is opened to expose the nerve roots of the cauda equina. Individual roots of the cauda equina are stimulated electrically during surgery while at the same time recording the pressure in the bladder to identify the anterior roots responsible for bladder contraction. Electrodes are then placed around these roots and connected to cables from the electrodes, which are brought through the dura and tunneled under the skin to a convenient site on the front of the body. There they are connected to a stimulator implanted though a separate incision. This stimulator is powered and controlled by radio transmission from a small battery-powered transmitter operated by the individual.

The posterior (sensory) roots are seen clearly during the operation for implantation of the electrodes and can be cut at that time or can be cut at their entry into the conus medullaris in a separate operation before or after the implantation.

RESULTS

The use of this technique in women has been included in reports from several countries in Europe (Brindley, Polkey, Rushton, & Cardozo, 1986; Colombel & Egon, 1991; Madersbacher, Fischer, & Ebner, 1988; Sauerwein, 1990). These have been reviewed in another study (Creasey, 1993).

Data have also been collected from many of the European centers in a questionnaire study by Van Kerrebroeck, Koldewijn, and Debruyne (1993). Information was obtained on 94 women from 10 countries. The women who underwent the procedures ranged in age from 17 to 75 years (Van Kerrebroeck et al., 1993). Table 1 shows the number of these who were using the device for micturition. The majority were using the device alone; a few sometimes supplemented it by intermittent catheterization (IC), and four reverted to using IC alone.

Residual volumes are shown in Table 2. All women using the stimulator had a residual volume of less than 60 ml. Low residual volumes of urine after voiding might be expected to lead to reduced urinary tract infection (UTI). In this study, a record was made of the presence or absence

Table 1. Methods of bladder emptying used by 94 women following implantation of Brindley electrical stimulator

Micturition	
Method	No. women
Stimulator alone	88
Stimulator and intermittent catheterization	2
Intermittent catheterization	4

Adapted from Van Kerrebroeck et al. (1993).

Table 2. Residual volumes in 94 women following implantation of electrical stimulator

Residual volumes	No. women
<30 ml	84
31–60 ml	6
61–200 ml	2
>200 ml[a]	2

Adapted from Van Kerrebroeck et al. (1993).
[a]The four individuals with residual volumes greater than 60 ml were women who were not using the stimulator.

of UTI with or without fever, before and after operation, and is shown in Table 3. Although this form of reporting is simplistic, it gives an indication of trends in symptomatic UTI that have been validated by other reports (Arnold, Gowland, MacFarlane, Bean, & Utley, 1986; Brindley & Rushton, 1990; Colombel & Egon, 1991; Madersbacher et al., 1988). Van Kerrebroeck also reported on a personal series of 22 patients with follow-up of at least 1 year, in whom the mean incidence of UTIs per year was reduced from 4.2 (range 2–12) to 1.4 (range 0–2) (Van Kerrebroeck, 1993).

As shown in Table 4, the majority of individuals who received the device became continent of urine. This is probably due mainly to posterior rhizotomy, which was carried out in the majority of the persons undergoing this procedure: 57 had complete posterior sacral rhizotomies from S2–S5, 14 had incomplete rhizotomies, and 3 had no rhizotomy; the rhizotomy status of 20 individuals was not recorded. The decrease of infection might also be expected to reduce stimulation of nonspinal bladder reflexes, and a reduction in residual urine allows greater time between the occasions when the bladder reaches its capacity.

Autonomic dysreflexia was present in 13 women before surgery and in 1 of these after surgery; none of the individuals in the study developed autonomic dysreflexia for the first time after surgery. A total of 3 women had signs of upper tract dilatation before surgery, and in all 3 improvement

Table 3. Infections as reported from 144 individuals (male and female) before and after use of implanted electrical stimulator

Status	No. with urine infection	
	Before	After
Infections	127	25
No infections	17	119

Adapted from Van Kerrebroeck et al. (1993).

Table 4. Continence of 94 women following implantation of electrical stimulator

Status	No. women
Fully continent	85
Mild stress incontinence	7
Severe stress incontinence	1
Reflex incontinence	1

Adapted from Van Kerrebroeck et al. (1993).

was seen postoperatively; one woman had ureteric reflux preoperatively, and this also improved after the procedure. None of the participants developed ureteric reflux or hydronephrosis following surgery with the implant.

Defecation is not usually produced during micturition because the time-course of contraction in the bowel is slower than that in the bladder. However, defecation can be produced in some individuals, after emptying the bladder, by a slower pattern of intermittent stimulation. In this series, 59 of the women used the stimulator to aid in defecation, but only 22 of these were able to defecate with the stimulator alone, and 21 required manual evacuation as well (Table 5).

Stimulation of the sacral parasympathetic fibers produces contractions of the bowel as far proximal as the distal transverse colon, as would be expected from the parasympathetic innervation of the bowel (Binnie, Smith, Creasey, & Edmond, 1990). Most individuals find that the regular stimulation of the sacral parasympathetic nerves used for micturition improves peristalsis in the colon, bringing stool into the rectum from whence it can be removed more readily (Binnie, Smith, Creasey, & Edmond, 1991). The time spent in bowel emptying was reduced in one group of men and women by 80% (MacDonagh, Sun, Smallwood, Forster, & Read, 1990).

Potential Complications

All procedures have a component of risk, and the development of a new technology may create unexpected complications, which as the procedures are perfected become less common.

Table 5. Use of electrical stimulator by 94 women to produce or assist defecation

Method	No. women	
Stimulator alone	22	⎫
Stimulator and medication	16	⎬ 63%
Stimulator and manual evacuation	21	⎭
Stimulator not used	15	
Not known	20	

Adapted from Van Kerrebroeck et al. (1993).

Follow-up of individuals for up to 15 years has shown that chronic nerve stimulation at levels used with these devices does not result in damage to the nerves. There is a possibility, however, that damage to the nerves themselves may occur during surgery. Such injury may result in some temporary loss of function, potentially delaying use of the stimulator for several months. With improved surgical approach and with surgeons' increased experience with the technique, the likelihood of such nerve injury becomes very small. Other complications, such as cerebrospinal fluid leakage (Brindley, 1981a; Brindley et al., 1986) and rate of infections of the implants (Rushton, Brindley, Polkey, & Browning, 1989), have been significantly reduced by subsequent developments in procedures and materials.

DISCUSSION

Detrusor-Sphincter Dyssynergia

It has sometimes been feared that the contraction of the sphincter at the same time as the bladder would produce dangerously high pressures in the bladder, possibly resulting in trabeculation of the bladder, ureteric reflux, and hydronephrosis. The pressures during voiding can be chosen by selection of the stimulation parameters and have usually been set to between 55 and 85 cm of water pressure (Cardozo, Krishnan, Polkey, Rushton, & Brindley, 1984; Creasey, 1993; Madersbacher et al., 1988; Van Kerrebroeck, Koldewijn, Wijkstra, & Debruyne, 1992). It has been found in several series (Brindley et al., 1986; Van Kerrebroeck et al., 1993) that reflux and hydronephrosis have more often tended to decrease than to increase, possibly because the posterior rhizotomy reduces bladder pressure during the storage of urine.

Nevertheless, many urologists would like to be able to reduce the resistance due to external urethral sphincter contraction. Reducing contraction of the external anal sphincter might also serve to improve defecation, because feces, being more viscous than urine, are more difficult to evacuate in the intervals between bursts of stimulation. Recent research in animals has shown that this may be possible. The lower motor neurons innervating the external urethral and anal sphincters are considerably larger than the parasympathetic fibers supplying the smooth muscle of the bladder and rectal wall. The large fibers are more readily depolarized near a cathode than smaller fibers, and it has usually not been possible to produce contraction of the bladder and rectum without contraction of the external sphincters. However, near an anode the large fibers are also more readily hyperpolarized than smaller fibers. It is thus possible, using a long-duration stimulus, to maintain sufficient hyperpolarization in large fibers at an anode to prevent propagation of action potentials generated at a cathode, while

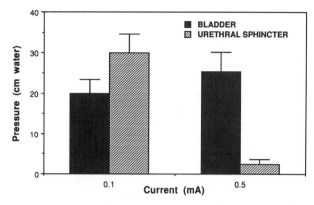

Figure 1. Pressure rise in the bladder and in the urethra at the level of the external sphincter, in response to 20 Hz trains of quasitrapezoidal stimuli of pulse width 500 microsec with exponential falling edge of time-constant 500 microsec, applied to the S2 anterior root unilaterally in acute dog experiment. Note that by increasing the stimulus amplitude to 0.5 mA, the sphincter contraction is blocked.

allowing propagation in smaller fibers to the bladder and rectum. This has been shown in animals to produce contraction of the bladder and rectum with little or no contraction of the external sphincters (Figures 1 and 2). This technique needs to be tested in humans for its ability to produce improved defecation and micturition.

Posterior Rhizotomy

Cutting the posterior sacral roots in patients with a hyperactive detrusor is probably the main reason for the reduction of incontinence. This interven-

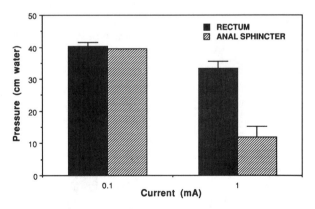

Figure 2. Pressure rise in the rectum and in the anal sphincter, in response to 20 Hz trains of quasitrapezoidal stimuli of pulse width 500 microsec with exponential falling edge of time-constant 500 microsec, applied to the S2 anterior root unilaterally in acute dog experiment. Note that by increasing the stimulus amplitude to 1 mA, the anal sphincter contraction is blocked.

tion is also considered to contribute to low-pressure storage and protection of the upper tracts. Previous experience with sacral rhizotomies was sometimes disappointing; a variety of different of forms of rhizotomy were performed, and often selectively nerve pathways were ablated (Manfredi & Leal, 1968; McGuire & Savastano, 1984; Toczek, McCullough, & Boggs, 1978). It now appears that provided a complete posterior rhizotomy is performed from S2 caudally, the results last at least 10 years and are probably permanent.

SELECTION OF SUBJECTS

This procedure can be considered for individuals with complete SCI at any time after initial rehabilitation, provided the bladder is capable of contracting in response to activity in the parasympathetic efferent fibers of the sacral anterior roots. A cystometrogram showing strong reflex contractions can provide sufficient evidence for such activity. However, when in doubt, the sacral parasympathetic nerves can be stimulated electrically by placing an electrode in the rectum (Brindley, 1981b) or by inserting needle electrodes via the posterior sacral foramina (Schmidt, Senn, & Tanagho, 1990).

Individuals with incomplete SCI should probably wait until at least 18 months after injury to allow any spontaneous recovery of function to occur. Thereafter it is important to determine whether the implant is likely to cause pain; pain sensation in the sacral dermatomes should be tested not only by pinprick of the sacral dermatomes but also by rectal probe electrical stimulation. Special implants are available for some individuals with preserved pain sensation (Brindley, 1991). If a person with preserved pain sensation agrees to undergo posterior rhizotomy, it is unlikely that the implant will cause pain.

The best subjects for the procedure are women with complete paraplegia, particularly those who are incontinent because of hyperactive bladder contractions. These women can become continent by posterior rhizotomy, and the stimulator then provides a method of voiding that is more convenient and probably less prone to infection than IC. Men with complete paraplegia are also suitable, but some may have reservations about the loss of reflex erection and reflex ejaculation entailed by posterior rhizotomy, even though other methods of producing erection and seminal emission are available.

Tetraplegic men have also benefited from the procedure, particularly in terms of reduction of infection, improvement of bowel function, and the abolition by posterior rhizotomy of autonomic dysreflexia. Those with higher levels of tetraplegia sometimes choose to continue to wear a condom and leg-bag to reduce the need to transfer to a toilet seat, in which case any improvement in continence is less of an asset.

Tetraplegic women who are incontinent because of a hyperreflexic bladder can be made continent by posterior rhizotomy. However, they will then need to decide which method of emptying the bladder will be best for them. The stimulator can be implanted if the person is able to use a urine collection device or to transfer to a toilet seat; otherwise a method such as IC may be used for voiding.

A few individuals with multiple sclerosis have benefited from the procedure; success, however, is dependent on the nature of neurological deficits and the motivation of the individual. Adults with myelomeningocele above the level of the sacral segments may also be able to benefit from this technology, but in children with spina bifida, there are likely to be difficulties associated with growth.

The device as sold in Great Britain cost approximately £1500 in 1994, to which must be added the costs of investigation and admission for surgery. A study by the Dutch government has indicated that, when the device is used under a research protocol, it is likely to pay for itself within 8 years (P.E.V. Van Kerrebroeck, personal communication, 1994). In clinical practice this period may be shorter.

CONCLUSIONS

Clinical Trials with Existing Technology

Clinical experience with approximately 1,000 cases in Europe since 1976 provides evidence of the safety and effectiveness of the device for improving bladder and bowel emptying in individuals with SCI. It appears that the combination of implantation with posterior rhizotomy is able to reduce the prevalence of ureteric reflux and hydronephrosis; the results of a large clinical study in Germany are expected to confirm these findings (D. Sauerwein, personal communication, 1994).

To improve both bladder and bowel management, further clinical research is needed

1. To allow bowel emptying to be produced in a higher proportion of individuals
2. To confirm the effects of complete posterior sacral rhizotomy alone (e.g., to provide continence to tetraplegic women who do not wish to void with the stimulator)
3. To investigate the relative merits of extradural and intradural approaches to implantation
4. To investigate the application of this technique to individuals with other diagnoses

Development of Further Technology

It has long been a goal of research in this area to produce contraction of the bladder and bowel without contraction of the external sphincters. Now that this has been demonstrated, it will be important to determine whether the interventions described in this chapter can be used to increase the proportion of individuals able to defecate using electrical stimulation and to produce continuous-stream micturition at low voiding pressures. Anodal block may also be applied to posterior sacral roots for selective activation and block of different sizes of afferent fibers. This might be used to initiate useful reflexes for voiding and continence and, potentially, to avoid posterior rhizotomy.

These attempts may require improved electrodes capable of accurate control of the electric field, and digitally controlled implanted stimulators capable of accurate production of refined stimulus waveforms.

The pursuit of clinical and technical research in parallel is likely to lead to useful collaboration and productive synergy.

REFERENCES

Arnold, E.P., Gowland, S.P., MacFarlane, M.R., Bean, A.R., & Utley, W.L. (1986). Sacral anterior root stimulation of the bladder in paraplegics. *Australian and New Zealand Journal of Surgery, 56*(4), 319–324.

Binnie, N.R., Smith, A.N., Creasey, G.H., & Edmond, P. (1990). Motility effects of electrical anterior sacral nerve root stimulation of the paraplegic supply of the left colon and anorectum in paraplegic subjects. *Journal of Gastrointestinal Motility, 2,* 12–17.

Binnie, N.R., Smith, A.N., Creasey, G.H., & Edmond, P. (1991). Constipation associated with chronic spinal cord injury: The effect of pelvic parasympathetic stimulation by the Brindley stimulator. *Paraplegia, 29*(7), 463–469.

Brindley, G.S. (1981a). A grommet for preventing cerebrospinal fluid from leaking along the outside of implanted tubes and cables. *Journal of Physiology, 320,* 1P.

Brindley, G.S. (1981b). Electroejaculation: Its technique, neurological implications and uses. *Journal of Neurology, Neurosurgery, and Psychiatry, 44,* 9–18.

Brindley, G.S. (1991). *The Finetech-Brindley bladder controller: Notes for surgeons and physicians.* Welwyn Garden City, Hertfordshire, England: Finetech Ltd.

Brindley, G.S., Polkey, C.E., Rushton, D.N., & Cardozo, L. (1986). Sacral anterior root stimulators for bladder control in paraplegia: The first 50 cases. *Journal of Neurology, Neurosurgery, and Psychiatry, 49*(10), 1104–1114.

Brindley, G.S., & Rushton, D.N. (1990). Long-term follow-up of patients with sacral anterior root stimulator implants. *Paraplegia, 28*(8), 469–475.

Cardozo, L., Krishnan, K.R., Polkey, C.E., Rushton, D.N., & Brindley, G.S. (1984). Urodynamic observations on patients with sacral anterior root stimulators. *Paraplegia, 22*(4), 201–209.

Colombel, P., & Egon, G. (1991). Electrostimulation of the anterior sacral nerve roots. An International Congress—Le Mans—24–25 November 1989. *Annals of Urology Paris, 25*(1), 48–52.

Creasey, G.H. (1993). Electrical stimulation of sacral roots for micturition after spinal cord injury. *Urology Clinics of North America, 20*(3), 505–515.

Levin, R.J., & MacDonagh, R.P. (1993). Increased vaginal blood flow induced by implant electrical stimulation of sacral anterior roots in the conscious woman: A case study. *Archives of Sexual Behavior, 22*(5), 471–475.

MacDonagh, R.P., Sun, W.M., Smallwood, R., Forster, D., & Read, N.W. (1990). Control of defecation in patients with spinal injuries by stimulation of sacral anterior nerve roots. *British Medical Journal, 300*(6738), 1494–1497.

Madersbacher, H., Fischer, J., & Ebner, A. (1988). Anterior sacral root stimulator (Brindley): Experiences especially in women with neurogenic urinary incontinence. *Neurourology and Urodynamics, 7,* 593–601.

Manfredi, R., & Leal, J. (1968). Selective sacral rhizotomy for the spastic bladder syndrome in patients with spinal cord injuries. *Journal of Urology, 100,* 17–20.

McGuire, E., & Savastano, J. (1984). Urodynamic findings and clinical status following vesical denervation procedures for control of continence. *Journal of Urology, 132,* 87–88.

Rushton, D.N., Brindley, G.S., Polkey, C.E., & Browning, G.V. (1989). Implant infections and antibiotic-impregnated silicone rubber coating. *Journal of Neurology, Neurosurgery, and Psychiatry, 52*(2), 223–229.

Sauerwein, D. (1990). Surgical treatment of spastic bladder paralysis in paraplegic patients: Sacral de-afferentation with implementation of a sacral anterior root stimulator. *Urologe A, 29,* 196–203.

Schmidt, R., Senn, E., & Tanagho, E. (1990). Functional evaluation of sacral nerve root integrity. *Urology, 35*(5), 388–392.

Toczek, S., McCullough, D., & Boggs, J. (1978). Sacral rootlet rhizotomy at the conus medullaris for hypertonic neurogenic bladder. *Journal of Neurosurgery, 48,* 193–196.

Van Kerrebroeck, P.E.V. (1993). *Clinical and experimental aspects of bladder stimulation in spinal cord injury* (Chapter 9, p. 125). Unpublished thesis. Catholic University, Nijmegen, the Netherlands.

Van Kerrebroeck, P.E.V., Koldewijn, E.L., & Debruyne, F.M.J. (1993). Worldwide experience with the Finetech-Brindley sacral anterior root stimulator. *Neurourology and Urodynamics, 12*(5), 497–503.

Van Kerrebroeck, P.E.V., Koldewijn, E.L., Wijkstra, H., & Debruyne, F.M.J. (1992). Urodynamic evaluation before and after intradural posterior sacral rhizotomies and implantation of the Finetech-Brindley anterior sacral root stimulator. *Urodinamica, 1,* 7–16.

PHYSICAL FITNESS AND WELL-BEING

Lynn H. Gerber

The following section on physical fitness in women with disabilities addresses several important issues. With great energy and insight, the authors describe various aspects of fitness and well-being. Turk (Chapter 30) raises the concern that our treatments must be specific to the individual and must also be selected with full knowledge of the nature of the disease, its natural history, and its influence on the organ and systems pertaining to a particular disability. Hicks (Chapter 31) stresses the need to establish a comprehensive program for rehabilitation. In her work with women with polymyositis, she has learned that exercise to strengthen muscles often must be coupled with range of motion, use of adaptive strategies for energy conservation, and adaptive equipment. Psychological and vocational support are also necessary to maximize outcome. DePauw (Chapter 32) discusses adapted physical activity and sport for women with disabilities. Physical activity is a key element in addressing quality of life issues. Roller (Chapter 33) who has helped to develop a community-based program for persons with disabilities, presents her analysis of the spa program she visited in Germany—a domiciliary program that reaffirms life in all its ramifications, including physical, emotional, aesthetic, and societal. The fundamental goal of the program is to promote health and wellness.

Acknowledgment was made of the importance of outcome measures that would apply to both objective and subjective assessments. It is critical to measure wellness and some of the outcomes that look at comprehensive function. Furthermore, these measures would have to assess a variety of populations; those that might be ethnically diverse, span different ages and life stages, and have a variety of living conditions.

As professionals working with women with disabilities, we have identified four major goals for developing a research agenda:

1. Development of good evaluation and outcome measures for this population. These should be broad-based and not confined to specific

measures of organ systems, but should evaluate the woman in the context of family and environment and society.

2. Identification of the kinds of treatments that are currently used and that need to be developed to promote fitness, good function, and wellness for women with disabilities (and possibly secondarily for children and men as well).

3. Methodical evaluation of the benefits of fitness and exercise in women with disabilities.

4. Identification of the factors that influence the degree of severity of disability or the perception that a disability is severe.

With respect to outcome measures, we all agree that we must be able to measure activity in women with disabilities. What are these women actually doing, and how close do they come to reaching their maximal potential for function based upon multifaceted parameters? The nature of the assessments could be questionnaires or be based on personal interviews and should be highly specific for a given disability. These measures should be sensitive to change over long periods of time and must be validated. They cannot be limited to measuring one or two (even major) organ systems. These outcome measures need to correlate a variety of factors, such as strength/endurance or endurance/function and reported perceptions of disability with some of the more "objective" measures. Furthermore, we need to know whether these measures predict ability to work either at home or outside of the home and how they correlate with important roles throughout the life span.

Treatment must be selected in accordance with the individual and her specific needs. These may change throughout the life span, as women age and their biology changes, but also as they pass through developmental stages (girlhood, adolescence, young adulthood, middle age, later years) and concomitant roles. In addition to age and developmental stages, we must be aware of the severity and chronicity of the disability, both of which are likely to moderate treatment efficacy. Because we know very little about how to sequence treatments and how to gauge when individuals may be most receptive and responsive to interventions, these treatments need to be evaluated. For example, in the woman with severe disabilities, should aerobic conditioning precede specific muscle strengthening exercises or vice versa? Which exercises and in which sequences promote the perception of progress and empowerment and enhance wellness and fitness? The woman with severe disabilities is often forgotten. This population should be targeted for study. How do we promote fitness in someone who cannot move? Does stress—physiological stress—promote fitness? Does pleasuring or sexual stimulation? After all, these activities do accelerate heart rate.

Measuring the impact of exercise on the woman with a disability should include anatomically based, individually based, and societally based measures. We need to challenge long-held beliefs that may actually be myths based on insufficient data. We should target some of our efforts to the three biggest life-threatening illnesses—cancer, heart disease, and stroke—in addition to the two most common disabling illnesses—osteoporosis and arthritis. What are the benefits of promoting fitness for women with disabilities? Does fitness or wellness produce secondary prevention strategies? Do we reduce comorbidities as a result of fitness and wellness programs? Does fitness in persons with disabilities convey some benefits that we can introduce to the general population? For example, does fitness improve disease resistance, help in recovery from viral disease or cancer, or otherwise affect the immune system and its regulation? Is early intervention a critical component to fitness and promotion of well-being in persons with disabilities, or is timing through the disability spectrum important in terms of early, middle, and late interventions? Are the strategies different at each stage of disability?

Finally, research is desperately needed to determine which factors influence disability or the perception of severity of disability. Many of these influences have been touched upon in other sections of this book, including age of onset of disability, stage in life, severity, chronicity, premorbid status, social network and supports, economic status, life values, and coping strategies, to name a few.

The writers in this section affirm the view that evaluations and interventions should be connected to reports of well-being, fitness, and empowerment. At the same time, these interventions should measure activity that is traditionally valued by individuals and society at work, home, or school. Fitness must be seen in the broadest possible context and must be related to performance. In addition, research should target specific populations among women with disabilities, including those with severe disabilities and minority women. As an adjunct to these efforts, consumer participation in research activity is appropriate. The level of participation could be at the collaborator or initiator level, as well as at the advisory level. We would like to see more women with disabilities in an advisory capacity to grant applicants and, for those who are qualified, to participate in the peer review process. Program evaluation and dissemination of results of supported research must be built into programs designed to measure or promote fitness, activity, and well-being in women with disabilities.

chapter 30

The Impact of Disability on Fitness in Women

Musculoskeletal Issues

Margaret A. Turk

Fitness indicates an optimal state of physical well-being; the term seldom appears in scientific or lay publications in reference to women with disabilities. With regard to musculoskeletal issues, fitness is defined by the measurable components of exercise and body composition. Musculoskeletal issues include osteoporosis and performance capability over the lifetime. The effect of exercise on persons with disabilities has become a popular topic of interest for research, publication, and practical application. Although the availability of information regarding exercise for persons with disabilities is increasing, information specifically pertaining to women is scant.

This chapter outlines the components of fitness and the benefits of exercise for persons with disabilities. Information from published literature provides a basis for understanding the role of exercise for women with disabilities. Suggested research areas are noted, including health promotion.

COMPONENTS OF FITNESS

The components of fitness related to exercise include flexibility, muscular strength and endurance, and cardiopulmonary conditioning. Flexibility refers to the range of motion around a joint, determined by bony structures and soft tissue elasticity. Stretching programs have become a strong component of exercise programs, with research data showing improved concentric contraction velocities and a decrease in overuse injuries (Saal, 1993). However, there are no data to promote flexibility to improve coordinated movements (O'Toole & Douglas, 1994). With regard to persons with disabilities, flexibility is a strategy used to manage spasticity. Anecdotally, persons with disabilities report that stretching exercises help to decrease the discomfort of spasticity, provide a short-lived decrease in episodes of spasticity, and allow better performance. However, no research data have been published to support these observations.

Strength is the maximal force generated by a muscle and can be static/isometric (force exerted against an essentially immovable object with no muscle length change) or dynamic/isotonic/isokinetic (various amounts of force or changes in muscle length). Dynamic strength can involve concentric contractions (shortening contraction with acceleration) and eccentric contractions (lengthening contractions with deceleration). Muscular endurance is the ability to continue an activity, and it relies on aerobic and anaerobic capacities. Muscle strength and endurance are related, but there is no evidence that endurance increases as strength increases. There is, however, a strong correlation between strength and ability to perform work (deLateur & Lehmann, 1990). Fatigue is a decrement in performance because of previous activities. The physiological endpoint is related to the contractile process, oxygen consumption, and therefore energy utilization. The concepts of strength, endurance, and fatigue have been determined through research, mainly in male subjects without disabilities. Women can improve their strength and endurance through training; however, women develop significantly less muscle hypertrophy than is noted in men.

Cardiopulmonary conditioning results in increased capacity of the heart and lungs to utilize and distribute oxygen, that is, increased maximal aerobic capacity. Important factors involved in this conditioning are maximal oxygen consumption (VO_2 max: maximum rate of O_2 utilization based on cardiac output, pulmonary function, and peripheral biochemical factors), mitochondrial density (cell-level organs involved in energy increases with endurance training in muscle fibers), performance efficiency (involves metabolic efficiency and technique), and body composition. Both women and men can improve their cardiopulmonary status, but sex-determined physiological differences influence performance in complex ways. Studies in populations without disabilities show that women's performance times are slower than men's in endurance sports events (Fahey, 1994).

Any discussion of fitness and exercise must include a discussion of training. Effective training induces a metabolic challenge to the system and results in an adaptive response to that challenge. Early improvements noted in exercise performance are related to improved coordination and synchronization of motor units. Additional performance improvements develop in the months after initiation of an exercise program, as a result of cellular adaptive changes. Because there is some specificity in the response to exercise (deLateur & Lehmann, 1990), the training program should reflect the desired improved performance capability. In choosing strengthening programs, it is important to note that improved isometric strength does not necessarily improve activities that require dynamic strength. However, exercise programs must be designed to consider existing pathology or disease states. In determining an activity or exercise program, issues of intensity (resistance) and rate (repetitions) must be considered. In the absence of time or motivational restraints, it is more effective to pace to fatigue, but is more efficient to continue to fatigue without a rest cycle (deLateur & Lehmann, 1990). It is also important to note that once improvements have been achieved with exercise, an ongoing maintenance exercise program is required to preserve gains.

For persons with disabilities, there are function-specific issues that apply to training programs. It has long been generally accepted that persons with disabilities who propel their wheelchairs or walk with crutches have significant strength and endurance, based on the exercise benefit of these tasks. These tasks obviously require more energy—that is, they are less efficient than is comparable standard gait. However, although these individuals may have the strength and endurance to perform that specific task, they do not develop general fitness from it. The body develops efficient means to perform the modified mobility, and the individuals are usually unable to routinely stress their motor system any more than can an unfit person without a disability. Therefore, despite facing daily tasks that require more energy than comparable tasks by individuals without disabilities, persons with disabilities need to consider exercise and activity programs as a means of maintaining a healthy fitness status. Exercise programs (acute rehabilitation, developmental programs, maintenance programs) should be designed to accomplish specific short- and long-term benefits and to recognize the risks of certain activities. It should also be remembered that the principles of exercise have been established through research involving mostly male subjects without disabilities. Although some generalizations can be made, some specific gender- and disability-based differences exist. Persons who have sustained spinal cord injuries (SCIs) have altered autonomic nervous system function; cardiac and peripheral vascular responses to endurance activities will be limited (Weber, 1993). Overwork weakness, although not a well-understood concept, should be avoided in persons who have weakness secondary to neuromuscular diagnoses (e.g., polio, Guillain-Barré syndrome, muscular dystrophies) (Milner-Brown & Miller, 1989). The exercise design must consider that persons with disabilities may have limited access to routine exercise sites, particularly persons with significant motor impairments. Most health clubs and exercise equipment are inaccessible. Lifetime physical therapy does not promote self-direction for persons with disabilities and has not been shown to be an effective strategy to maintain function for persons with lifelong disabilities. Attitudinal barriers may also limit women with disabilities' access to exercise. There are no studies showing specific outcome information to direct exercise in persons who have severe motor impairment.

BENEFITS OF EXERCISE

The benefits of exercise and activity have been noted throughout this book. Known physical benefits for women to exercise are similar to those for men and include improved aerobic capacity, improved performance, improved cardiovascular responses (heart rate, blood pressure), improved weight control, modified aging responses (less age-related decline in peak performance and maximal aerobic capacity), and possible prevention of osteoporosis in certain circumstances (O'Toole & Douglas, 1994). Improvement in psychological health and quality of life are also reported. Exercise is suspected to contribute to prevention of coronary artery disease (Haskell, 1984) and in promoting longevity.

Some of the aforementioned benefits may apply to women with physical disabilities, but specific information is lacking. However, there is a positive relationship between physical fitness and gainful employment for persons with paraplegia (Noreau & Shephard, 1992).

DISABILITY-SPECIFIC ISSUES

A literature review (1986–1995) suggests that, although the number of studies reported are limited, there is a growing interest in exercise for persons with disabilities. Studies of individuals with mild to moderate impairments tended to report similar physiological and psychological benefits for persons with disabilities as are noted for persons without disabilities. Some reports suggested activity and exercise strategies for specific disability groups. Women were represented in most studies reporting gender, and they were the majority of study subjects in arthritis studies. Women were less well represented in study populations of persons who sustained SCIs. There were no studies that evaluated exercise in a group with severe motor impairments, and there were no studies about attitudinal issues for women, their support systems, or their health care providers regarding participation in exercise programs.

Neuromuscular Diseases

Strengthening exercise protocols for persons with neuromuscular diseases can be found in the literature. Traditionally, persons with progressive diseases have been advised against active exercise. Newer studies have changed this concept, although limited activity for very weak muscles is still advocated. Study groups in this research topic are small, with women subjects participating.

Studies using defined exercise protocols have been reported for small groups for specific etiologies, including persons with fascioscapulohumeral muscular dystrophy, myotonic dystrophy, Becker muscular dystrophy, limb-girdle muscular dystrophy, spinal muscular dystrophy, and idiopathic polyneuropathy. Improved muscle strength was objectively noted in exercise programs of high-resistance weight training (Milner-Brown & Miller, 1988), low-resistance weight training with electrical stimulation (Milner-Brown & Miller, 1988), and moderate-resistance weight training (Aitkens, McCrory, Kilmer, & Bernauer, 1993). These reports pertain only to individuals with slowly progressive forms of the disease, and they recommend that muscles that are greater than 15% of normal strength be exercised. Persons with mild to moderate myasthenia gravis also showed objective strength improvement in a moderate, progressive exercise program (Lohi, Lindberg, & Anderson, 1993). No functional measures were used in the studies to determine effect on daily activities. Subjective reports were of improved endurance and general well-being. No long-term studies have been reported. Hicks (Chapter 31) details an exercise protocol for persons with inflammatory myopathy.

Fatigue is the limiting factor in prescription of exercise for persons with neuromuscular diseases. Overwork weakness (overuse) has been difficult to analyze, but is better understood using maximal voluntary force, calculated fatigue indices, and recovery time to previous strength level (Milner-Brown, Mellenthin, & Miller, 1986). Persons with neurogenic weakness fatigue more quickly than their counterparts without disabilities (Milner-Brown & Miller, 1989). Consequently, exercise programs should be designed that incorporate this principle.

Late Effects of Polio

Persons who had polio have reported problems with increasing weakness, fatigue, and pain as they age. Reasons for these sequelae continue to be sought, but there is a growing belief that disuse, overuse (overwork weakness), and weight gain contribute to these complaints (Agre, Rodriquez, & Tafel, 1991). Strengthening and conditioning exercises are now promoted for polio survivors to improve their functioning and well-being.

Exercise protocols for persons many years after their acute illness have included "nonfatiguing" exercise (Feldman & Soskolne, 1987), high-resistance, short-duration exercise (Einarsson, 1991; Milner-Brown, 1993), and high-resistance, low-repetition exercise (Perry, Young, & Barnes, 1987). Upper-extremity aerobic training has also been reported for cardiopulmonary conditioning (Kriz et al., 1992). All studies showed improvement in parameters tested. Functional measures for improved outcome were not reported other than subjective responses of improved performance.

Again, fatigue is an important factor. Paced intermittent isometric activity has been recommended to avoid fatigue effects (Agre & Rodriquez, 1991).

Spinal Cord Pathology

Past discussions of exercise for persons with paraplegia or quadriplegia have been in the context of rehabilitation following the acute injury or as developmental activities for children with congenital spinal cord pathology (spina bifida). Persons living with SCI, whether for years or for a lifetime, note pain, fatigue, weight gain, or changes in function (Dunne, Gingher, Olsen, & Shurtleff, 1984; Gerhart, Berstrom, Sharlifue, Menter, & Whiteneck, 1993). They have more musculoskeletal complaints, particularly related to shoulders (Sie, Waters, Adkins, & Gellman, 1992) and there is conflicting information regarding whether activity or inactivity is a cause for pain (Bayley, Cochran, & Sledge, 1987; Wylie & Chakera, 1988). More recent research in exercise has been directed toward postinjury exercise or newer techniques of exercise. Studies cited are those that included women participants.

In the literature, strengthening exercises for persons with incomplete quadriplegia (at least 1 year postinjury) have been evaluated by comparing traditional supervised therapy and two newer exercise techniques: neuromuscular stimulation and electromyographic feedback (Klose et al., 1990). Improvement was found for all three modalities in strength, self-care, and mobility following this 16-week training program, suggesting that postacute rehabilitation exercise is valuable. Strengthening exercises in SCI directed toward improving expiratory muscles as a means of prevention for pneumonia showed improved strength, but no documentation of effectiveness as a prevention strategy (Roth, Oken, Primack, Fisher, & Powley, 1990).

Conditioning programs for persons with SCI have traditionally used upper limb ergometry. Improvements in fitness have been noted for persons with paraplegia (Davis, 1993). Although improvements are noted for persons with quadriplegia (Whiting, Dreisinger, & Dalton, 1983), upper limb exercise unfortunately can provide only limited forces to improve cardiopulmonary conditioning significantly. More attention has been paid to functional neuromuscular stimulation (FNS) in quadriplegia as a means of exercising for cardiopulmonary conditioning, using paralyzed muscles. SCI also modifies responses to exercise: Cardiac response is lower (heart rate, cardiac output); blood pressure responses can be erratic in quadriplegia; extremity venous return is decreased; and lack of sweating in quadriplegia below the level of the lesion limits temperature control and thus exercise (Weber, 1993). These limited responses also limit the training response.

However, FNS has been shown to improve aerobic capacity and to be a relatively safe mode of exercise training (Pollack, Haas, & Ragnarsson, 1986; Pollock et al., 1989; Hooker et al., 1990). FNS in combination with arm ergometry increases the conditioning response in quadriplegia (Figoni, 1993). Long-term effectiveness in changing function or health outcome has not been established.

Brain Injury

For purposes of this chapter, we define brain injury as traumatic onset at any age (TBI), congenital onset (cerebral palsy [CP]), mental retardation (MR), or stroke. Persons with brain injury may exhibit motor impairment with or without some degree of cognitive impairment. The motor impairment may include a spastic (increased tone) component, an involuntary movement disorder, incoordination and/or balance problems, low muscle tone (hypotonia), and inability to initiate or maintain muscle contraction. The motor impairment may require use of a wheelchair, braces or walking aids or may not require assistive devices for mobility. The degree of the motor impairment can limit the use of exercise equipment. Cognitive issues are important in exercise programs for safety reasons and motor planning ability to use existing exercise equipment. Because of the wide variation in motor function and the possibility of other associated conditions, information regarding exercise is often difficult to generalize to a broadly recognized disability group.

The presence of significant spasticity leads many health professionals to avoid recommending strengthening programs. When recommended, the design emphasizes isolated muscle group activities for strengthening in order to strengthen antagonist muscles to oppose the spastic movements and to avoid triggering abnormal muscle movements (Laskowski, 1994). In hypotonic individuals, the recommendation is often to push strengthening exercises. There is no objective experimental evidence to support or refute either of these theoretically derived strategies.

Persons with CP have demonstrated a lower physical work capacity than their peers without disabilities (Lundberg, 1978; Fernandez, Pitetti, & Bentzen, 1990), and they require more energy for ambulation (Rose, Medeiros, & Parker, 1985). Deconditioned states are also documented for persons after TBI (Jankowski & Sullivan, 1990) and with MR (Fernhall, Tymeson, Millar, & Burkett, 1989). Cardiopulmonary function has been measured using a variety of equipment, including treadmills, bike ergometers, wheelchair ergometers, and arm ergometers. Training programs have been effective for persons with CP (Fernandez & Pitetti, 1993), MR (Schurrer, Weltman, & Brammel, 1985), TBI (Jankowski & Sullivan, 1990), and stroke (Potempa et al., 1995).

Arthritis

The arthritis disability group involves persons with noninflammatory arthritis and inflammatory arthritis. The inflammatory group often has other systemic manifestations that must be considered in discussions of exercise and are beyond the scope of this chapter. For purposes of this chapter, osteoarthritis (OA) and rheumatoid arthritis (RA) are used as representative groups. Population surveys indicate that in people 45 years and older, women are more often and more severely affected by OA. The general prevalence of RA is two to three times higher in women than in men (Hicks & Gerber, 1993).

Muscle strength and conditioning are decreased at least in part because of inactivity secondary to joint pain and deformities. Fitness can be compromised by systemic manifestations of a connective tissue disease (RA) as well as inactivity. Exercise programs are tailored to the individual medical and mechanical joint-related needs. Goals target improving function through a progressive program. During acute exacerbations, pain relief and limited joint movements are emphasized (isometric exercises). In general, progressive resistive exercises and isokinetic exercises are not recommended for persons with arthritis because of the stresses placed on the joint. Instead, low-weight, low-intensity prolonged exercise taken to fatigue is recommended to increase muscle strength and endurance and to avoid joint pain (deLateur & Lehmann, 1990). Limitation in the number of repetitions is also recommended. An isokinetic program for persons with mild OA and RA was suggested to be safe (Hicks & Gerber, 1993). Progressive home strengthening programs have been effective in increasing strength and function in women with OA (Fisher, Pendergast, & Gresham, 1990), and the benefits have remained for up to 2 years following completion of the exercise program in 55% of women (Fisher & Pendergast, 1992). Aerobic exercises have been shown to increase aerobic capacity in persons with OA and RA (Minor, Hewett, Webel, Anderson, & Kay, 1989).

Aerobic cardiopulmonary conditioning activities (biking, swimming, gardening) accompanied by dynamic low-repetition, low-resistance isotonic exercise (light weights through a short arc of motion) can produce improved strength and conditioning. Individually adapted training programs have proven successful for elderly persons with RA on steroids, with no increase in disease or joint manifestations (Lynberg, Harreby, Bentzen, Frost, & Danneskiold-Samsoe, 1994).

Other exercise or activity programs that have been beneficial for persons with arthritis include aquatic therapy (McNeal, 1990), recreational exercise (Hicks & Gerber, 1993), dance (Van Duesen & Harlowe, 1987), and low-impact aerobics (Hicks & Gerber, 1993).

Multiple Sclerosis

Multiple sclerosis (MS) is more prevalent in women and usually is progressive with changing constellations of impairments and disabilities. The principle motor impairment can vary among spasticity, ataxia, fatigability, deconditioning, and weakness. Issues of fatigue, heat intolerance, and abnormal autonomic nervous system responses (heart rate, blood pressure, sweating) must be taken into account when considering exercise programs. Consequently, time of day, temperature of exercise room or pool, and clothing used during exercise must be considered (Cobble, Dietz, Grigsby, & Kennedy, 1993).

Research data have shown that persons with mild MS may have similar responses to exercise as their peers without disabilities (Ponchitera-Mulcare, 1993) and that in general exercise can improve muscle performance (Gehlsen, Grigsby, & Winant, 1984). Persons with MS can participate in conditioning programs, and those with a more significant disability and who exercised for shorter periods achieved a lower intensity and lower maximal oxygen uptake (Shapiro, Petajan, Kosich, Molk, & Feeney, 1988). The incorporation of rest intervals in exercise programs has been recommended (Brar & Wangaard, 1985).

Osteoporosis in Disability

Osteoporosis is a recognized health problem for women without disabilities and is not covered in this chapter. Secondary osteoporosis related to immobility is likely to be an issue for women with motor impairments. There are few published data regarding diagnosis and recognition of secondary osteoporosis in disability groups and even less information about interventions (see also Chapter 6).

It is logical that secondary osteoporosis exists in women with motor impairments—they experience a lack or limitation of muscle contraction and mechanical loading, and both factors are known to be required to promote bone formation. There may be other factors producing secondary osteoporosis (medication, lack of estrogen, nutrition) in women with a motor impairment; however, there is no information regarding the combined impact of multiple factors on the degree of osteoporosis.

The literature regarding persons with SCI and osteoporosis is the best developed. In SCI, secondary osteoporosis is believed to represent limited bone density from immobility and dysfunction of the sympathetic nervous system. No intervention is known to reverse the osteoporosis in SCI, unlike that seen in the general population. Fractures of long bones occur as a result of osteoporosis, and there are anecdotal reports that positively relate fracture incidence to exercise. However, in a recent report, the authors reported less-than-expected bone loss following FNS exercise in persons with SCI (Weber, 1993; Hangartner, Rodgers, Glaser, & Barre, 1994). Therefore, there may be a potentially positive effect of FNS exercise in relation to secondary osteoporosis in SCI. No literature supports the traditional strategies of supported standing and non–weight-bearing strengthening activities as effective in preventing this secondary osteoporosis.

CONCLUSIONS

Fitness is a component of health and a feeling of well-being. As has been noted, strengthening and conditioning exercises have been shown to have some beneficial element for women with a variety of disabilities. Recommendations for specific training programs have been noted, taking into account disability-specific risk factors for complications. Benefits have been described in terms of strength and some activity changes, but little information has been offered regarding impact on functional daily activities, general well-being, or health outcome. Reported benefits also are short term and do not reflect the need for maintenance or ongoing programs. Long-term musculoskeletal effects of a motor impairment have been noted; however, the impact of exercise and fitness on these complaints is unknown. Therefore, although there is literature to support some positive effect of exercise in defined conditions in women with disabilities, there are significant gaps in knowledge in the following areas:

1. Outcome measures—Standard exercise outcome measures of increased strength and aerobic capacity need to have better applicability to the function of persons with disabilities. Quality of life issues need to be addressed (handicap measures) as well as impairment and disability measures.
2. Longitudinal studies—Benefits of exercise are reported as short-term effects. Long-term issues, need for maintenance, or the effect of aging (years with a disability) have not been addressed. Age at which to consider beginning training programs and maintenance programs for those with congenital or childhood onset disabilities is not known.
3. Degree of disability—In existing studies, the degree of disability is often not noted. Description of motor impairment (e.g., spasticity, ataxia, incoordination), degree of involvement, and function would improve applicability of information, particularly for persons with brain injury and MS.
4. Attitudinal issues—Women with disabilities have traditionally refrained from exercise. Although there may be attitudinal barriers regarding exercise participation, it can originate with the woman with the disability, her support system, or her health care providers. Knowing how to target education requires knowing where attitudinal changes need to begin.

5. Environmental barriers—Even assuming desire to participate in exercise programs, a person with a disability may have difficulty joining health clubs or using exercise equipment. This may also include lifestyle changes involving transportation. The impact of environmental barriers on exercise participation is unknown.

6. Cross-disability issues—Considering the prevalence of certain disabilities, study groups may be enhanced by bringing disability groups together, based on common issues. This could include gender, age, impairment, lifestyle, or other commonalities. Cross-disability studies may also offer insights into specific disability group responses.

7. Significant motor impairment groups—Women with severe motor impairments have little information regarding their participation in exercise either for fitness or for direct effect of focused exercise (e.g., exercises to improve respiratory muscle strength).

8. Benefits of exercise—Standard muscular and cardiopulmonary benefits have been documented for exercise in some disability groups. However, the more global responses to exercise (psychological) or medically directed benefits (obesity, osteoporosis, relationship to coronary heart disease) need to also be evaluated.

9. Secondary conditions—A secondary condition is an impairment, disability, functional limitation, handicap, or injury that may occur any time throughout the disability continuum. The primary disabling condition can be a risk factor for that condition or may alter the management or prevention strategy used for that condition. For persons with motor impairments (across disabilities), the common complaints that may indicate secondary conditions are pain, fatigue, or changes in function (Seekins, personal communication, 1994). These same complaints have been noted in persons with SCI (Gerhart, Bergstrom, Sharlifue, Menter, & Whiteneck, 1993) and CP (Turk, 1994). The effect that exercise and fitness may have on these complaints either as prevention or intervention strategies is unknown.

10. Health promotion—The level of fitness, exercise, and activity participation may have an effect on long-term function and quality of life (Shephard, 1991). Aerobic exercise does lead to improved fitness (Santiago, Coyle, & Kinney, 1993). Exercise may also be a prevention strategy for onset of secondary conditions (Turk, 1994). However, there need to be longitudinal studies to evaluate exercise or recreational activity programs as prevention strategies.

REFERENCES

Agre, J.C., & Rodriquez, A.A. (1991). Intermittent isometric activity: Its effect on muscle fatigue in postpolio subjects. *Archives of Physical Medicine and Rehabilitation, 72,* 971–975.

Agre, J.C., Rodriquez, A.A., & Tafel, J.A. (1991). Late effects of polio: Critical review of the literature on neuromuscular function. *Archives of Physical Medicine and Rehabilitation, 72*, 923–931.

Aitkens, S.G., McCrory, M.A., Kilmer, D.D., & Bernauer, E.M. (1993). Moderate resistance exercise program: Its effect in slowly progressive neuromuscular disease. *Archives of Physical Medicine and Rehabilitation, 74*, 711–715.

Bayley, J.C., Cochran, T.P., & Sledge, C.B. (1987). The weight-bearing shoulder. The impingement syndrome in paraplegics. *Journal of Bone and Joint Surgery (U.S.), 69*, 676–678.

Brar, S.P., & Wangaard, C. (1985). Physical therapy for patients with multiple sclerosis. In F.P. Maloney, J.B. Burks, & S.P. Ringel (Eds.), *Interdisciplinary rehabilitation of multiple sclerosis and neuromuscular disorders* (pp. 364–391). Philadelphia: J.B. Lippincott.

Cobble, N.D., Dietz, M.A., Grigsby, J., & Kennedy, P.M. (1993). Rehabilitation of the patient with multiple sclerosis. In J.A. DeLisa (Ed.), *Rehabilitation medicine: Principles and practice* (2nd ed., pp. 861–885). Philadelphia: W.B. Saunders.

Davis, G.M. (1993). Exercise capacity of individuals with paraplegia. *Medicine and Science in Sports and Exercise, 25*(4), 423–432.

deLateur, B.J., & Lehmann, J.F. (1990). Therapeutic exercise to develop strength and endurance. In F.J. Kottke, G.K. Stilwell, & J.F. Lehman (Eds.), *Krusen's handbook of physical medicine and rehabilitation* (4th ed., pp. 480–519). Philadelphia: W.B. Saunders.

Dunne, K.B., Gingher, N., Olsen, L.M., & Shurtleff, D.B. (1984). *A survey of the medical and functional status of members of the adult network of the Spina Bifida Association of America.* Unpublished manuscript.

Einarsson, G. (1991). Muscle conditioning in late poliomyelitis. *Archives of Physical Medicine and Rehabilitation, 72*, 11–14.

Fahey, T.D. (1994). Endurance training. In M.M. Shangold & G. Mirkin (Eds.), *Women and exercise: Physiology and sports medicine* (2nd ed., pp. 73–88). Philadelphia: F.A. Davis.

Feldman, R.M., & Soskolne, C.L. (1987). The use of non-fatiguing strengthening exercise in post-polio syndrome. *Birth Defects, 23*, 335–341.

Fernandez, J.E., & Pitetti, K.H. (1993). Training of ambulatory individuals with cerebral palsy. *Archives of Physical Medicine and Rehabilitation, 74*, 468–472.

Fernandez, J.E., Pitetti, K.H., & Bentzen, M.T. (1990). Physiological capacities of individuals with cerebral palsy. *Human Factors, 32*(4), 457–466.

Fernhall, B., Tymeson, G.T., Millar, A.L., & Burkett, L.N. (1989). Cardiovascular fitness testing and fitness levels of adolescents and adults with mental retardation including Down syndrome. *Education and Training in Mental Retardation, 24*, 133–138.

Figoni, S.F. (1993). Exercise responses and quadriplegia. *Medicine and Science in Sports and Exercise, 25*(4), 433–441.

Fisher, N.M., & Pendergast, D.R. (1992). Two-year follow-up of the effects of muscle rehabilitation in patients with osteoarthritis of the knees [Abstract]. *Archives of Physical Medicine and Rehabilitation, 73*, 972.

Fisher, N.M., Pendergast, D.R., & Gresham, G.E. (1990). Progressive, quantitative rehabilitation of patients with osteoarthritis [Abstract]. *Archives of Physical Medicine and Rehabilitation, 71*, 762.

Gehlsen, G.M., Grigsby, S.A., & Winant, D.M. (1984). Effects of an aquatic fitness program on the muscular strength and endurance of patients with multiple sclerosis. *Physical Therapy, 64*, 653–657.

Gerhart, K.A., Bergstrom, E., Sharlifue, S.W., Menter, R.R., & Whiteneck, G.G. (1993). Long-term spinal cord injury: Functional changes over time. *Archives of Physical Medicine and Rehabilitation, 74,* 1030–1034.

Hangartner, T.N., Rodgers, M.M., Glaser, R.M., & Barre, P.S. (1994). Tibial bone density loss in spinal cord injured patients: Effects of FES exercise. *Journal of Rehabilitation Research and Development, 31*(1), 50–61.

Haskell, W.L. (1984). Cardiovascular benefits and risks of exercise: The scientific evidence. In R.H. Strauss (Ed.), *Sports medicine* (pp. 57–76). Philadelphia: W.B. Saunders.

Hicks, J.E., & Gerber, L.H. (1993). Rehabilitation of the patient with arthritis and connective tissue disease. In J.A. DeLisa (Ed.), *Rehabilitation medicine: Principles and practice* (2nd ed., pp. 1047–1081). Philadelphia: W.B. Saunders.

Hooker, S.P., Figoni, S.F., Glaser, R.M., Rodgers, M.M., Ezenwa, B.N., & Faghri, P.D. (1990). Physiologic responses to prolonged electrically stimulated leg-cycle exercise in the spinal cord injured. *Archives of Physical Medicine and Rehabilitation, 71,* 863–869.

Jankowski, L.W., & Sullivan, S.J. (1990). Aerobic and neuromuscular training: Effect on the capacity, efficiency, and fatigability of patients with traumatic brain injuries. *Archives of Physical Medicine and Rehabilitation, 71,* 500–504.

Klose, K.J., Schmidt, D.L., Needham, B.M., Brucker, B.S., Green, B.A., & Ayyar, D.R. (1990). Rehabilitation therapy for patients with long-term spinal cord injuries. *Archives of Physical Medicine and Rehabilitation, 71,* 659–662.

Kriz, J.L., Jones, D.R., Speirer, J.L., Canine, J.K., Owen, R.R., & Serfass, R.C. (1992). Cardiorespiratory responses to upper extremity aerobic training by postpolio subjects. *Archives of Physical Medicine and Rehabilitation, 73,* 49–54.

Laskowski, E.R. (1994). Rehabilitation of the physically challenged athlete. *Physical Medicine and Rehabilitation Clinics of North America: Sports Medicine, 5*(1), 215–233.

Lohi, E.-L., Lindberg, C., & Anderson, O. (1993). Physical training effects in myasthenia gravis. *Archives of Physical Medicine and Rehabilitation, 74,* 1178–1180.

Lundberg, A. (1978). Maximal aerobic capacity of young people with spastic cerebral palsy. *Developmental Medicine & Child Neurology, 20,* 205–210.

Lynberg, K.K., Harreby, M., Bentzen, H., Frost, B., & Danneskiold-Samsoe, B. (1994). Elderly rheumatoid arthritis patients on steroid treatment tolerate physical training without an increase in disease activity. *Archives of Physical Medicine and Rehabilitation, 75,* 1189–1195.

McNeal, R.L. (1990). Aquatic therapy for patients with rheumatic disease. *Rheumatologic Diseases Clinics of North America: Exercise and Arthritis, 16*(4), 915–929.

Milner-Brown, H.S. (1993). Muscle strengthening in a post polio subject through a high resistance weight-training program. *Archives of Physical Medicine and Rehabilitation, 74,* 1165–1167.

Milner-Brown, H.S., Mellenthin, M., & Miller, R.G. (1986). Quantifying human muscle strength, endurance, and fatigue. *Archives of Physical Medicine and Rehabilitation, 67,* 530–535.

Milner-Brown, H.S., & Miller, R.G. (1988a). Muscle strengthening through electric stimulation combined with low-resistance weights in patients with neuromuscular disorders. *Archives of Physical Medicine and Rehabilitation, 69,* 20–24.

Milner-Brown, H.S., & Miller, R.G. (1988b). Muscle strengthing through high-resistance weight training in patients with neuromuscular disorders. *Archives of Physical Medicine and Rehabilitation, 69,* 14–19.

Milner-Brown, H.S., & Miller, R.G. (1989). Increased muscular fatigue in patients with neurogenic muscle weakness: Quantification and pathophysiology. *Archives of Physical Medicine and Rehabilitation, 70,* 361–366.

Minor, M.A., Hewett, J.E., Webel, R.S., Anderson, S.K., & Kay, D.R. (1989). Efficacy of physical conditioning exercise in patients with rheumatoid arthritis and osteoarthritis. *Arthritis and Rheumatology, 32,* 1396–1405.

Noreau, L., & Shephard, R.J. (1992). Return to work after spinal cord injury: The potential contribution of physical fitness. *Paraplegia, 30,* 563–572.

O'Toole, M.L., & Douglas, P.S. (1994). Fitness: Definition and development. In M.M. Shangold & G. Mirkin (Eds.), *Women and exercise: Physiology and sports medicine* (2nd ed., pp. 3–23). Philadelphia: F.A. Davis.

Perry, J., Young, S., & Barnes, G. (1987). Strengthening exercise for post-polio sequela (abstract). *Archives of Physical Medicine and Rehabilitation, 68,* 660.

Pollack, S., Axen, K., Spielholz, N., Levin, N., Haas, F., & Ragnarsson, K.T. (1989). Aerobic training effects of electrically induced lower extremity exercises in spinal cord injured people. *Archives of Physical Medicine and Rehabilitation, 70,* 214–219.

Pollack, S., Haas, F., & Ragnarsson, K.T. (1986). Endurance training by functional electrical stimulation of muscles paralyzed by spinal cord injury [Abstract]. *Archives of Physical Medicine and Rehabilitation, 67,* 658.

Ponichtera-Mulcare, J.A. (1993). Exercise and multiple sclerosis. *Medicine and Science in Sports and Exercise, 25*(4), 451–465.

Potempa, K., Lopez, M., Braun, L.T., Szidon, P., Fogg, L., & Tincknell, T. (1995). Physiologic outcomes of aerobic exercise training in hemiparetic stroke patients. *Stroke, 26*(1), 101–105.

Rose, J., Medeiros, J.M., & Parker, R. (1985). Energy cost index as an estimate of energy expenditure of cerebral-palsied children during assisted ambulation. *Developmental Medicine & Child Neurology, 27,* 485–490.

Roth, E.J., Oken, J.E., Primack, S., Fisher, M., & Powley, S. (1990). Expiratory muscle training in spinal cord injury: Preliminary results [Abstract]. *Archives of Physical Medicine and Rehabilitation, 71,* 796.

Saal, J. (1993). Rehabilitation of the injured athlete. In J.A. DeLisa (Ed.), *Rehabilitation medicine: Principles and practice* (2nd ed., pp. 1131–1164). Philadelphia: J.B. Lippincott.

Santiago, M.C., Coyle, C.P., & Kinney, W.B. (1993). Aerobic exercise effect on individuals with physical disabilities. *Archives of Physical Medicine and Rehabilitation, 74,* 1192–1198.

Shapiro, R.T., Petajan, J.H., Kosich, D., Molk, B., & Feeney, J. (1988). Role of cardiovascular fitness in multiple sclerosis. *Journal of Neurologic Rehabilitation, 2,* 43–49.

Shephard, R.J. (1991). Benefits of sport and physical activity for the disabled: Implications for the individual and for society. *Scandinavian Journal of Rehabilitation Medicine, 23,* 51–59.

Schurrer, R., Weltman, A., & Brammel, H. (1985). Effects of physical training on cardiovascular fitness and behavior patterns of mentally retarded adults. *American Journal of Mental Deficiency, 90,* 167–170.

Sie, I.H., Waters, R.L., Adkins, R.H., & Gellman, H. (1992). Upper extremity pain in the postrehabilitation spinal cord injured patient. *Archives of Physical Medicine and Rehabilitation, 73,* 44–48.

Turk, M.A. (1994). Attaining and retaining mobility: Clinical issues. In D.J. Lollar (Ed.), *Preventing secondary conditions associated with spina bifida or cerebral palsy: Proceedings and recommendations of a symposium* (pp. 42–53). Washington, DC: Spina Bifida Association of America.

Weber, R.J. (1993). Functional neuromuscular stimulation. In J.A. DeLisa (Ed.), *Rehabilitation medicine: Principles and practice* (2nd ed., pp. 463–476). Philadelphia: J.B. Lippincott.

Whiting, R.B., Dreisinger, T.E., & Dalton, R.B. (1983). Improved physical fitness and work capacity in quadriplegics by wheelchair exercise. *Journal of Cardiac Rehabilitation, 3,* 251–255.

Wylie, E.J., & Chakera, T.M.H. (1988). Degenerative joint abnormalities in patients with paraplegia of duration greater than 20 years. *Paraplegia, 26,* 101–106.

Van Duesen, J., & Harlowe, D. (1987). The efficacy of the ROM dance program for adults with rheumatoid arthritis. *American Journal of Occupational Therapy, 41*(2), 90–95.

chapter 31

Treatment Strategies for Patients with Inflammatory Muscle Disease
A Model for Exercise and Activity

Jeanne E. Hicks

Idiopathic inflammatory myopathy (IIM) represents a progressive and multisystem disease process that affects women more than men, manifests in a variety of ways, and can account for a variety of permanent (and sometimes progressive) disabilities. Thus, various aspects of acute management, rehabilitation, and long-term issues can be incorporated into a model for exercise and activity in a specific disease process. This chapter describes this disease process medically, considers diagnosis and acute medical issues, and outlines comprehensive rehabilitation strategies over the progression of the disease.

CLASSIFICATION OF POLYMYOSITIS AND DERMATOMYOSITIS

Inflammatory muscle disease can be divided into polymyositis (PM) and dermatomyositis (DM). PM is an inflammatory disorder of still unknown etiology that primarily affects skeletal muscle, causing infiltration of inflammatory cells (lymphocytes) into the muscle, degeneration of muscle, and weakness. Secondarily, it may affect other body organs. It occurs by itself or in association with other diseases. DM is inflammatory muscle disease with skin involvement. Primarily, the skin of the face, chest, arms, and hands is involved with a violaceous purple rash. Certain firm diagnostic

The author wishes to acknowledge the assistance of Lula Russell, Rehabilitation Medicine Department, the National Institutes of Health, in the preparation of text, diagrams, and figures associated with this chapter.

criteria must be present to make a definite diagnosis of PM or DM (Table 1). For a diagnosis of PM, three of the first four criteria listed in Table 1 must be present. For a diagnosis of DM, the fifth criteria (skin involvement) must also be present.

The differential diagnosis in this disease is extensive (Plotz, Leff, & Miller, 1993). It is very important to determine the initial diagnosis early. Many of the diseases in the differential diagnosis are amenable to medical management, and PM and DM have a better overall outcome (as noted by Medsger & Oddis, 1994) if diagnosed and treated early in the course of the disease.

The type of PM/DM has a definite impact on the disease prognosis and outcome. Therefore, there is an official classification of the types of PM and DM. These types are as follows: Type I, primary adult idiopathic polymyositis; Type II, primary adult idiopathic dermatomyositis; Type III, PM/DM associated with malignancy; Type IV, PM/DM of childhood; Type V, PM/DM associated with other rheumatic diseases—rheumatoid arthritis (RA), systemic lupus erythematosus (SLE), progressive systemic sclerosis (PSS), Sjögren's syndrome (SS), and mixed connective tissue disease (MCTD); and Type VI, inclusion body myositis (IBM).

Incidence

PM and DM usually have a gender incidence of 2:1—there are twice as many women with this disease as there are men. However, IBM is more common in men and is a slowly progressive disease. In terms of race, there is a 5:1 occurrence ratio, with the disease being 5 times more common among African Americans.

Etiology

Although no definite etiology has yet been established for PM/DM, studies thus far reveal it to be associated with a number of immunological abnormalities on both the cellular and humoral levels. Also, drugs and toxins, infectious agents, and genetic factors have been implicated (Plotz et al., 1993). Diagnosis is made through muscle biopsy, electrodiagnosis laboratory studies and evidence of muscle weakness.

Table 1. Diagnostic criteria for polymyositis/dermatomyositis

Polymyositis
  Symmetrical proximal muscle weakness
  Muscle inflammation by biopsy
  Abnormal electromyogram with small motor unit potentials
  Elevated creatine phosphokinase

Dermatomyositis—need three of the above criteria, plus
  Skin rash (face, chest, hands)

Problems Associated with PM/DM

There are a number of problems associated with PM/DM that affect an individual's mobility, activities of daily living, and ability to work. Hicks (1984) mentions a number of these problems: muscle weakness, decreased range of motion (ROM) of joints, muscle soreness, decreased static endurance of muscle, decreased aerobic capacity, difficulty swallowing, fatigue, arthritis, and skin disease.

MUSCLE WEAKNESS

Muscle weakness is the hallmark of this disease. It occurs in a proximal distribution only in the majority of cases. About 20% of individuals with Types I–IV may have both proximal and distal weakness. According to Dalakas (1992), distal weakness is more common in the IBM subtype and can be present in up to 50% of individuals. The trunk and spinal muscles are also commonly affected and cause problems with posture, balance, and neck control. Involvement of the respiratory muscles can cause decreased lung vital capacities. Interstitial lung disease can occur due to the disease itself or methotrexate. Ocular and face involvement is uncommon. Myocardial involvement has been found to be present in about 35% of patients and includes arrhythmia and pericardial effusions; this also has an impact on endurance.

Muscle atrophy resulting from the disease itself and steroid use is frequently seen, particularly in long-standing disease and in persons with IBM (Figure 1). The atrophy occurs in the proximal and distal muscles of the upper and lower extremities.

Thornton, Egan, Parks, Hicks, and Vargo (1994) have noted that muscle weakness causes specific problems in the hand. Decreased flexor strength leads to decreased ability to close the hand and grasp objects. Intrinsic muscle weakness contributes to the latter problem. Ligamentous laxity causes hyperextension at the proximal interphalangeal joints and some hyperflexion at the distal interphalangeal joints, causing swan neck-like deformities as pronounced as those seen in RA (Figure 2). Forearm extensor weakness leads to decreased wrist extension.

There are also characteristic speech problems due to weakness of the pharyngeal muscles. These include, according to D. Scheib (personal communication, April 1, 1994), weakness of the oral motor area and the tongue, neck muscles, and pharyngeal constrictor muscles. Aspiration of food is rare but can occur in serious cases. We have also seen esophageal dysmotility and reflux.

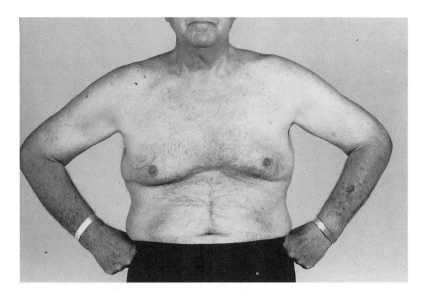

Figure 1. A patient with atrophy of the proximal upper extremity muscles.

JOINT MOTION PROBLEMS

Decreased motion of joints often occurs because of weak muscles and inability to move joints through their full ROM. The joints most commonly affected are the shoulders, elbows, knees, and ankles. In addition, children with DM often have deposits of calcium in the soft tissue around their joints, which are painful and further restrict joint motion. Some persons with PM/DM have arthritis, particularly of the hands, which also restricts joint motion.

Assessment of Function and Disease Activity

Medical tests to assess disease activity include muscle enzyme levels of creatine phosphokinase (CPK) and aldolase, electromyography (EMG), and magnetic resonance imaging (MRI) as described by Fraser, Frank, Dalakas, Miller, and Hicks (1991). Tests of function, such as the Manual Muscle Test (MMT) and activities of daily living (ADL) tests, are also used to assess the activity of the disease. The latter two tests (MMT and ADL), along with the MRI are now considered most useful in assessing disease activity. The MMT and ADL tests are useful in following outcome on drug treatment regimens. Although a muscle biopsy can reveal inflammation, it reveals only a small segment of muscle. The MRI can check for disease activity in entire muscle groups and is also often used to determine the best site for a muscle biopsy.

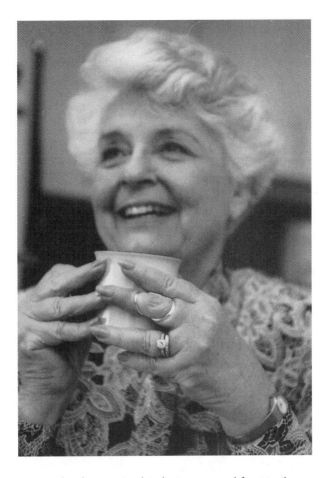

Figure 2.   A patient with polymyositis and PIP hyperextension deformities (hyperextension at the proximal interphalangeal joint and flexion at the distal interphalangeal joint). A Silver Ring Splint® is used in this figure to correct the deformity.

To measure functional deficits in these patients we use some simple measures of assessing joint ROM with goniometric techniques. We use an MMT graded on a 0–5 scale: 0 being no strength and 5 showing full resistance in a full range of motion.

At the National Institutes of Health (NIH) we use an ADL assessment, which is a questionnaire called a modified Convery questionnaire. It contains 14 items in areas of ambulation, dressing, transfers, and reaching. It is graded on a global scale from dependent to independent. We also use some timed tests, timing patients as they get in and out of a chair and dress themselves. This can also be a test of endurance, in addition to strength and mobility of joints.

The MMT correlates well with ADL testing in most PM patients. Hicks et al. (1991) has noted in those patients with significant interstitial lung disease with reduced forced expiratory volume (FEV) and diffusion capacity, causing decreased endurance, correlation with ADL testing is poor. The problem of altered endurance must be considered in functional testing to help facilitate a better correlation between activities and muscle strength.

There are other ways to measure strength besides the MMT. For measuring hand grasp and finger pinch, dynamometry is available. We can also measure endurance of specific muscle groups on a Biodex isokinetic machine as well as the isometric and isokinetic strength (peak torque). Aerobic capacity can be measured by bicycle ergometry.

In our assessment at NIH, we look carefully at the MRIs of muscles because they can tell us a lot about the muscle bulk and inflammation. When a biopsy of a muscle is performed, the picture is focused to a very small section. When an MRI is employed, the ratio of the muscle itself to the fatty and soft tissue is noted. This can provide more general information about disease activity and functional strength. Two patient examples follow:

1. An MRI of a patient with early active PM will show good muscle bulk and little fat and areas of inflammation that show up as white areas. There are also areas of no muscle involvement.
2. An MRI of a patient with chronic IBM shows severe atrophy of muscle (small muscles), with a large soft tissue component around the muscles.

At NIH, Buczek, Leff, Hicks, and Gerber (1994) have studied the gait of a patient in our motion analysis laboratory. Many PM patients fall, particularly the IBM patients, and it is important to determine the cause of their falling. Falls may occur because of a foot clearance problem or a friction problem with the floor surface. Assessment of function is also important in the speech and language pathology area. A number of tests have been developed and quantified to assess oral motor and swallowing function.

Medical Treatment

Treatment first consists of medical management of muscle inflammation. High-dose corticosteroids are the first line of management in PM and DM. Often an immunosuppressive drug such as methotrexate is added to the regimen when the patient is not responding completely to steroids. The addition of methotrexate often allows the reduction of the steroid dose. This is advantageous because steroids are associated with many side effects that can impair the individual's function (myopathy, avascular necrosis of bone, cataracts, and serious life-threatening infections). Other immunosuppressive medication usage has been described by Kagen (1994). These drugs may be associated with fetal abnormalities and infertility. They are sometimes used in combination. In a controlled study, Miller et al. (1992) described leukophoresis, which revealed no benefit over placebo treatment. Immunoglobulin was reported by Dalakas et al. (1993) to result in a significant improvement in some patients with dermatomyositis.

Prognosis

The prognosis of the disease as noted by Medsger and Oddis (1994) and Plotz and Miller (1994) has been linked to certain factors. A poorer prognosis is linked to the presence of malignancy, other connective tissue diseases, pulmonary diseases, dysphagia, severe weakness, older age, delayed treatment, and cardiac involvement. IBM seems to have the worst functional prognosis because of its slow downhill course and resistance to all medical treatments. Presence of certain autoantibodies is also correlated with a poor prognosis in terms of length of survival and disability.

Rehabilitation Treatment

The literature before 1983 had virtually nothing about the rehabilitation management of persons with IIM. Rest seemed to be the most typical advice these patients were given. Exercise was avoided for fear of stressing muscles and exacerbating the inflammatory disease. We now know that persons with IIM need rehabilitation evaluation and interventions—and they need them early in the course of the disease. To delay the course of some interventions, including exercise, is thought to be associated with more disability and poorer response to rehabilitative treatment regimens.

Rehabilitation for persons with IIM involves a comprehensive effort. This effort utilizes a team approach, early intervention, ongoing treatment, periodic reassessment, and patient and family involvement. After a careful assessment of the person's problem, goals and an individualized treatment plan are set up. Main goals may be restorative (return of lost function), maintenance (preserve current function), or preventive (advert functional decline). Most individuals with IIM have some restorative functional goals. Those individuals with significant muscle atrophy may have only maintenance or preventive goals. Specific goals also need to be addressed. Some specific rehabilitation goals for individuals with PM include increasing joint motion and strength, decreasing muscle pain, increasing overall endurance (aerobic capacity), conserving energy, protecting joints, improving gait and mobility, improving ADL, enhancing vocational performance, and promoting self-esteem.

The rehabilitation treatment armamentarium utilized in the management of persons with IIM includes rest; exercise; modalities of heat, cold, and transcutaneous electrical nerve stimulation (TENS) for pain management; assistive devices, adaptive aids, and orthotics; speech therapy; and counseling.

EXERCISE

Stretching exercises and ROM exercises are very important for these individuals. Motion is commonly lost in the shoulder, and an over-the-door pulley system is useful to maintain motion. Studies by Hicks, Miller, Plotz, Chen, and Gerber (1989) at NIH note that in some persons with PM or DM, isometric exercises can significantly improve muscle strength. The program lasts for 1 month, with 3-times-a-week exercise sessions. PM patients with stable active disease and a normal or mildly reduced peak muscle torque and MMT of 4–5 increase their muscle strength. If these individuals start the program with significant muscle atrophy, they do not increase their strength significantly.

Hicks et al. (1993) also noted that, when CPK is measured at the beginning and the end of the exercise program, there may be transient increased CPK levels at 2, 4, and 24 hours, but these return to normal at 48 and 72 hours postexercise. So there is no sustained inflammation of muscle caused by this type of exercise. Hicks and Fromhertz (1987) also found decreased local muscle endurance ratios of muscle in PM patients at the NIH.

Based on the outcome of their exercise study, PM patients at NIH begin with an isometric exercise program. They are progressed to an isotonic exercise program, lifting light 1- to 2-pound weights just to the point of fatigue when the disease is stable for several months on the same dose of medication. When the CPK is normalized, patients are instructed in an aerobic program of low intensity (60% VO_2MAX).

Pool exercises are good for these patients because they can do ROM and strengthening and aerobic exercises with much greater ease. The water helps relieve the pain in their muscles, and the effect of gravity is reduced, putting less stress across muscles and joints. Exercise is one of the key treatments for these individuals.

ASSISTIVE DEVICES

PM and DM individuals with shoulder girdle problems and difficulty reaching and grooming. Long-handled devices such as toothbrushes, hairbrushes, and reachers are very appropriate for dressing, as are long-handled shoe horns for putting on shoes. Clothes with Velcro closures make dressing easier. PM patients have difficulty getting up from seats, and they use strategies of leaning forward and rocking back and forth or pushing up from the seat with their hands. Cushions used on seats effectively raise the height of the chair and help them get up from the seat. The spring-assist cushion is the easiest to use and is most effective (Figure 3). Elevated toilet seats are important as well as appropriate bathroom equipment, such as a shower chair. A collar with a cosmetic cover can be used for weak neck musculature. Mobility devices, such as canes and walkers, are needed for safe ambulation with weak hip muscles. We use an ankle foot orthoses (short leg brace) when the quadriceps are very weak (MMT 2/5), using ankle angle changes to control knee stability.

If the individual cannot walk after all of the treatments, power mobility devices (scooter, power wheelchair) are recommended for independent mobility in the home or for longer community distances.

EDUCATION

Instructions in conservation of energy are critical and help these individuals carry out their functional activities. Small rest periods during the day should be encouraged as well. Consultation with a vocational rehabilitation counselor may be necessary if job retraining is needed.

Disease Stage-Specific Treatments

Acute Phase Hicks (1994) reports that in the acute stage of the disease, the patient may have such profound weakness that hospitalization may be required. The rehabilitation at this phase is at first limited. Although medical therapy is being initially instituted to control the muscle inflammation, rehabilitation goals may be preserving joint motion, proper positioning in bed, splinting of some joints to avoid contractures, and appling heat and massage to relieve painful muscles. If respiratory muscles are compromised, chest physical therapy may be needed.

Subacute Phase (Directed Therapy) As the muscle inflammation reduces on medical treatment and the muscle strength begins to improve, other rehabilitation interventions may be added. These may include use of the tilt table to acclimate the body systems to the upright posture again; work on reeducating muscle; active assisted ROM in gravity-eliminated positions; work on balance and posture; and use of assistive devices such as a long-handled comb, toothbrush sponge, and reacher. At this time, bathroom ADL is evaluated and appropriate equipment such as elevated toilet seats, a shower chair, and a long-handled shower hose is dispensed. An isometric strengthening program is started when the person can contract muscle and move it against some resistance. As muscle strength improves to the antigravity level, work is begun on ambulation in the parallel bars and then outside the bars with a walker. The person may be allowed to be transferred to a rehabilitation facility at this stage, where

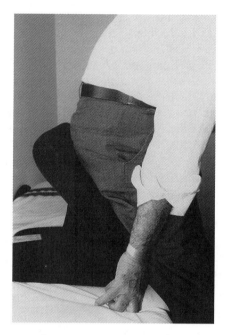

Figure 3. The spring-assist cushion.

working on strength, water exercise, mobility, balance, and ADL will continue. Some light isotonic exercises may be added as well as low-intensity, low-duration aerobic exercise after the muscle strength has improved on medication and on an isometric strengthening program.

Chronic Phase (Activity Programs) Often inflammation may either continue at a low level or cease. However, the muscle usually has residual atrophy from the disease process itself or due to steroid use. The strengthening program should be started early in the disease course and continued as long as the muscle is strong enough to do these programs. ROM programs should continue throughout the course of the disease, particularly in persons with muscles below the 4/5 range, as joint contractures frequently occur in these persons. Use of a light inexpensive pulley system attached to a door or wand exercise are very helpful. Use of ROM and strengthening exercise in the pool is also useful. The warm water feels good on sore muscles and the effect of gravity is reduced, making movement easier. If the quadriceps muscles are at the 3/5 level or lower, these patients often begin to fall. As noted earlier, a brace can be adjusted to maintain knee stability. Speech and swallowing problems often persist. Dysphagia is common; speech pathologists can give advice about appropriate food textures, positioning, swallowing strategies, and pharyngeal and neck muscle strengthening. Sometimes neck muscles are in the 2+/5 level or less, making it impossible to extend the neck. A collar assists in holding up the neck.

CONCLUSIONS

Idiopathic inflammatory myopathy is an example of a progressive disease process in women that can restrict function and interfere with mobility and daily living activities. Early medical diagnosis, drug intervention, and rehabilitation programs help to assure a better functional outcome. Delay in diagnosis and treatments is likely to be associated with a poorer outcome. A comprehensive rehabilitation approach can assure a plan for all phases of the disease process. Exercise and fitness are an important part of the rehabilitation plan.

Further research is needed to understand the effect of different types of strengthening exercise programs on the ability to increase strength and function as the disease progresses in these individuals. Also, studies are needed that document the degree of aerobic deconditioning in the various disease types and stages. The effect of aerobic training programs on the aerobic capacity and function of persons with PM has not been studied yet. Studies to better delineate the impact of the disease on vocational, educational, and social pursuits should be identified more clearly in adults and children. Finally, a study on the impact of a comprehensive organized rehabilitation program on the functioning of persons with PM should be undertaken.

REFERENCES

Buczek, F.L., Leff, R.L., Hicks, J.E., & Gerber, L.H. (1994). A study of falling: Slips and trips in a patient with muscle weakness due to myositis. In J. Vossoughi (Ed.), *Biomedical engineering—Recent developments. Proceedings of the Thirteenth Southern Biomedical Engineering Conference* (pp. 559–562). Washington, DC: University of the District of Columbia Press.

Dalakas, M.C. (1992). Clinical immunopathologic and therapeutic considerations of inflammatory myopathies. *Clinical Neuropharmacology, 15*(5), 327–351.

Dalakas, M.C., Illa, I., Dambrosia, J.M., Soueidan, S.A., Stein, D.P., Otero, C., Dinsmore, S.T., & McCrosky, S. (1993). A controlled trial of high-dose intravenous immune globulin infusions as treatment for dermatomyositis. *New England Journal of Medicine, 329*, 1993–2000.

Fraser, P., Frank, J., Dalakas, M., Miller, J., & Hicks, J. (1991). Magnetic resonance imaging in the idiopathic inflammatory myopathies. *Journal of Rheumatology, 18*, 11.

Hicks, J. (1984). Comprehensive rehabilitation management of patients with polymyositis/dermatomyositis. In M. Dalakus (Ed.), *Polymyositis* (pp. 284–304). London: Butterworth.

Hicks, J. (1994). Rehabilitation of patients with polymyositis. In J. Klippel & P. Dieppe (Eds.), *Rheumatology* (Section 6:15.4-6). St. Louis: C.V. Mosby.

Hicks, J., Miller, F., Plotz, P., Chen, T.H., & Gerber, L. (1989). Response of po-lymyositis patients to an isometric exercise program. *Arthritis and Rheumatism, 32*(Suppl. I), 149.

Hicks, J., Miller, F., Reyburn, T., Plotz, P., Richardson, D., & Gerber, L. (1991). Correlation of a functional assessment tool for idiopathic inflammatory myopathy with CPK, MMT and aldolase values. *Arthritis and Rheumatism, 34*(Suppl. 5), R31.

Hicks, J.E., & Fromhertz, W. (1987). Cybex II strength and endurance testing in normals and polymyositis patients. *Archives of Physical Medicine and Rehabilitation, 68*, 661.

Hicks, J.E., Miller, F., Plotz, P., Chen, T.H., & Gerber, L. (1993). Isometric exercise increases strength and does not produce sustained CPK rises in a patient with polymyositis. *Annals of Rheumatic Disease, 20*, 1399–1401.

Kagen, L.J. (1994). Management of inflammatory muscle disease. In J. Klippel & P. Dieppe (Eds.), *Rheumatology* (Section 6:14.1-4). London: C.V. Mosby.

Medsger, T.A., & Oddis, C.V. (1994). Inflammatory muscle disease: Clinical features. In J. Klippel & P. Dieppe (Ed.), *Rheumatology* (Section 6, 12.1-14). London: C.V. Mosby.

Miller, F., Leitman, S., Cronin, M.E., Hicks, J.E., Leff, R.L., Dalakas, M., Wesley, R., Fraser, D.D., & Plotz, P.H. (1992). Controlled trial of plasma exchange and leukapheresis in polymyositis and dermatomyositis. *New England Journal of Medicine, 326*, 1380–1384.

Plotz, P.H., Leff, R.L., & Miller, F.W. (1993). Inflammatory and metabolic myopathies. In J. Klipple (Ed.), *Primer of rheumatic diseases*. Atlanta, GA: Arthritis Foundation.

Plotz, P.H., & Miller, F.W. (1994). Etiology and pathogenesis of inflammatory muscle disease. In J. Klippel & P. Dieppe (Ed.), *Rheumatology* (Section 6, 13.1-10). St. Louis: C.V. Mosby.

Thorton, B., Egan, M., Parks, B., Hicks, J., & Vargo, M. (1994). *Rehabilitation treatment of inclusion body myositis.* Harrisonburg, VA: Inclusion Body Myositis Association.

chapter 32

Adapted Physical Activity and Sport

Karen P. DePauw

Civil rights for all citizens have been sought throughout U.S. history. By the 1960s, nondiscrimination on the basis of race and gender had become the law of the land. Nondiscrimination on the basis of "handicap" was first legislated in the Rehabilitation Act of 1973, Section 504, but the civil rights movement for individuals with disabilities (disability rights movement) gained momentum with the passage of the Americans with Disabilities Act, PL 101-336, in 1990.

Since then, increasing public attention has been directed toward issues of health and well-being, particularly among women. This chapter provides a brief introduction to adapted physical activity, summarizes relevant research on physical activity and sport with individuals with disabilities—especially girls and women with disabilities—and offers recommendations for future research. The traditional research paradigm for physical activity, sport, and exercise has tended to emphasize the study of Caucasian males without disabilities. As a result, few studies have been conducted with women, members of ethnic minority groups, and individuals with disabilities as subjects; fortunately, these studies are on the rise. However, the physiological functioning and health-related physical activity of girls and women with disabilities are virtually unstudied to date.

BACKGROUND
Physical Activity

Physical activity, an umbrella term that encompasses sport, fitness, physical education, exercise, recreation, and dance, is an essential ingredient for a healthy lifestyle and a feeling of well-being. Physical activity designed for individuals with disabilities is often described with different terminology: adapted physical activity, adapted physical education, therapeutic recreation, and disability sport, for example. Adapted physical education is perhaps the most familiar program because of its location in the public schools and relationship to special education.

In the United States, adapted physical education refers to school-based programs of physical activity for individuals with disabilities. Professionals and scholars throughout the world engaged in physical activity–based programs have encouraged the expansion of adapted physical education beyond the confines of public school education and appropriately retitled the discipline as adapted physical activity. Specifically, *adapted physical activity* is defined as a cross-disciplinary body of knowledge directed toward the identification and solution of motor problems throughout the life span, development and implementation of advocacy and attitude theories in support of access to sport and active lifestyle, and innovation and cooperative home-school-community service delivery and empowerment systems (DePauw & Sherrill, 1994).

Disability

It is important to define the population of individuals under discussion here—women with disabilities. Perhaps the most common definition of disability is "a loss or reduction of functional ability and/or ability" (World Health Organization [WHO], 1980). Within this definition, it is speculated that 10% of all children, 30% of adults, and 50% of those over the age of 65 years have a disability (see Figure 1). To date, published statistics are not reported by gender. As expected, the types and severity of disability vary and include sensory, physical, and mental impairments.

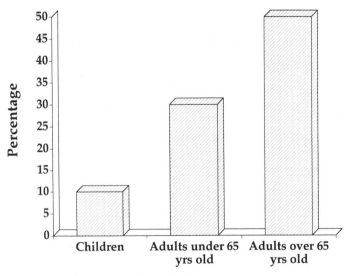

Figure 1. Percentage of population with a disability, by age.

The WHO definition of disability has roots in the medical model (Chappell, 1992) that places emphasis upon a disability-specific, categorical approach and explains disability as an individual problem (Barnes, 1990). Disability is the presence of a functional limitation resulting from an impairment (loss of an organ or organ system function). Given this definition, disability is viewed as a form of deviance and emanates from labeling theory (e.g., Hanks & Poplin, 1981) and stigma (e.g., Brown & Smith, 1989; Goffman, 1963).

The disability rights movement has challenged us to revisit the previous definition of disability and to consider disability not as an "individual" problem but rather in the context of social relationships (Chappell, 1992; Hanks & Poplin, 1981), as a social role that becomes legitimized over time (e.g., Lemert, 1951; Haber & Smith, 1971; Shapiro, 1993). It is important not only to understand disability as social construction (defined by those with power), but also to undertake emancipatory research (Morris, 1992) that challenges old notions of disability.

RESEARCH

Historical Perspectives

Research on adapted physical activity has been conducted since the early 1900s (Broadhead, 1986; DePauw, 1988; Pyfer, 1986; Stein, 1983). Throughout the 20th century, research questions have continued to evolve, research designs and methodology have improved, and numbers and groupings of individuals have increased. Prior to the 1960s, adapted physical activity research described the growth and development of individuals with specific types of primary disabling conditions, identified postural disorders, and determined specific motor characteristics. The populations studied included those with mental retardation, mental illness, and sensory impairment (auditory and visual) primarily from institutional settings.

Research conducted in the 1960s and 1970s examined the initial effects of fitness and exercise as well as perceptual motor programs for individuals with disabilities. Early intervention programs and program effectiveness, including mainstreaming, behavior management approaches, and assessment/evaluation, were studied during this time. In addition, the motor characteristics of selected disability groupings were identified. Groupings included autism, asthma, cerebral palsy (CP), deafness, emotional disturbance, learning disability, mental retardation, obesity, and visual impairment.

During the 1970s, research on sport for individuals with disabilities was studied for the first time. Physiological (fitness, response to exercise) and biomechanical (wheelchair propulsion) aspects of sport performance were the two primary topics studied in the early days of disability sport research. These initial sport investigations were conducted with males with spinal cord injury (SCI) or postpolio from rehabilitation settings. Disability sport research has progressed from investigations of sport for rehabilitation to research on athletes with disabilities. Sport research has become sport specific, disability specific, performance related, and sport subdiscipline specific (e.g., sport psychology, sport physiology, sport biomechanics, sport sociology, sport medicine) (DePauw, 1988).

Adapted physical activity research of the 1980s and 1990s has provided increased knowledge and understanding, which can be grouped in four general areas:

1. Scientific bases for motor performance
2. Effects of physical activity
3. Teaching and learning of physical activity
4. Influences upon physical activity (DePauw, 1992)

The adapted physical activity research literature is contained in journals such as the *Adapted Physical Activity Quarterly, Palaestra, Physician and Sports Medicine, Research Quarterly for Exercise and Sport, Rehabilitation Yearbook, Journal of Teaching Physical Education, Medicine and Science in Sport and Exercise, Physical Educator, Physical Education Review, Journal of Biomechanics, Journal of Applied Physiology* and other journals that emphasize special education, rehabilitation, therapy (physical, occupational) and recreation. In addition, adapted physical activity research has been reported in volumes of compiled research, such as *Completed Research in Health, Physical Education, Recreation & Dance, Abstracts of Research Presentations at American Alliance for Health, Physical Education,* and *Recreation & Dance Convention.* For an excellent overview review of adapted physical activity research, see Shephard (1990).

Much of this research supports the benefits of physical activity and sport for individuals with disabilities including the physical, mental, social, psychological, functional, vocational, and recreational aspects as well as the effectiveness of instructional training programs. These benefits include the following:

1. Individuals with disabilities have demonstrated physiological responses to exercise similar to those of athletes without disabilities. Differences that exist are identified with differences in functional muscle mass due to factors such paralysis, amputation, or osteoporosis in paralyzed limbs and the severity of the physical impairment or are based on difficulties of comprehension, initiation, or mechanical efficiency related to specific types of primary disabling conditions (e.g., mental retardation, CP) (Shephard, 1990). In some cases, it remains

unclear whether the differences in physiological responses are due to differences in physiological functioning or assessment techniques.

2. Although a specific disability may affect the degree of intensity, duration, and frequency of exercise, evidence suggests that physiological training effects can be achieved with individuals with disabilities. For example, type of activity (endurance vs. strength) influences maximum oxygen consumption (e.g., wheelchair athletes who compete in track and swimming events have larger maximum oxygen intake than those who compete in strength events).

3. Wheelchair propulsion for movement efficiency has been studied in terms of rim diameter, stroke frequency, seat height, technique, speed, level of impairment, and sporting event (sprint vs. distance). With the decrease in the mass of the chair in addition to individual adaptations of seat height and inclination, camber of the wheels and variations in handrim sizes, athletic performance (movement efficiency) has increased substantially.

4. Training or instructional programs were found to be effective but dependent upon the specific type of program provided (e.g., fitness, balance, flexibility, motor skills). Improvements in self-concept and social interaction were found as byproducts of intervention programs, although on a limited basis.

5. Inclusion or integration of individuals with disabilities with persons without disabilities was found to be effective in enhancing learning and motor performance as well as increasing appropriate behavior and improving social interaction. In addition, positive changes in attitudes toward individuals with disabilities were found.

Research about Women with Disabilities

Our limited understanding of physical activity and health issues for women with physical disabilities stems from results of the disability sport research initially conducted in the 1970s and 1980s. Because emphasis was placed upon performance and understanding physiological responses to exercise, most of the investigators used a sport classification system in an attempt to distinguish among degree and extent of disabling condition. It is important to note that the subjects for investigations are primarily males with SCI who used wheelchairs. Through 1993, a total of 13 studies have been conducted on body composition of individuals with SCI. The majority of these studies used males as subjects and none used females exclusively. Although more males than females with SCI are available as subjects, this fact alone should not eliminate research on women. The studies of pulmonary function were conducted with males; only one study included women. This pattern seems to have been repeated with studies of cardiovascular response, handgrip, and forearm cranking. Only a few studies (n = 3) included females among the subjects, and none have focused upon women with disabilities or gender-specific phenomena in particular. In general, the subjects also tended to be drawn from an active (and athletic) population.

Research on active males with SCI has obvious limited application to all women with physical disabilities, but this research constitutes the largest body of knowledge presently available about the physiological functioning of individuals with disabilities. Among the findings of these and other studies (including males and females) are the following points (adapted from Shephard, 1990):

1. Normal wheelchair propulsion does not prove sufficient stimulus to maintain physical condition.
2. Amputation and muscle atrophy due to impairment may restrict lean body mass and adversely influence accurate measures of body composition and prediction of ideal body mass.
3. Resting oxygen consumption and cardiac output may be lessened due to physical impairment (e.g., limb paralysis).
4. Increase in heart rate with exercise among spinally injured tetraplegics is less than that found among able bodied individuals.
5. Regular participation in wheelchair sport increases cardiac stroke volume.
6. Shoulder and elbow strength among wheelchair users is greater than among able-bodied individuals.
7. Maximum oxygen intake is more limited in spinally injured tetraplegics than in paraplegics; wheelchair athletes have the advantage of peak oxygen intake and peak power output relative to their inactive peers.
8. Higher values for isometric and isokinetic muscle force data are found among wheelchair athletes; males with disabilities were found to be stronger than females with disabilities.

These findings offer a general sense of the biological responses of individuals with disabilities but fall short of considering the experience of women with SCI or the experience of other women with physical disabilities such as CP.

Findings of training studies indicate the beneficial effects of training programs (Rimmer, 1994; Shephard, 1990). The majority of these studies were undertaken in the following six areas: wheelchair ergometry, arm cranking, swimming, sport/physical activity, resistance training, and calisthenics (see Figure 2). As shown, the majority of training studies have also been conducted with males.

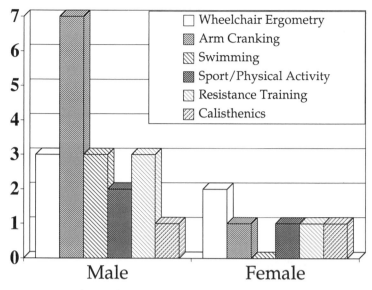

Figure 2. Training studies conducted with individuals with disabilities, by sex and type of training.

Physical Activity Patterns

Physical activity is important for each of us. Data exist about general physical activity patterns of women, but little is known about the physical activity patterns of girls and women with disabilities. Because no data were found about the physical activity patterns of women with disabilities in the United States, a selected sample of the findings from a comprehensive study conducted by Fitness Canada Women's Program (n.d.) are presented here.

In Canada, 40% of the women with disabilities were reported as inactive, 28% somewhat inactive, and 31% as quite or very active (see Figure 3). It was found that women with disabilities participate in physical activity at a lower rate than women without disabilities. The current and preferred types of settings for physical activity among the sample of women with disabilities is shown in Figure 4. Overall, it appears as if the women sampled would "prefer to participate at a higher level than their current one," but as much as possible in noncompetitive, organized settings.

Among other topics, the Canadian study queried the respondents about their primary reasons for being active and the barriers to participation. The results indicated that these women sought physical activity primarily to relax and reduce stress, to improve or maintain fitness, for pleasure or fun, and to feel better. Contrary to common assumptions, the respondents did

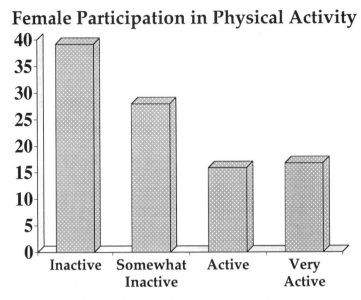

Figure 3. Participation levels of females with disabilities in Canada.

not participate primarily for medical or therapeutic reasons. These reasons reported in this study are similar to reasons for participation in physical activity found among women in general.

The respondents reported six common barriers to participation in physical activity: the timing of programs, nature of programs, accessibility

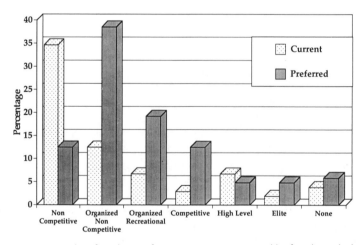

Figure 4. Current and preferred type of activity programs reported by females with disabilities in Canada.

of facilities, transportation, lack of knowledgeable instructors, and lack of available information. It is interesting to note that these barriers are all changeable. Program planners and service providers should explore the implications of the reasons for and the barriers to participation in physical activity identified in the study and plan accordingly.

Research Directions

In preparing for and addressing health concerns of women with disabilities, professionals must accept specific roles and responsibilities for research and programming in the area of physical activity. Of primary importance is emphasizing emancipatory activities and programs as well as emancipatory research. In other words, programs should be designed for and with females with disabilities and not just simply modified from the able-bodied model. At the same time, research should be undertaken that is useful and meaningful to females with disabilities and that serves as a basis for empowerment and independence. Thus, a paradigm shift is critical, a shift away from a traditional medical model that presumes there is a "problem in the person" and emphasizes professional concerns over individual concerns to a perspective that respects and stresses the individual rather than the disability. In adopting a human rights and dignity perspective, professionals need to listen to the voices of those with disabilities and work collaboratively to dispel myths and stereotypes, eliminate labels, and understand the social meaning of our programs and research in the broader societal context.

As discussed previously, the results of prior research are not necessarily generalizable to females with disabilities. More research is needed that specifically addresses health-related issues of women with physical disabilities. Specifically, the biological responses and adaptations to exercise must be examined. There are biological responses that are gender and disability independent—responses that result regardless of one's sex or physical impairment: Men and women respond the same to a given stimulus (e.g., increase in heart rate with increase in energy expenditure). On the other hand, there are biological responses and adaptations to exercise that are gender or disability dependent (e.g., maximum heart rate, stroke volume)—responses that are influenced by one's gender and/or disability. This is conceptualized in Figure 5. The overlapping portions of the circles represent the biological responses that are independent (e.g., overlap between male and female; intersection of male, female, and disability). In this schematic representation, only one circle is used to depict disability; in reality, disability could also be divided, as was gender. It is important to understand that specific types of impairments may also influence one's response to exercise, the particulars of which are not known currently.

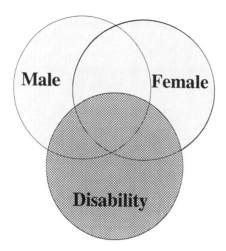

Figure 5. Schematic representation of the interaction of sex and disability for research on biological responses and adaptations to exercise.

To understand fully the performance of women with disabilities, it is important to identify and understand the biological responses or adaptations to exercise that are gender and disability independent, but especially those that are gender and disability dependent and those that result from the interaction of sex and disability. In addition to the biological responses to exercise, research must consider other biological factors such as age, ethnicity, and race within the social context of the human experience, including factors such as class, education, family, motivation, socialization, and the sociopsychological perspectives of gender, race, disability, and sexual orientation.

Given a model of gender- and disability-independent and dependent responses and adaptations to exercise framed within the broader societal context, four general topics are proposed for research on health concerns for women with physical disabilities. These topics are meant to apply across age groups (youth, adults, and older adults with disabilities), geographic region and setting (urban and rural), and race and ethnicity:

1. Physical activity patterns of girls and women with disabilities, including types and accessibility of physical activity programs; reasons for participation in physical activity; barriers to participation; frequency, type, and duration of activity or exercise; attitudes toward physical activity; and socialization into physical activity programs.

2. Exercise-related concerns of females with disabilities and biological responses and adaptations to exercise, including isotonic activity (explosive power, anaerobic power, anaerobic capacity, aerobic power, prolonged exercise); muscular performance (peak isometric force, iso-

metric endurance, isotonic power output, isotonic endurance, eccentric force and endurance, isokinetic force and endurance); anaerobic and aerobic performance (anaerobic capacity, aerobic power, anaerobic power); respiration and performance (ventilation, oxygen cost of breathing, pulmonary diffusion); cardiovascular performance (cardiac output, oxygen difference); fitness and health (body composition and percent body fat, flexibility, blood pressure); mechanical efficiency and biomechanics; and training response.

3. Specific exercise concerns such as aging and osteoporosis, nutrition, and exercise and immune function.

4. Contraindications of physical activity and exercise for females with disabilities, including injury prevention and treatment.

5. Appropriate treatment programs and strategies—school-based or community-based programs, rehabilitation programs, disease prevention and health promotion programs, and specific training and instructional programs.

CONCLUSIONS

The general direction of research is to understand the relationship among health, physical activity (exercise, fitness, recreation, sport), and disability within the female population. The challenge facing researchers is the need to balance perceived scientific rigor and merit with relevance to the experience of females with disabilities. To be successful, research must be conducted in collaboration and cooperation with females with disabilities and framed within the societal context (i.e., family, school, community). That is, research needs to be applicable and meaningful to the female with a disability as an individual and appropriate to the societal context in which she functions.

REFERENCES

Americans with Disabilities Act of 1990 (ADA), PL 101-336. (July 26, 1990). Title 42, U.S.C. 12101 et seq.: *U.S. Statutes at Large, 104*, 327–378.

Barnes, C. (1990). *Cabbage syndrome: The social construction of dependence.* Basingstoke, England: Falmer Press.

Broadhead, G.D. (1986). Adapted physical education research trends: 1970–1990. *Adapted Physical Activity Quarterly, 3*, 104–111.

Brown, H., & Smith, H. (1989). Whose "ordinary life" is it anyway? *Disability, Handicap & Society, 4*(2), 105–119.

Chappell, A.L. (1992). Towards a sociological critique of the normalization principle. *Disability, Handicap & Society, 7*(1), 35–50.

DePauw, K.P. (1988). Sport for individuals with disabilities: Research opportunities. *Adapted Physical Activity Quarterly, 5*, 80–89.

DePauw, K.P. (1992). Current international trends in research in adapted physical activity. In R. Williams, L. Almond, & A. Sparkes (Eds.), *Sport and physical activity: Moving toward excellence.* London: E & FN SPON.

DePauw, K.P., & Sherrill, C. (1994). Adapted physical activity: Present and future. *The Physical Education Review, 17*, 6–13.

Goffman, E. (1963). *Stigma: Notes on the management of spoiled identity.* Englewood Cliffs, NJ: Prentice Hall.

Haber, L.D., & Smith, R.T. (1971). Disability and deviance: Normative adaptations of role behavior. *American Sociological Review, 36*, 87–97.

Hanks, M., & Poplin, D.E. (1981). The sociology of physical disability: A review of literature and some conceptual perspectives. *Deviant Behavior: An Interdisciplinary Journal, 2*, 309–328.

Lemert, E.M. (1951). *Social pathology.* New York: McGraw-Hill.

Morris, J. (1992). Personal and political: A feminist perspective on researching physical disability. *Disability, Handicap & Society, 7*, 157–166.

Fitness Canada Women's Program. (n.d.). *Physical activity and women with disabilities: A national survey.* Ottawa, ON, Canada: Canada Women's Program.

Pyfer, J.L. (1986). Early research concerns in adapted physical education. *Adapted Physical Activity Quarterly, 3*, 95–103.

Rehabilitation Act of 1973, PL 93-112. (September 26, 1973). Title 29, U.S.C. 701 et seq.: *U.S. Statutes at Large, 87*, 355–394.

Rimmer, J.H. (1994). *Fitness and rehabilitation programs for special populations.* Dubuque, IA: Brown & Benchmark.

Shapiro, J. (1993). *No pity: People with disabilities forging a new civil rights movement.* New York: Times Books.

Shephard, R.J. (1990). *Fitness in special populations.* Champaign, IL: Human Kinetics.

Stein, J.U. (1983). Bridge over troubled waters—research review and recommendations for relevance. In R.L. Eason, T.L. Smith, & F. Caron (Eds.), *Adapted physical activity* (pp. 189–198). Champaign, IL: Human Kinetics.

World Health Organization. (1980). *International classification of impairments, disabilities, and handicaps: A manual of classification relating to the consequence of disease.* Geneva, Switzerland: Author.

chapter 33

Health Promotion for People with Chronic Neuromuscular Disabilities

Sunny Roller

As an educator, support group leader, manager of the Post-Polio Research and Training Program at the University of Michigan Medical Center, and one of the many persons with postpolio symptoms, I have personally experienced and observed among my peers the interplay of aging and long-term disability. We are moving into our middle and late years and have begun to experience the effects of normal aging. Our uniqueness as people with disabilities, however, stems from the fact that our expected aging challenges have been combined and complicated with the newly recognized late effects of polio. These could become even more seriously complicated by the effects of disuse and new disease.

The polio population serves disability researchers. We are the first who have been identified as having the late effects of neuromuscular impairment. People with spinal cord injury (SCI), spina bifida, and cerebral palsy (CP) are also now reporting similar late effects. Since the mid-1980s, increasing numbers of polio survivors with progressive new weakness, severe disabling fatigue, and a variety of pain management problems have sought medical attention.

In our 1991 study of 120 polio survivors (56% of whom were women) at the University of Michigan, we found that 82% had a treatable musculoskeletal problem of some kind (Maynard, 1991). Modern rehabilitation methods can bring people back to satisfactory levels of functioning. New braces, for example, could support legs that are weakening. Strengthening exercises could alleviate some pain problems. A shoe lift could relieve hip pain and enhance walking endurance. But 35% of the polio survivors in this study were obese; 36% had an elevated cholesterol level; and 35% had a comorbidity such as diabetes, gastrointestinal disease, and heart trouble (see Table 1). Sixty-two percent had an exercise capacity below the expected and achievable levels. Based on these findings, prevention efforts that focus on improved diet and individually designed exercise plans were medically recommended.

To avoid depression and reduce stress, people with the late effects of polio must be continually encouraged to use creative approaches to reduce their physical problems, many of which may be preventable. Because of their special vulnerabilities to new health problems such as pain, weakness, and fatigue, polio survivors need intensive instruction, coaching, and support to learn how to apply general health promotion practices to their unique conditions and circumstances. But often, because of very limited wellness opportunities, they have been at a disadvantage because they cannot work out on the local health club machines that are meant for members without neuromuscular disabilities. Many weight loss centers do not even have a scale that is wheelchair accessible. Swimming classes are not often given in pools that are warm enough or accessible enough, and adapted coaching by the instructor is not generally provided.

Polio survivors and our counterparts who have similar disabilities justly desire and deserve to maintain lifestyles that are as fully functional, diverse, and independent as possible. As we begin to cope with the late effects of our disease, new questions arise. "What can I do to feel good?

Table 1. Secondary pathologies found in postpolio sample

Condition	Percent of subjects with condition
Anemia	7%
Elevated cholesterol ratio	36
Hypertension	8
Obesity	35
Other significant medical comorbidity (one or more from list below)	35
Diabetes	2.5
Respiratory diseases (COPD/asthma)	7.5
Heart trouble	8
Circulation trouble in limbs	5
Gastrointestinal disease (e.g., gall bladder problems or stomach ulcers)	8
Urinary tract disorder (e.g., infections, stones, or prostate problems)	4
Rheumatoid arthritis	3
Non-polio nerve/muscle disorders causing weakness or paralysis	9

From Maynard, F., et al. (1991). *The late effects of polio: A model for identification and assessment of preventable secondary disabilities.* Alexandria, VA: National Technical Information Services, U.S. Department of Commerce.

*Judged to be serious enough to potentially affect functional capacity.

Could I ever feel as well as an athlete looks? Must I be condemned to struggle from one medical crisis to the next in future years, or is there something I can do along the way to prevent new problems? Can I possess a sense of harmony and pleasant satisfaction with who I am and the life I am living? Is it possible to have a disability, feel less pain, be more rested, and have more energy for the activities I want to participate in?" We want to stay strong and pain free, prevent injury, stay out of the hospitals, and contribute on the job until we choose to retire, and we need insurance coverage that will support our commitment to staying healthy and productive.

Because more and more women with chronic neuromuscular disabilities are living longer, our society needs to address the long-term needs of this growing population. Health promotion programs that help people stay well could fill a gap in our health care system and eliminate unnecessary spending connected with the devastating effects of poor health and functional decline among people with disabilities.

With these factors in mind, I advocate two health promotion models. The first is the residential model developed in Europe, which I have studied in Germany. The second is a commuter model described in the book *Stay Well* (Roller & Maynard, 1991). Both models of health care provision are unique because they prescribe a holistic set of treatments in one accessible location. A one-stop shopping mode of program delivery would meet our serious need for convenient therapies. Some therapies would lead to maintaining sound health. Other therapies could lead to the prevention of new problems. Depending on their quantity, duration, and intensity, the same therapies could be used for either maintenance or prevention. The importance of a holistic wellness program is that it considers the whole person as a unit with interlaced parts, each of which has a dramatic effect on the others. This approach is appealing because as women, we have unique needs in a variety of areas—as described in detail throughout this book—mental, physical and spiritual needs. Also, for those of us with very limited physical function, if we could not succeed at exercise, there would be other wellness interventions to learn and participate in that include the areas of nutrition or general lifestyle enhancement. Thus, such a comprehensive menu would provide us with more choices and opportunities to improve our health.

RESIDENTIAL MODEL

In 1992, the World Institute on Disability awarded me a grant to do a descriptive study of the health spa system in Germany. In November of that year, my collaborator, Eva Wortz, and I flew to Bavaria to visit three spas. Our purpose was to investigate unique techniques and methods of support for helping people with long-held neuromuscular disabilities stay well and prevent new disabilities as they grow older. In the United States, our mental picture of a spa is a building that houses equipment and pools. Very healthy people go to these spas to get more healthy. A spa might also mean a tanning salon. Or a spa may simply be another word for a hot tub. In Germany, spas are like small towns. They are made up of hotels, restaurants, churches, and shops. There are clinics and various treatment centers that house swimming pools and specially equipped treatment rooms. Spas have parks, tennis courts, lakes, and concert halls. Many doctors and therapists have offices on the spa grounds. People take part in their own customized holistic wellness programs. This residential concept entices the participant to live at the facility for a length of time to focus full time on maximizing health. Individuals go to the spa to rejuvenate their health and to prevent further deterioration. These visits require a doctor's prescription in order to be covered by insurance.

The required elements of the spa's unique holistic approach include a residential time away from home; a relaxed and aesthetically delightful environment; a group of individualized exercise, nutritional, and recreational treatments; an individualized health education program; and a time to set goals for long-term follow-up of health-enhancing behaviors. Some of these elements are described in the following paragraphs.

Residential time away provides participants with disabilities a unique opportunity to fully focus on health rejuvenation. As one woman polio survivor, a German spa participant, remarks:

> I would rather choose such an inpatient treatment plan than outpatient treatment. The community of patients is psychologically supportive and helps one forget one's own pains. In such a treatment plan, one is there only for one's body—one is taken care of in every respect. In an outpatient treatment plan, one must also go home and take care of the family afterwards. This is less successful.

Upon entering a German spa, one cannot help but become engulfed in the health-promoting surroundings. The relaxed and aesthetically delightful environment was obvious and alluring to us. The scenic beauty, the peaceful pools and lakes, the glittering elegance in the small shop windows, and the contented humming chit-chat of strolling spa guests all coalesced to lift spirits and create positive attitudes that lead to good health. All of the spa directors and physicians that we met emphasized that a spa should never look or feel like a hospital. "It must be fun," one of the therapists stressed, with serious enthusiasm. Hospitals are designed for sick people. Spas are built to intensify health promotion and invite the well-being of the visitors.

The accessible spa clinics we visited looked like hotels and offered a long list of treatments. We learned that these clinics would be ideal places for people with severe disabilities to participate in a holistic wellness program because all treatments could be completed in this one barrier-free and accessible building. People who are able to walk longer distances over more difficult terrain could stay at a regular spa hotel and walk from building to building to receive treatments.

Everyone who goes to the spa must first be evaluated by a physician. At the spas we visited, participants staying at the spa clinics must receive a battery of tests to assess strengths and deficits. Physicians then collaborate with therapists and the participant to set up an individualized program. The customized treatments must take into consideration the late effects of the neuromuscular disability—like polio or SCI. The daily schedule must include all the appropriate rest breaks, for example. That is a key to success demonstrated at Bad Griesbach, one German spa we visited.

The treatments include physical and occupational therapy; speech therapy; psychotherapy; group treatments, including stress reduction techniques, cognitive treatments, independent living training, and diet counseling and participation; and complementary medical treatments, such as massage, mud baths, and aroma and herbal therapy. An important part of the spa experience is the educational programming that accompanies the actual therapies. Participants who make a serious commitment to learning new attitudes to end self-defeating health behaviors attend lectures and workshops on various health topics—from how to quit smoking to how to cook nutritious meals. Commitment is expressed through attendance at all therapies and scheduled lectures, which are mandatory. Avoiding any of these activities may mean that the participant is discharged from the spa and is charged with all costs of treatment, rather than receiving insurance reimbursement.

It was explained that a long-term follow-through therapy plan is laid out and discussed with spa participants as part of their educational program. Therapists meet with participants to let them know what treatments they need to do when they return home and how often they must be done. Most of the people we interviewed agreed that, for people with disabilities, the full benefit of the 4- to 5-month good feeling that comes after the stay at the spa would likely require a return visit, perhaps annually.

Most spas are not aggressive in attracting people with disabilities, but all three spa directors we interviewed revealed that with proper preplanning they could accommodate special needs. Anyone who goes to a spa for treatments will have various amounts of reimbursement provided if they first receive a prescription from their physician. Typically, an eligible person would wait for 3–5 weeks and receive a certain amount per day for food, lodging, and all treatments. The average spa visitor goes once every 3 years for 3–4 weeks.

Because the spa treatments—or "Kur," as the Germans describe it—will help keep a person healthy in general and fit and able to work, preventing premature medical retirement, the person's visit is reimbursed by one of the state insurance programs or private health insurance. There is a German Spa Association that coordinates research on spa treatment and effectiveness. They have been quoted as saying that for every mark spent on a stay at the spa, 3 marks go back to the German society (R. Hasselberger, personal communication, November 29, 1992).

If a person with a disability lives close enough to a spa and is in need of treatment, he or she can qualify to have three or four "Kurs" per week. This becomes a German version of a community-based health promotion program that people travel to regularly, rather than the live-in arrangement, which is more common at the German spas.

We believe that the German health spa model could be adapted and used in the United States. This model supports the concept of prevention as well as the independent living philosophy of personal empowerment because it promotes self-care after the stay and is dedicated to the prevention of new disabilities that could ultimately inhibit a person's ability to function freely. It appears that Franklin D. Roosevelt participated in his own version of a spa-like health promotion program here in the United States when he vacationed at Warm Springs, Georgia, during his later years to swim, eat right, and feel rejuvenated. Based on that small American tradition and on the success of the German health spa concept, U.S. health care professionals and consumers could assess their local/regional facilities, professional resource pool, and community interest and need for potential wellness programming opportunities that are accessible to people with disabilities. Adapted variations on the spa programs and practices could be established based on their findings.

COMMUTER WELLNESS PROGRAM

A second model, called the commuter wellness program, lays out a plan for a comprehensive and integrated program that would offer a range of treatments all in one location that is within driving distance of the person's home.

"Stay Well!" is an example of a commuter program that introduces polio survivors to new tactics that can be customized to their needs. Generated from consumer-reported requests for self-education and based on a pilot program codesigned and conducted by polio survivors and health care professionals in Michigan, "Stay Well!" is an expanded and untested community health promotion program. Its design is worthy of serious consideration. The program strives to help participants

1. Alleviate, manage, and prevent a variety of secondary conditions that are associated with long-term muscle impairments
2. Promote good health and wellness
3. Introduce new health promotion tactics customized to individual needs
4. Facilitate long-term adoption of health-enhancing behaviors

This is a modular program designed to be established at an accessible and convenient community location and led by a committed group of community members, including consumers with disabilities, health care professionals, and others. As stated in the handbook, *Stay Well! The Polio Network's Manual for a Health Promotion Program* (Roller & Maynard, 1991), the program contains three major content or curriculum areas. These include sound nutritional practices, individualized physical exercises, and general lifestyle enhancement techniques. Each curriculum section should be adapted to meet the priorities of potential program participants.

The nutrition section teaches participants to identify and adopt a diet that can optimize total well-being. Often people with the late effects of polio are faced with having to conserve energy to maintain optimal health. This necessary change in lifestyle can create new weight problems. Because many people with polio have limited physical activity, we often should not exceed a 1200-calories-per-day diet.

As part of "Stay Well!", participants are encouraged to 1) discover the "New American Diet" and its potential benefits, 2) decrease fat intake, 3) achieve and maintain optimal weight, 4) achieve a gradual and moderate increase of dietary fiber, 5) reduce overall sodium intake, and 6) recognize the importance of adequate intake of calcium-rich foods to prevent osteoporosis.

The exercise section teaches that, by individualizing and practicing the principles of fitness, exercise, relaxation, pacing, and utilization of local community resources for exercise equipment, it is possible to stay optimally healthy with a postpolio disability. Participants are taught that this can be accomplished by defining and practicing the principles of 1) a stretching program for flexibility, 2) a strengthening program, 3) a cardiovascular fitness training program, and 4) aquatic exercise. The principles of proper posture and back care, body mechanics, and joint protection are also taught, and participants are introduced to guidelines for using community resources.

The overall goal of the lifestyle enhancement section is to give participants an opportunity to enhance their repertoire of strategies for conducting daily activities. It teaches that this can be accomplished by learning how to 1) increase personal levels of self-acceptance and self-confidence; 2) identify and cope more effectively with stress; 3) apply the principles of assertive behavior, including coping with anger; 4) connect with available community service resources such as postpolio groups, government agencies, and other health care services; 5) develop satisfying leisure-time activities; and 6) tap available personal resources, which include our internal coping skills and values as well as external resources such as friends, a nurturing home environment, and financial resources.

"Stay Well!" is a model health promotion program that could provide convenient opportunities for polio survivors and people with similar disabilities to learn how to apply general health promotion practices to their unique conditions and circumstances. It is dedicated to preventing the unnecessary progression of disability and encouraging its participants to get well and stay well for years to come.

CONCLUSIONS

As we consider both residential and commuter health promotion program models for people with disabilities, some unanswered questions remain. Will health care insurance cover the costs of such preventive health care activities in the United States? Could an interdisciplinary conference among American health promotion specialists and professionals from abroad be held to discuss and design wellness programming for people with disabilities? Could grant funding be provided to groups of health care professionals and consumers to conduct research on the outcomes of wellness program protocols and the most successful modes of program delivery? What can we learn and apply through wellness programs that will address the specific needs of women who have physical disabilities?

Further research is needed on the effectiveness of complementary therapies, such as some of those practiced at the German spas, in preventing secondary disabilities; the feasibility of establishing regional spas for people with chronic disabilities at national facilities such as Warm Springs, Georgia; the conceptual, philosophical, or physical barriers to creating health promotion programs for people with disabilities existing in our local communities that need to be recognized and addressed; the resources that are already in place in our communities that could be utilized to build a health promotion program; the possibility of sharing resources that already exist among agencies and organizations; and funding sources that could be accessed to support a health promotion program for people with chronic neuromuscular disabilities.

We know that accessible, holistic, live-in wellness programs are being provided for people with disabilities in Germany. A holistic commuter program like "Stay Well!" offers us another model that might be even more quickly adaptable in U.S. community structures. These models can give us a new vision for lifelong wellness for women with disabilities in the United States.

REFERENCES

Maynard, F., et al. (1991). *The late effects of polio: A model for the identification and assessment of preventable secondary disabilities.* Alexandria, VA: National Technical Information Services, U.S. Department of Commerce.

Roller, S., & Maynard, F. (1991). *Stay Well! The Polio Network's manual for a health promotion program.* Ithaca, MI: Polio Network, Inc.

Conclusion

Margaret A. Nosek,
Margaret A. Turk, and Danuta M. Krotoski

A broad range of issues of concern to women with physical disabilities is presented in the preceding chapters. The focus is on four general topics: sexuality, bowel and bladder management, stress, and physical fitness. The information transmitted, however, can have a far-reaching impact on every aspect of living for women, their families, and the health care professionals who serve them. We would like to conclude by touching on some over-arching themes identified by the participants in the conference that generated this volume and by offering some observations about directions we would like to see taken with this information and the future studies it might inspire. We address issues in research methodology, clinical practice, dissemination of new information, and the participation of women with disabilities in the research process.

We are witnessing a paradigm shift along many dimensions in how society regards women with disabilities. Although the image of people with disabilities in general has made a quantum leap since the post–World War II era, as seen in media portrayals and the passage of strong civil rights legislation, the image of women with disabilities has begun to emerge from the asexual stereotype only in the late 1990s. With the increased interest in women's health and the rise of women in research and health care professions and policy-making positions, we see a shedding of old paradigms for the role of women in society and a gradual abandonment of standards and definitions developed for men. There is a new understanding of wellness and sexuality for women in general, and, as expressed in this volume, the door has cracked open to include women with disabilities. We need to promote actively the new definitions of *wellness* and *fitness* in the context of disability, a new definition of *sexuality* that includes psychological and social as well as physical aspects, and a new definition of *functioning* that addresses the ability to fill social roles and deal with the stress that accompanies living with disability. In response to these new definitions, we need new methods and tools for measuring these constructs and clinical practices for implementing them.

RESEARCH METHODOLOGY

The literature to date consists mostly of small-scale studies that are largely anecdotal in nature. In order to understand better the life experiences of women with disabilities and to develop interventions that will meet their real needs, large-scale epidemiological studies need to be conducted. These studies should offer a clearer picture of the incidence of secondary conditions and other problems related to disability and should enable the examination of risk factors. In connection with studying the status of women with disabilities in general, we must also look at strategies for preventing secondary conditions and interventions for resolving existing health conditions and psychosocial problems. Longitudinal studies will add considerable depth of knowledge to the field, but they require extensive resources and collaboration to be successfully implemented.

A number of research methodologies should be used in research on women with disabilities. One such approach is the use of population-based studies, that is, studies that sample a broad representation of individuals. Instead of looking only at populations of women with disabilities, we must look at women with disabilities within the context of the population of women in general. This approach will strengthen our efforts to apply the same standards and definitions to women with disabilities as we do to all women. It will enable us to obtain better statistics on the incidence and relevance of certain conditions compared to women in general. An example of a collaborative effort in such types of studies is the supplement given by the NICHD National Center for Medical Rehabilitation Research to a national multicenter study of the menopause transition sponsored by the NIH Office of Research on Women's Health, the National Institute on Aging, and the National Institute of Nursing Research. This supplement will enable the women with disabilities enrolled in the study to be identified based on functional limitations. Little is known about menopause in women with disabilities. Participation in this study will provide information on the natural history of this process within the context of disability. In addition, by being part of a large study, the data obtained should point to potential risk factors and consequences that may be disproportionately experienced by women with disabilities.

The techniques of qualitative research are also important tools for examining complex phenomena related to the experiences of women with disabilities. In addition to providing valuable insights into these phenomena, the results of qualitative research can also be used as grounding for larger-scale quantitative investigations. Topics such as abuse and reactions to stress would be better served by looking at the interrelationship of factors in women's lives as expressed by the women themselves, not by looking only at numbers. Although a hallmark of good research is focus, efforts must also be taken to draw together information from the perspective of basic, biomedical, psychosocial, and behavioral science to construct a more holistic understanding of the experiences of women with disabilities. Much attention has been paid to the effect of the environment, including adaptive equipment, on the physical and social functioning of people with disabilities, especially by the World Health Organization in their efforts to distinguish impairment from disability from handicap. We still have quite a distance to go in operationalizing environmental variables and including them in medical and behavioral studies.

An issue of fundamental importance in research methodology is sampling. The selection of women to participate in studies determines and limits the applicability of the results of the research. Certain sampling techniques pose serious limitations on the generalizability of findings, such as consecutive admissions to hospitals, clinics, or educational programs; solicited volunteers; or recruitment through residential programs or consumer organizations. Although population-based sampling is not always feasible, researchers must, to the greatest extent possible, construct samples that are maximally representative of the population in question. When only restricted samples are available, documentation must state clearly the limitations in interpreting the results. The literature contains many excellent examples of research on people with certain types of disabilities. We encourage the expansion of types of disabilities examined and a focus on segments of the population of women with disabilities who have not often been the subject of research. We encourage efforts similar to those that resulted in the conference that generated this book to address the health needs of women with disabilities other than physical disabilities. The extraordinary barriers faced by women with sensory or mental impairments as they attempt to gain access to health information and health care systems also have not received the attention they deserve.

Because of the low incidence of certain disabilities among women, such as spinal cord injury and neuromuscular disorders, collaboration among researchers in multicenter studies is necessary to achieve adequate sample sizes. We must also take extra steps to include women in research studies who may be harder to identify, such as women with very rare disabilities and women with combinations of disabilities. In constructing samples, we must bring to a halt the traditional exclusion of institutionalized women, that is, women who reside in skilled nursing facilities, developmental centers, or other publicly or privately funded congregate living arrangements. Women occupy a majority of the beds in skilled nursing facilities. Many of these women are not elderly and are placed in these facilities for a variety of reasons, including lack of environmental accessibility and personal assistance resources. We must be mindful of exclusion criteria that are based on convenience for the researchers and not on scientific integrity. The federal government has recognized the design inadequacy of studies conducted only on men and samples that do not include members of racial or ethnic minorities. The U.S. Public Health Service, which includes the National Institutes of Health and the Centers for Disease Control and Prevention, requires that all studies using human subjects clearly describe the efforts that will be undertaken to ensure inclusion of women and minorities. These plans are reviewed by initial review groups, National Advisory Councils, and federal program administrators, and the plans must be found adequate before funding can take place.

The use of control or comparison samples needs to be expanded and refined in the study of women with disabilities. This is not a simple task. On the one hand, we must hold women with disabilities to the same standard as all women; on the other hand, we must be sure that we are making fair comparisons. An NIH-funded national survey of women with physical disabilities (Nosek et al., 1995) constructed a comparison sample by asking every participant to recruit an able-bodied female friend to complete the survey as well. This technique allowed the comparison of women from similar geographic and socioeconomic backgrounds on a variety of psychological, behavioral, developmental, and interpersonal relationship variables, but had certain limitations when differences in demographic variables were studied. Many other techniques exist for constructing valid control or comparison samples. Researchers are encouraged to explore all available and feasible options for including this in their research designs.

In studying the effect of interventions, it is important to include nontreatment control groups. As obvious as this precaution seems, it is too often overlooked in rehabilitation research. Because disability is such a diverse phenomenon, with widely varying types of disabilities, ages at onset, prognoses, and levels of functional limitation, it is essential that samples be as homogeneous as possible and that comparisons be made on groups of similar disability characteristics appropriate to the topic.

In order to achieve a higher level of excellence in the study of women with disabilities, it is important that we advance the technique of investigating outcomes. Many current interventions in the field of medical rehabilitation have resulted not from a research and development base, but rather from service provision. This is particularly true for women with disabilities, as discussed in earlier chapters. Thus, there is a need to develop a strong research base on which to identify treatment interventions. Furthermore, in the field of disability, there are few adequate measures for determining the effectiveness of interventions that are currently being used. There is a need for valid, reliable, and sensitive measures for comparing the effectiveness of interventions, systems of care, methods of financing, and consumer satisfaction and preferences (Fuhrer, 1995). Finally, outcomes have to be redefined to reflect the expectations of persons with disabilities. To date, outcomes have been measured according to standards that reflect traditional definitions and paradigms. For example, the vocational rehabilitation closure category of homemaker has always been acceptable for women with disabilities; indeed, it was sometimes more common than attainment of salaried employment. This does not reflect the increasing numbers of women with disabilities in postsecondary education or the increasing percentage of women in the labor force. New efforts must be undertaken to ensure that outcome assessment keeps pace with the new definitions and paradigms that we are promoting.

CLINICAL PRACTICE

Most early research on health and function issues of persons with disabilities has been based in clinical practice. Clinical settings have offered occasions for descriptive studies and studies to document the response to preventive or intervention strategies. As noted, design and methodology of studies are of significant importance. The domains of intervention strategies and outcome measures must be expanded beyond traditional biomedical evaluation. In the mid-1990s, there has been a greater awareness of health services research. Changes in the delivery of health care may have a significant impact on persons with disabilities. Also, the knowledge base of health professionals regarding issues of persons with disabilities has often been noted by consumers and other professionals to be limited. As a consequence, clinical practice continues to provide an opportunity for much-needed research and education.

The nature of clinical practice has taken dramatic new turns in the 1990s. Managed care organizations, health systems management, and the federal government have provided different foci, restraints, and structure on providers and consumers. Consumers of health care are becoming more vocal and educated regarding their needs. Several chapters herein issue a strong call for a partnership between women and their physicians. We hear a demand that priority be set on wellness and the prevention of secondary conditions. We hear of many general health needs, such as reproductive health, fitness training, and stress management, that should be available to women with disabilities. How to provide the best opportunity for a woman with a disability to receive optimal health care has yet to be determined. A health care delivery system must offer a knowledgeable principal caregiver who collaborates with a knowledgeable specialist in partnership with a woman with a disability. Methods of communication between consumer and health care provider, accessibility of environment, education of providers and consumers, and documentation of medical history are all challenges to the system. A model of delivery, the efficacy of a model for the consumer, and the effectiveness of a model for managed care organizations all need to be better described and researched. We must develop new models of service delivery that are better equipped to meet the health care needs of women with physical disabilities.

Education of health care providers regarding issues of women with physical disabilities is also of importance. Most undergraduate curricula in health care fields devote little time to women's issues, particularly women with disabilities. Issues of general prevention strategies, secondary conditions, aging, multiculturalism, and psychological health are often neglected. Furthermore, general disability-related biases are also usually addressed in a limited fashion, including issues such as attitudinal barriers and environmental barriers. The U.S. Congress recognized the need for improved training in women's health and commissioned the NIH Office on Women's Health to develop a medical school curriculum in this area. This curriculum includes a chapter on the specific health needs of women with disabilities. All health professionals—not only physicians—should have issues of women with disabilities addressed in the curricula.

The challenge before us is substantial. Concerns of health care delivery and education of health care professionals are of a national scope. We must begin a powerful movement to convince health care policy makers that women with disabilities have important but neglected health care needs. Improvements in the areas of education and health care delivery may result in early recognition of treatable or preventable health issues, with a long-term effect of improvement in the health and functional status of women with disabilities.

DISSEMINATION

Vast new opportunities are opening up before us in the communication of information. Advances in electronic communication databases, including the Internet and telemedicine, offer unprecedented outlets for creativity in packaging information and targeting it to diverse audiences. New funding sources are appearing, such as the National Telecommunications and Information Administration, that serve to advance the application of these new technologies. As the state-of-the-art progresses, however, we must be vigilant to ensure that important segments of the population are not left out of the information loop for lack of technological sophistication. Although many people with disabilities have found computers to be a new vehicle for integration into society, many others find that computer technology is still beyond their means. We must initiate new and creative methods for bringing technology of all types within their financial reach. Computer technology is also not part of the active vocabulary of many practicing clinicians. In addition to offering training opportunities that will raise their level of computer competence, we must create incentives for them to learn. Until we achieve a more computer-literate society, it is important that we continue to expand efforts to disseminate information via a multitude of avenues, including academic journal articles, summaries, and fact sheets, as well as press releases to the print and broadcast media, a primary information resource for consumers and professionals alike. A variety of formats and accessible media are necessary to reach all segments of the population who can benefit from this information.

In the study of health needs of women with physical disabilities, the challenge is an issue not only of dissemination but also of public education. Our educational mission is not only one of spreading knowledge but also one of changing attitudes. Our targeted learners include 1) medical professionals; 2) policy makers, including medical directors and administrators in public and private facilities; 3) deans and other administrators of training programs for health care professionals; and 4) women with disabilities and their friends, families, and acquaintances. The first and most potent educator is the family, yet it is typical of families, as it is of all society, to hold very protective attitudes toward girls and women with disabilities. By reaching mothers and fathers, we can influence their attitudes about their children with disabilities and help them gain access to the many resources available. Incorporating disability information in primary and secondary school health curricula empowers youth to understand their bodies better and to go beyond stereotypes and prejudice in relating to their peers with disabilities.

It is amazing how little current information filters down to consumers themselves. All women face barriers in gaining access to the most current information about their health and the availability of new health care techniques; for women with disabilities, barriers resulting from environmental inaccessibility, financial limitations, knowledge gaps, and negative attitudes compound this problem. Women who received medical services for their disability in the 1960s and 1970s and are not followed regularly by disability specialists have little access to the means of dissemination traditionally used by researchers. Even those who have received services more recently may not have access to current information if they are not connected with major medical centers. Those whose disabilities are relatively stable may have no need to see rehabilitation professionals and may have the majority of their medical needs met by primary care physicians. For some women, their early experiences in medical and rehabilitation settings were negative, even traumatic or abusive, and consequently they have deliberately avoided contact with disability-related health services. Public health educators and funding agencies should put a priority on educating the general public and consumers with disabilities about ways to obtain current medical information related to disability, including the many issues contained in this volume.

Informing and educating medical professionals require some different strategies. The vehicle of the continuing education seminar can be used very effectively to transmit information in practical terms. Appropriate documentation and follow-up can enhance learning and offer an accessible information resource that can be used on an individual basis. We would like to issue a challenge to the field to create networks of information sharing. This concept has been extensively discussed, but remains little more than a fragmented conglomeration of pockets of expertise. Serious efforts must be undertaken to draw together these pockets in combination with the vast literature and other resources available through the Internet and telemedicine to produce a viable, easily accessible, well-known network of information related to disability.

CONSUMER PARTICIPATION

Personal experience with disability constitutes a qualification of inestimable value for researchers and clinical practitioners, particularly in understanding the psychological and social impact of disability. We support the principles of participatory action research, in which the population of interest is integrally involved in every step of the research process, from problem identification through design conceptualization, implementation, interpretation of findings, and finally outcome evaluation. One of the best ways to ensure high-quality, relevant research is to increase the number of women with disabilities who are trained as researchers and clinical practitioners. This cadre of women would also be available to be involved in research projects and grant review panels and to hold policy-making positions in health care and research funding. Strategies for achieving this include 1) urging vocational rehabilitation counselors to encourage gifted female students with disabilities to pursue careers in the sciences, 2) creating scholarship incentives for pursuing such studies, 3) offering sponsorship for participation in scientific meetings and conferences (including coverage of disability-related expenses), 4) creating a comprehensive list of women with disabilities trained in research and medical practice, 5) circulating such a list among public and private research funding agencies and encouraging them to recruit women with disabilities to serve on grant review panels, and 6) urging placement agencies for positions in medical administration to pursue qualified women with disabilities for such positions.

We chose four areas of focus for this volume, and, in doing so, we have opened discussion on hundreds of other related topics. We hope this work will be a catalyst for exploration of the breadth and depth of the many questions that have been raised herein. The purpose of this volume will be well served if the many recommendations for research and practice given in each chapter motivate individual researchers, clinicians, and consumers to engage in passionate campaigns to bring about change within their own sphere of influence to improve the health and quality of life of women with disabilities.

REFERENCES

Fuhrer, M.J. (1995). Conference report: An agenda for medical rehabilitation outcomes research. *American Journal of Physical Medicine and Rehabilitation, 74,* 243–248.

Nosek, M.A., Rintala, D.H., Young, M.E., Howland, C.A., Foley, C.C., Rossi, C.D., & Chanpong, G. (1995). Sexual functioning among women with physical disabilities. *Archives of Physical Medicine and Rehabilitation, 77*(2), 107–115.

Author Index

Subject Index

Page numbers followed by "f" or "t" indicate figures or tables, respectively.